Parasite Life Cycles

Dickson D. Despommier
John W. Karapelou

Parasite Life Cycles

With 49 Life Cycle Drawings

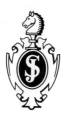

Springer-Verlag
New York Berlin Heidelberg
London Paris Tokyo

Dickson D. Despommier, Ph.D.
Professor of Public Health
  and of Microbiology
Division of Tropical Medicine
Columbia University
New York, N.Y. 10032, USA

John W. Karapelou
Chief Medical Illustrator
Center for Biomedical Communications
College of Physicians and Surgeons
Columbia University
New York, N.Y. 10032, USA

Library of Congress Cataloging-in-Publication Data
Despommier, Dickson D.
  Parasite life cycles / Dickson D. Despommier, John W. Karapelou.
      p.   cm.
  Bibliography: p.
  ISBN 0-387-96486-X
  1. Protozoa.   2. Helminths.   3. Parasites.   I. Karapelou, John W.
II. Title.
QL366.D47 1987

Typeset by Arcata Graphics/Kingsport, Kingsport, Tennessee.
Printed and bound by Arcata Graphics/Halliday, West Hanover, Massachusetts.
Printed in the United States of America

9 8 7 6 5 4 3 2 1

ISBN 0-387-96486-X Springer-Verlag New York Berlin Heidelberg
ISBN 3-540-96486-X Springer-Verlag Berlin Heidelberg New York

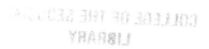

To Joan and Sam, and to
Nancy, John and Christina

Acknowledgments

We thank Larry Carter for his vision and belief in this project from its inception. We thank Drs. Philip A. D'Alesandro, Suzanne Holmes Giannini, William C. Campbell, Bernard Fried, Larry Roberts, and Meredith Behr for reviewing various aspects of the book. We especially thank Drs. Harold W. Brown and Kathleen Hussey for amassing an outstanding collection of parasite material from which we derived much of what is illustrated throughout the book. We thank Mrs. Terri Terilli for pushing us when we had to be pushed and for encouraging us to continue. We also thank her for her skillful handling of the typing of the manuscript.

Contents

Part 3 Trematoda

Part 4 Nematoda

Introduction

The concept of parasitism has fascinated scientists for centuries, and over the last one hundred years, the field of parasitology has assumed its place as a full member of the ecological sciences. In the early days of parasitology research, the life cycles of these interesting organisms were the focal point of studies, thereby revealing the ways in which they complete their often complex journeys from one stage to the next.

A central theme has emerged from the now extensive life cycle literature; namely that each developmental stage is dependent upon environmental cues in order for it to progress to the next stage. Elucidation of the precise conditions needed to elicit stage-specific behavior has often taken years of laboratory and field work. Thus, we have come to appreciate the complexities of each parasite through these many efforts.

Life cycles of protozoan and helminthic parasites continue to hold the attention of a small but hearty group of biologists, so that our knowledge of parasite life styles continues to unfold.

Many species of parasitic protozoans and helminths occupy, sequentially, several microenvironments and invertebrate vectors during their development to reproductive adulthood. One need only review the life cycle of the fish tapeworm, *Diphyllobothrium latum,* in order to fully comprehend the term "complex" life cycle. The numerous sites selected by parasitic organisms infecting the human as the definitive host is reflected in the rich diversity of organisms that have evolved and prospered at our expense. In contrast, plasmodia, the causative agent of malaria, are actually parasites of the female anopheline mosquito, with the human serving as the intermediate host. In other cases, such as with trichinella, humans are but one of many species of mammalian hosts susceptible to infection.

In the text that follows, we have attempted to distill out and present the essentials of the life cycles of parasites that infect the human host without detracting from the complexities of them.

We decided that this is best done with a maximum of detailed illustrations and a minimum of words.

We have tried to depict each step of the process of infection in such a way that both the uninitiated and experienced biologist can gain insight into the host-parasite relationship. The selected reading list provided at the back of the text is intended to lead the interested reader to more complete biological information. Monographs on specific parasites are particularly useful, especially those written after 1980, and we have striven to list most of them.

The text, itself, is organized in such a way that the reader is introduced first to the general concepts of the major group (e.g., Protozoa, Nematoda, etc.). Next, the classification of each group is listed, at least as far down in the classification scheme as Family. In some cases, only Orders are listed, due to constraints of space. For classifications down to species, monographs dealing with each Family must be consulted. Most parasites in each phyla which infect the human host are presented pictorially, accompanied by a short text describing the essentials of their life cycle. Each illustration is a synthesis derived from information gathered from a wide variety of sources, including histopathological tissue sections, whole mounted material and gross specimens. Finally, the complete classification of each parasite depicted is given.

It is our hope that having the life cycles of all major protozoan and helminthic parasites that infect the human host illustrated in a single volume will stimulate interest in them among those not yet familiar with them, and serve as a ready source of information to those whose job it is to transmit the excitement of the field of parasitology to the rest of the scientific community.

Dickson D. Despommier
John W. Karapelou

1 Protozoa

General Characteristics of the Protozoa

Approximately 66,000 species of protozoans have been described; about 10,000 of these are parasitic. Protozoans are single-celled organisms, exhibiting extensive diversity in all aspects of their biology. For example protozoans vary in their means of locomotion, and, to a great extent, this is the basis for their classification. They all exhibit some form of motility, often utilizing specialized organelles for that purpose (e.g., cilia and flagella). It is not known which motility mechanism(s) are employed by *Plasmodium* or the coccidae, since they do not possess any obvious locomotor organelles. Most species of protozoa are free-living and occupy niches as extreme as bottom sediments in deep marine trenches and geothermal springs. Similarly, parasitic protozoa show a wide variety of patterns for host selection and for site selection within a given host. Many are vectorborne—parasites in both cold-blooded and warm-blooded hosts. Literally every available niche within the human host can be parasitized.

All protozoa, be they free-living or parasitic, must carry out growth and replication within the confines of their unit membranes. Because of this, protozoans have been naturally selected for having uniquely solved various problems related to food-gathering and food-processing. Thus, their cytoplasm, depending upon the species, may contain highly specialized organelles that aid them in either aerobic or anaerobic energy metabolism.

Morphologically, protozoa vary in size from 1.5 μm to 50 mm in diameter. Division is accomplished by a wide variety of related mechanisms, with binary fission being the most common. Sexual reproduction also is a frequent reproductive strategy, and is particularly important for the coccidae and plasmodia. Protozoans parasitic for humans include representatives from 4 of the 7 groups, namely, Sarcomastigophora, Apicomplexa, Microspora, and Ciliophora. For brevity, and for relevance to the parasites in question, the classification presented here does not include suborder or family designations. However, the complete taxonomy for each parasite is given to aid readers when they consult the appropriate literature on a particular taxon.

Classification

Bold type indicates orders represented in book by parasites

Kingdom: Protista
  Phylum: Sarcomastigophora
    Subphylum: Mastigophora
      Class: Phytomastigophorea
        Order: Cryptomonadida
        Order: Dinoflagellida
        Order: Euglenida
        Order: Chrysomonadida
        Order: Heterochlorida
        Order: Chloromonadida
        Order: Prymnesiida
        Order: Volvocida
        Order: Prasinomonadida
        Order: Silicoflagellida
      Class: Zoomastigophorea
        Order: Choanoflagellida
        Order: Kinetoplastida
        Order: Proteromonadida
        Order: Retortamonadida
        Order: Diplomonadida
        Order: Oxymonadida
      Superorder: Parabasalidea
        Order: Trichomonadida
        Order: Hypermastigida
    Subphylum: Opalinata
      Class: Opalinatea
        Order: Opalinida
    Subphylum: Sarcodina
      Superclass: Rhizopoda
      Class: Lobosea
        Subclass: Gymnamoebia
        Order: Amoebida
        Order: Schizopyrenida
        Order: Pelobiontida
        Subclass: Testacealobosia
        Order: Arcellinida
        Order: Trichosida
      Class: Acarpomyxea
        Order: Leptomyxida
        Order: Stereomyxida
      Class: Acrasea
        Order: Acrasida
      Class: Eumycetozoae
        Subclass: Protostelia
        Order: Protosteliida
        Subclass: Dictyosteliia
        Order: Dictyosteliida

        Subclass: Myxogastria
        Order: Echinosteliida
        Order: Liceida
        Order: Trichiida
        Order: Stemonitida
        Order: Physarida
      Class: Plasmodiophorea
        Order: Plasmodiophorida
      Class: Filosea
        Order: Aconchulinida
        Order: Gromiida
      Class: Granuloreticulosea
        Order: Athalamida
        Order: Monothalamida
        Order: Foraminiferida
      Class: Xenophyophorea
        Order: Psamminida
        Order: Stannomida
      Superclass: Actinopoda
        Class: Acantharea
        Order: Holacanthida
        Order: Symphyacanthida
        Order: Chaunacanthida
        Order: Arthracanthida
        Order: Actineliida
        Class: Polycystinea
        Order: Spumellarida
        Order: Nassellarida
        Class: Phaeodarea
        Order: Phaeocystida
        Order: Phaeosphaerida
        Order: Phaeocalpida
        Order: Phaeogromida
        Order: Phaeoconchida
        Order: Phaeodendrida
        Class: Heliozoea
        Order: Desmothoracida
        Order: Actinophryida
        Order: Taxopodida
        Order: Centrohelida
  Phylum: Labyrinthomorpha
    Class: Labyrinthulea
        Order: Labyrinthulida
  Phylum: Apicomplexa
    Class: Perkinsea
        Order: Perkinsida
    Class: Sporozoea

Subclass: Gregarinia
    Order: Archigregarinida
    Order: Eugregarinida
    Order: Neogregarinida
Subclass: Coccidia
    Order: Agamococcidiida
    Order: Protococcidiida
    Order: Eucoccidiida
Subclass: Piroplasmia
    Order: Piroplasmida
Phylum: Microspora
  Class: Rudimicrosporea
    Order: Metchnikovellida
  Class: Microsporea
    Order: Minisporida
    Order: Microsporida
Phylum: Ascetospora
  Class: Stellatosporea
    Order: Occlusosporida
    Order: Balanosporida
  Class: Paramyxea
    Order: Paramyxida
Phylum: Myxozoa
  Class: Myxosporea
    Order: Bivalvulida
    Order: Multivalvulida
  Class: Actinosporea
    Subclass: Actinomyxia
Phylum: Ciliophora
  Class: Kinetofragminophorea
    Subclass: Gymnostomatia
      Order: Prostomatida
      Order: Pleurostomatida

      Order: Primociliatida
      Order: Karyorelictida
    Subclass: Vestibuliferia
      Order: Trichostomatida
      Order: Entodiniomorphida
      Order: Colpodida
    Subclass: Hypostomatia
      Superorder: Nassulidea
      Order: Synhymeniida
      Order: Nassulida
      Superorder: Phyllopharyngidea
      Order: Crytophorida
      Order: Chonotrichida
      Superorder: Rhynchodea
      Order: Rhynchodida
      Superorder: Apostomatidea
      Order: Apostomatida
    Subclass: Suctoria
      Order: Suctorida
  Class: Oligohymenophorea
    Subclass: Hymenostomatida
      Order: Hymenostomatida
      Order: Scuticociliatida
      Order: Astomatida
    Subclass: Peritrichia
      Order: Peritrichida
  Class: Polymenophorea
    Subclass: Spirotrichia
      Order: Heterotrichida
      Order: Odontostomatida
      Order: Oligotrichida
      Order: Hypotrichida

Trypanosoma Cruzi

1a The infective stage of *Trypanosoma cruzi* is the metacyclic trypomastigote. It is 15 μm in length and possesses a single nucleus and flagellum. The flagellum is continuous with the undulating membrane, and originates at the kinetoplast, a large organized collection of extranuclear DNA.

1b Transmission of *T. cruzi* from person to person occurs in many ways. The most frequent way is by the triatomid insect vector (the "kissing" bug). Many species of "kissing" bugs are vectors, the most common of which belong to the genera *Panstrongylus, Triatoma,* and *Rhodnius.* Infection occurs shortly after an infected bug takes a blood meal. During the feeding process, the insect defecates on the host's skin near the bite wound. Its feces contain the infective trypomastigotes.

2 When the bug leaves the site, the host experiences a mild itching sensation and rubs the trypomastigotes into the bite wound. If the bug bites on the face near the eye or mouth, then organisms can infect through mucous membranes. Other ways of acquiring *T. cruzi* include blood transfusions, transplacental infection and sexual intercourse.

3a Trypomastigotes enter a wide variety of cells at the site of the bite wound and transform into amastigotes. The amastigote is 3-5 μm in diameter and does not possess an external flagellum. The intracellular amastigotes replicate by binary fission.

3b The host becomes hypersensitive to the parasite as the result of the extensive cellular destruction at the site of initial infection.

4a Some amastigotes transform into trypomastigotes within dying host cells. After being released into the peripheral blood, trypomastigotes infect other sites in the body.

4b At this point in the infection any tissue may harbor parasites, including heart muscle (shown here) and nervous tissue (e.g., myenteric plexus). Transformation from amastigotes to trypomastigotes can occur at any site.

4c The trypomastigotes penetrate new cells, transform to amastigotes, and begin the replication process again.

5 The triatomid bug becomes infected when it takes a blood meal from an individual containing trypomastigotes.

6 Trypomastigotes rapidly transform into dividing epimastigotes within the midgut of the bug, resulting in thousands of new parasites. Epimastigotes differentiate into metacyclic trypomastigotes within the hindgut. This is the infective stage of the parasite.

7 All mammals are susceptible to infection and can serve as reservoir hosts. The sloth, the oppossum, and various rodents, are important in maintaining the sylvatic cycle.

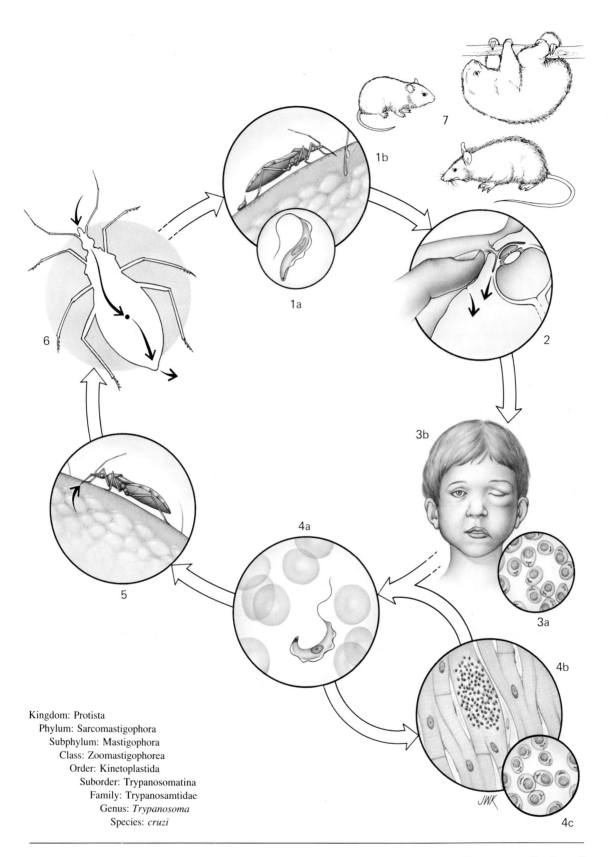

Kingdom: Protista
Phylum: Sarcomastigophora
Subphylum: Mastigophora
Class: Zoomastigophorea
Order: Kinetoplastida
Suborder: Trypanosomatina
Family: Trypanosamtidae
Genus: *Trypanosoma*
Species: *cruzi*

Trypanosoma Brucei Gambiense

1a   The infective stage of *Trypanosoma brucei gambiense* is the metacyclic trypomastigote. This stage is about 12–15 μm in length, and it possesses a single nucleus and a flagellum. The flagellum is continuous with the undulating membrane and originates at the kinetoplast.

1b   Transmission of *T. b. gambiense* occurs when an infected tsetse fly takes a blood meal. The metacyclic trypomastigotes are injected into the bite wound along with the fly's salivary secretions. The metacyclic trypomastigote rapidly transforms into the bloodstream trypomastigote and begins to replicate by binary fission. Tsetse flies in the genus *Glossina* are capable of transmitting *T. b. gambiense; G. palpalis* and *G. tachinoides* are the most common ones.

2   A primary chancre develops at the site of the bite wound, with trypomastigotes being found extracellularly in various fluid spaces within it. This stage of the infection can last for several weeks to several months.

3   The trypomastigotes eventually find their way into the bloodstream and lymphatic system, where they continue to replicate by binary fission. They spend their entire life cycle extracellularly. The host responds to the infection by producing antibodies. The surface antigenic determinants are glycoproteins in the outer coat of the trypanosomes. The antibodies directed against them destroy, by agglutination and lysis, all antigenically identical organisms. A few trypanosomes with different surface antigens escape destruction. These variants multiply and replace those that were destroyed. The host again responds by producing antibodies against the new antigenic variant. In turn, a third variant arises. Thus yet another brood of trypanosomes takes over, the host responds once more, and this tug-of-war continues until the host is eventually overcome. Invasion of the central nervous system also occurs at this time, but is not part of the life cycle.

4   A tsetse fly becomes infected when it ingests a blood meal containing bloodstream trypomastigotes.

5   The bloodstream trypomastigotes transform into procyclic trypomastigotes in the midgut, where they then divide over a 10-day period, producing hundreds of new individuals. The procyclic trypomastigotes then leave the midgut for the salivary glands and transform into epimastigotes. More division occurs at this site, ultimately resulting in the production of thousands of metacyclic trypomastigotes, the infective stage for the human host. The entire process takes about 25–50 days to complete. Tsetse flies remain infective throughout their life. There are no known reservoir hosts for *T. b. gambiense*.

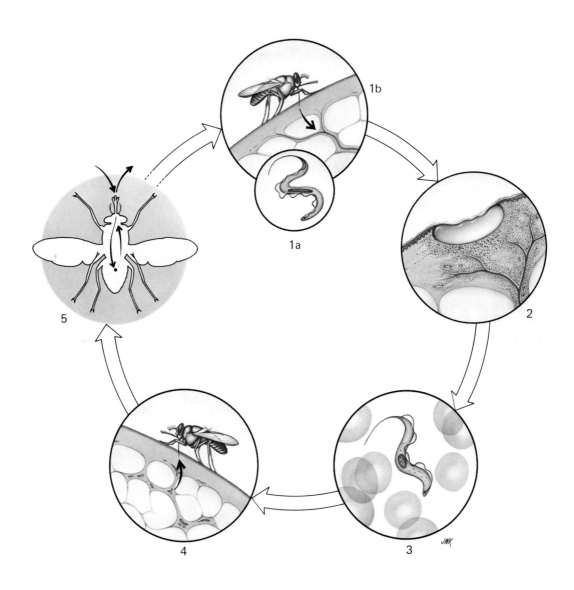

1a
1b
2
3
4
5

Kingdom: Protista
  Phylum: Sarcomastigophora
    Subphylum: Mastigophora
      Class: Zoomastigophorea
        Order: Kinetoplastida
          Suborder: Trypanosomatina
            Genus: *Trypanosoma*
              Species: *brucei*
                Subspecies: *rhodesiense*

Trypanosoma Brucei Rhodesiense

1a The life cycle of *Trypanosoma brucei rhodesiense* is similar to that of *T. b. gambiense*. The infective stage is the metacyclic trypomastigote, which lives within the salivary glands of the tsetse fly. This stage is approximately 15–20 μm in length, and it possesses a single nucleus, a flagellum attached to an undulating membrane, and a subterminal posterior kinetoplast.

1b Infection occurs when an individual is bitten by an infected tsetse fly. The organisms are introduced into the skin of the host along with the salivary secretions of the infected insect. Important vectors of *T. b. rhodesiense* include *Glossina morsitans* and *G. pallidipes*.

2 The metacyclic trypomastigotes rapidly transform into bloodstream trypomastigotes within the extracellular spaces in the subcutaneous tissues. There, the parasites replicate by binary fission. A primary chancre is produced as the result of their presence.

3 The trypomastigotes eventually find their way into the bloodstream and the lymphatics, where they continue the replication cycle. Antigenic variation is a main feature of the life cycle of *T. b. rhodesiense*. Invasion of the cerebrospinal fluid of the central nervous system also occurs during this phase of the infection, but does not contribute to the life cycle.

4 The tsetse fly becomes infected when it ingests the trypomastigote while taking a blood meal from an infected individual.

5 The trypomastigote transforms within the lumen of the midgut into the procyclic trypomastigote. After several cycles of cell division, the procyclic trypomastigote migrates to the insect's salivary glands, where it differentiates further into the epimastigote and resumes division. Epimastigotes develop within the salivary gland into metacyclic trypomastigotes, the infective stage for the mammalian host.

6 Hartebeest and zebu cattle are important reservoir hosts for *T. b. rhodesiense*. Other mammals in East Africa also become infected with this parasite.

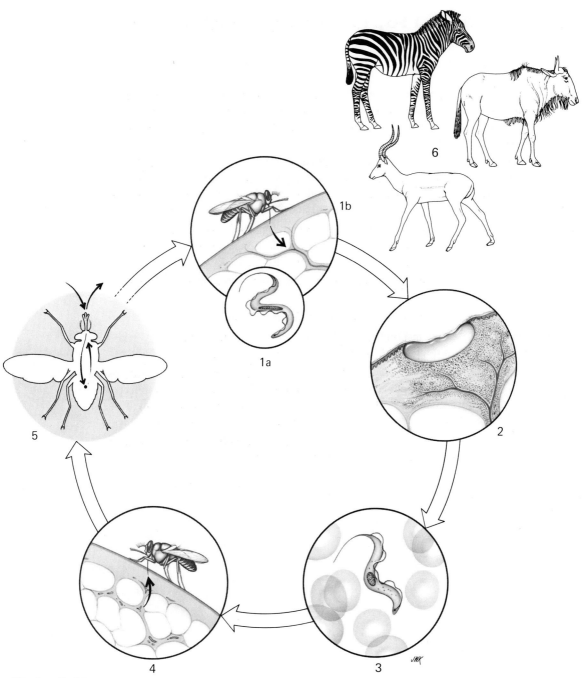

Kingdom: Protista
Phylum: Sarcomostigophora
Subphylum: Mastigophora
Class: Zoomastigophorea
Order: Kinetoplastida
Suborder: Trypanosomatina
Family: Trypanosamtidae
Genus: *Trypansoma*
Species: *brucei*
Subspecies: *gambiense*

Leishmania Tropica and L. Mexicana

1a The infective stage of *Leishmania tropica* and *L. mexicana* is the promastigote. This form of the organism lives in the midgut and mouthparts of the infected sand fly. It possesses a single nucleus, a flagellum, and a prominent subterminal anterior kinetoplast.

1b *L. tropica* and *L. mexicana* are transmitted from person to person by the bite of an infected sand fly. Sand flies in the genus *Phlebotimus* are the most common vectors in Europe, the Middle East, and Asia, whereas *Lutzomyia* commonly transmits *L. mexicana* throughout Central and South America.

2a Once the promastigote is injected into the skin, it is phagocytosed by a macrophage and rapidly transforms to the amastigote stage. Infection is limited to the cutaneous and subcutaneous tissues near the original site of infection.

2b The amastigotes replicate within each macrophage by binary fission. Lysis of the host cell ensues.

2c The reproductive cycle is repeated many times in the skin.

3a,b Amastigotes within macrophages are ingested by sand flies when they take a blood meal from the infected margin of the ulcer.

4 Once inside the sand fly midgut, the amastigotes are freed from infected host cells by digestion. The parasites then transform into promastigotes, the infective stage for the mammalian host. Promastigotes undergo several cycles of division, then migrate to the proboscis where they await the taking of another blood meal.

5 *L. tropica* and *L. mexicana* can infect other animals, as well as man, with rodents and dogs serving as important reservoir hosts for both species.

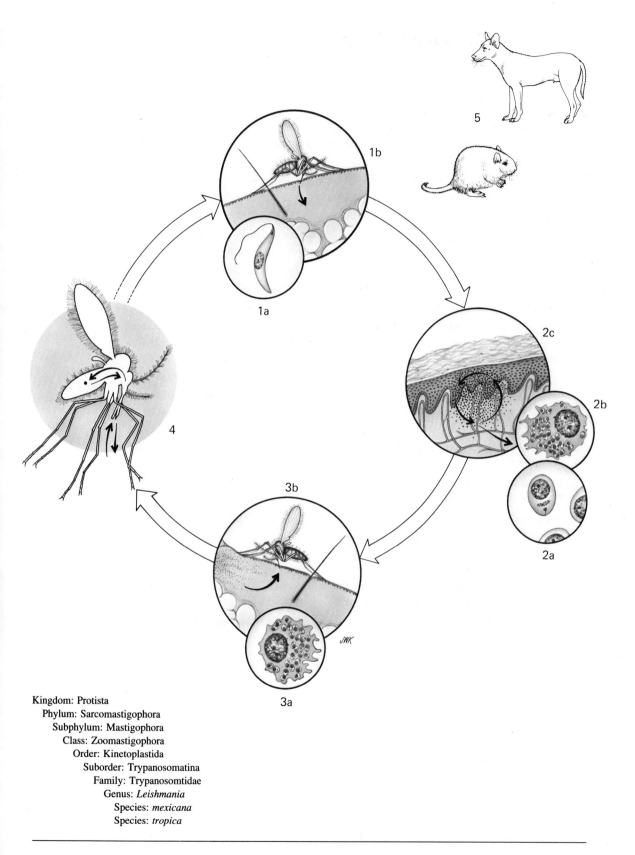

Kingdom: Protista
  Phylum: Sarcomastigophora
    Subphylum: Mastigophora
      Class: Zoomastigophora
        Order: Kinetoplastida
          Suborder: Trypanosomatina
            Family: Trypanosomtidae
              Genus: *Leishmania*
                Species: *mexicana*
                Species: *tropica*

Leishmania Braziliensis

1a The infective stage of *Leishmania braziliensis* is the promastigote. Promastigotes are 10–15 μm in length, and they possess a single nucleus, a flagellum, and a subterminal anterior kinetoplast. Sand flies in the genus *Lutzomyia* are the vectors of this parasite.

1b Infection occurs when an infected sand fly takes a second blood meal. The parasites enter the bite wound with the salivary secretion.

2a The promastigotes round up and lose their flagellum, becoming amastigotes.

2b Transformation from promastigote to amastigote occurs within the parasitophorous vacuoles of macrophages shortly after the phagocytes ingest the parasites.

2c The entire infection is limited to the subcutaneous tissue, with the growth and division of the parasites resulting in the death of the macrophages.

3a The infected macrophages continue to die, releasing more amastigotes.

3b Increased infection in the subcutaneous tissue near the bite wound leads to destruction of tissue, resulting in a craterform ulcer. Organisms are found at the edge of the lesion in living tissue.

3c Infected macrophages can travel via the bloodstream to other parts of the body before dying and releasing their parasites. However, only macrophages at mucocutaneous junctions are susceptible to infection. Such metastases can lead to erosion of the soft palate.

3d Infection at the mucocutaneous junction of the urogenital and anal regions can also occur.

4a Infected macrophages at the margins of ulcers at any infection site can serve as the source of infection for sand flies.

4b Sand flies acquire their infection during the taking of a blood meal.

5 Within the sand fly, the infected macrophages are digested in the midgut of the insect, liberating the amastigotes. The parasites rapidly transform into promastigotes, the infective stage for the mammalian host. After many replication cycles in the midgut, the promastigotes migrate into the proboscis of the insect and await the taking of another blood meal by the sand fly.

6 There are many reservoir hosts, including the sloth and several varieties of rodents.

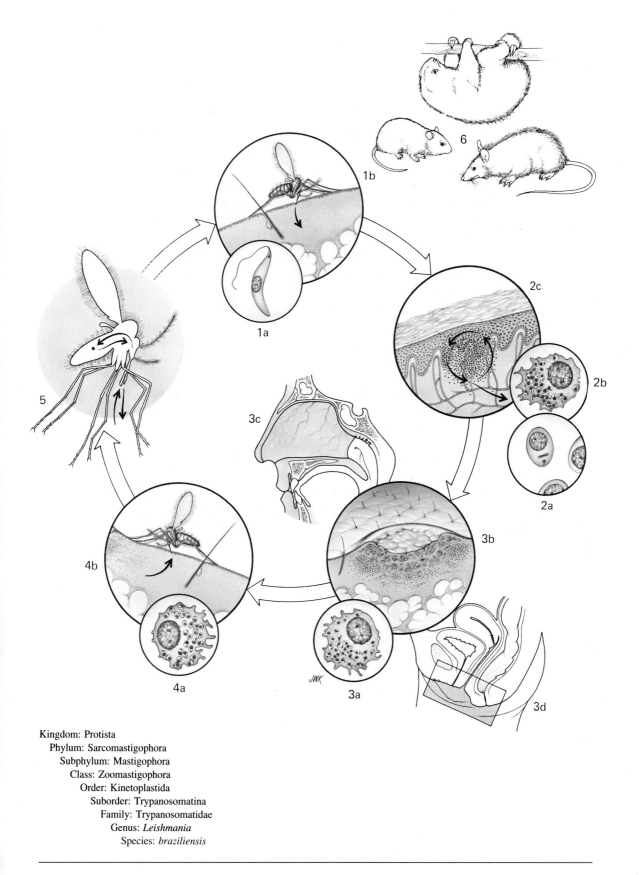

Kingdom: Protista
Phylum: Sarcomastigophora
Subphylum: Mastigophora
Class: Zoomastigophora
Order: Kinetoplastida
Suborder: Trypanosomatina
Family: Trypanosomatidae
Genus: *Leishmania*
Species: *braziliensis*

Leishmania Donovani

1a   The promastigote is the infective stage for humans. It lives within the lumen of the proboscis of its vector, the sand fly.

1b   The infected sand fly transmits *L. donovani* from person to person by injecting the promastigotes into the skin of the mammalian host, along with salivary secretions, during the taking of a blood meal. Sand flies in the genus *Phlebotomus* are common vectors in Africa, the Middle East, and Asia, while *Lutzomyia* transmits *L. donovani* in Central and South America.

2a   The promastigotes are rapidly phagocytosed in the skin by macrophages.

2b   The promastigotes then transform to amastigotes. In contrast to *L. tropica*, *L. mexicana*, or *L. braziliensis*, the amastigotes are not restricted to skin, but are carried throughout the viscera, where they infect a wide variety of fixed and wandering macrophages.

3a-3c   Subsequent replication and host cell death results in widespread distribution of the infection within the reticuloendothelial system (e.g., spleen, 3a; bone marrow 3b; and liver 3c).

4   The sand fly acquires its infection by ingesting an infected macrophage during the taking of a blood meal. Infected macrophages can be ingested from any bite wound site on the body, since infected cells are present throughout the peripheral circulation.

5   The amastigote transforms into the promastigote in the midgut of the sand fly. The parasites undergo several division cycles before migrating into the lumen of the proboscis, thereby completing the life cycle.

6   Many reservoir hosts exist in nature, the most important of which are the dog and the gerbil.

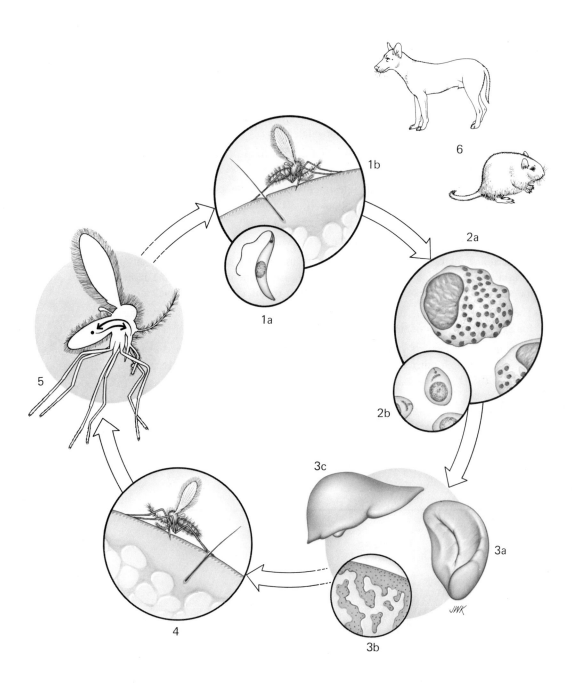

Kingdom: Protista
  Phylum: Sarcomastigophora
    Subphylum: Mastigophora
      Class: Zoomastigophorea
        Order: Kinetoplastida
          Suborder: Trypanosomatina
            Family: Trypanosomatidae
              Genus: *Leishmania*
                Species: *donovani*

Giardia Lamblia

1a   The infective stage of *Giardia lamblia* is the cyst, which is approximately 15 μm long by 5 μm wide, and possesses four nuclei.

1b   The cyst must be ingested in feces-contaminated food or water for the life cycle to begin.

2   Excystment occurs in the small intestine, with a single cyst giving rise to two trophozoites. Each trophozoite is about 10–20 μm long by 7–10 μm wide and possesses six flagella.

3   The trophozoites live upon the surface of the villi in the small intestine.

4   *G. lamblia* adheres to the columnar cells by means of a disklike depression on its ventral surface, which functions as a sucker. Encystment occurs in the lumen of the small intestine, resulting in the production of infectious quadrinucleate cysts.

5   The cysts pass into the environment with the fecal mass where they can survive for extended periods of time.

6   Both dogs and beavers have been identified as important reservoir hosts for *G. lamblia,* although other mammals, such as deer, can also become infected.

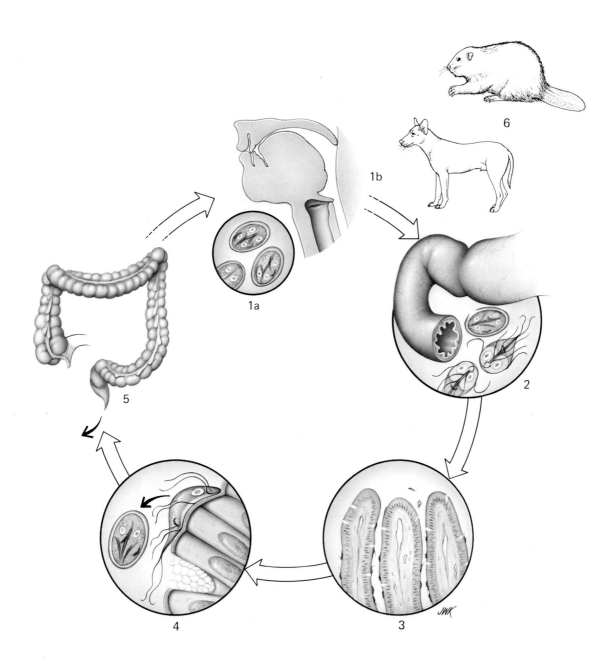

Kingdom: Protista
  Phylum: Sarcomastigophora
    Subphylum: Mastigophora
      Class: Zoomastigophorea
        Order: Diplomonadida
          Suborder: Diplomonadina
            Family: Hexamitidae
              Genus: *Giardia*
                Species: *lamblia*

Trichomonas Vaginalis

1a   There is only one stage of *Trichomonas vaginalis,* namely, the trophozoite. It measures approximately 10–25 μm in diameter. *T. vaginalis* possesses a single undulating membrane and four flagella. In addition, its cytoplasm contains various subcellular particles, one of which, the hydrogenosome, plays an important role in anaerobic metabolism. *T. vaginalis* lives on the surface of the epithelium of the urogenital tract where it derives its energy through anaerobic metabolic pathways, secreting molecular hydrogen as one of its waste products.

1b   *T. vaginalis* is transmitted from person to person most commonly by sexual intercourse. Infection of the newborn female can occur by passage through the infected birth canal of the mother. In such cases, infections remain quiescent until puberty. There are no reservoir hosts for this infection.

2   In the male, the most commonly infected site is the epithelium of the urethra in the region of the prostate gland. The prostate gland itself may also harbor organisms.

3   Adults become infected during sexual intercourse with an infected partner.

4   Trophozoites only infect the surface epithelium of the vaginal tract and cervix in the female. They never invade the surface of the uterus or fallopian tubes. Trophozoites reproduce by binary fission.

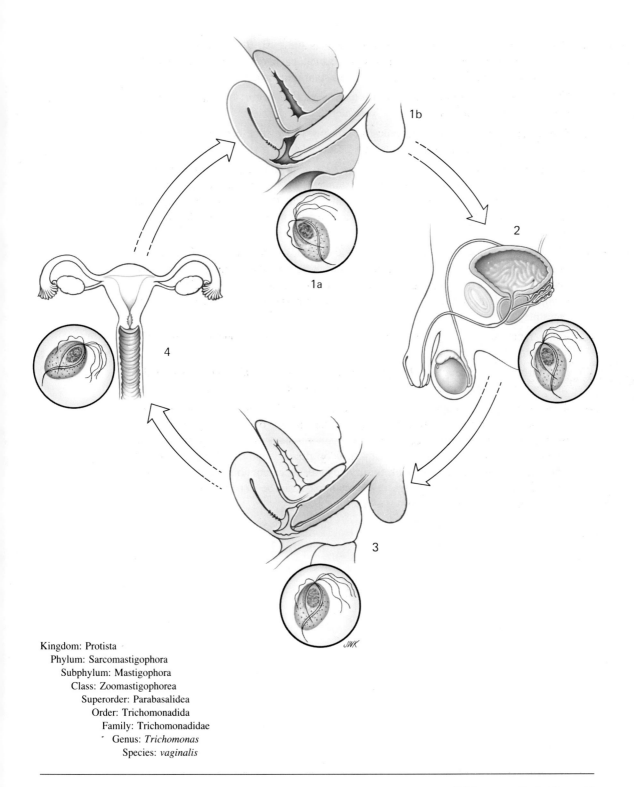

Kingdom: Protista
Phylum: Sarcomastigophora
Subphylum: Mastigophora
Class: Zoomastigophorea
Superorder: Parabasalidea
Order: Trichomonadida
Family: Trichomonadidae
Genus: *Trichomonas*
Species: *vaginalis*

Entamoeba Histolytica

1a The infective stage of *Entamoeba histolytica* is the cyst. The nonmotile cyst is 10–15 μm in diameter and contains four nuclei, each of which has a centrally located karyosome. It is surrounded by a resistant outer wall.

1b The cyst must be swallowed in order for the life cycle to begin. Cysts are commonly ingested in feces-contaminated food or water.

2 Excystment occurs in the small intestine, during which time each nucleus divides once. Thus eight motile trophozoites are produced from a single cyst.

3a The trophozoite varies in size from 20 to 30 μm in diameter. Its single nucleus contains a centrally located karyosome surrounded by even-sized and spaced chromatin at its periphery. The nucleus thus assumes the pattern of a bullseye. Ingested red cells may also be present in food vacuoles throughout the cytoplasm of *E. histolytica*.

3b The trophozoites of *E. histolytica* live in the tissues of the large intestine where they feed on living cells and replicate by binary fission. The trophozoites can also take up residence in other organs, but in this case are unable to participate in the completion of the life cycle, since they cannot return to the lumen of the large intestine.

4a Encystment occurs in the lumen of the large intestine. The trophozoite begins the process by "rounding up."

4b The early cyst is characterized by the presence of the cyst wall, one or two nuclei and smoothe ended chromatoidal bars (ordered arrays of ribosomes).

4c Cyst formation is complete when all four nuclei are present. Chromatoidal bars are usually not present in the cytoplasm of the mature cyst. Cysts pass out into the environment with the fecal mass and are resistant to a variety of physical conditions. In addition, they are not killed by dilute solutions of many types of chemicals. Therefore, they are able to survive in the feces-contaminated environment up to 1 month. While many species of mammals can be experimentally infected with *E. histolytica*, none serves as a reservoir host.

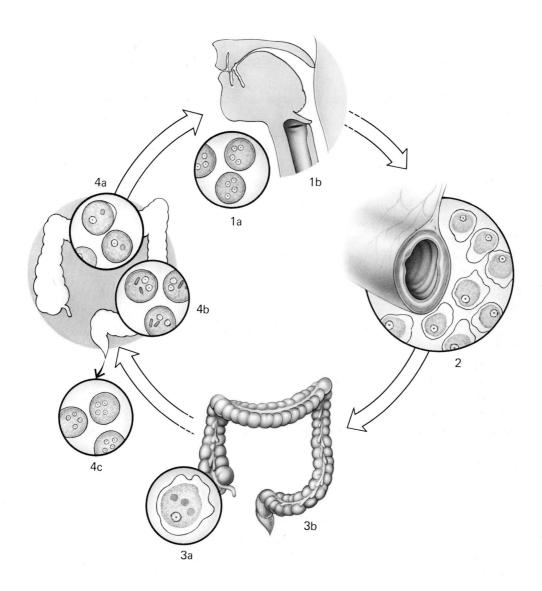

Kingdom: Protista
Phylum: Sarcomastigophora
Subphylum: Sarcodina
Superclass: Rhizopoda
Class: Lobosea
Subclass: Gymnamoebia
Order: Amoebida
Suborder: Tubulina
Family: Entamoebidae
Genus: *Entamoeba*
Species: *histolytica*

Toxoplasma Gondii

Asexual cycle

1a The infective stage of *T. gondii* for the human host is the pseudocyst. The pseudocyst is 30 μm to 100 μm in diameter, and contains hundreds to thousands of infectious units termed bradyzoites. *T. gondii* is an obligate intracellular parasite.

1b Infection is frequently initiated by ingestion of pseudocysts contained in raw or undercooked unfrozen meats. In addition, infection can occur by ingestion of oocysts (5d) in the feces of cats experiencing active intestinal infection.

2a The wall of either the pseudocyst or oocyst is broken down in the small intestine by host digestive enzymes releasing the bradyzoites or sporozoites, respectively, that then penetrate the columnar epithelium.

2b It is probable that bradyzoites or sporozoites reach the liver by the hematogenous route where they are ingested by Küpffer cells. Once inside a cell, the organisms are referred to as tachyzoites. Liver parenchymal cells also become infected. Replication immediately follows entry into host cells.

3a Macrophages transport *T. gondii* throughout the body. *T. gondii* survives and replicates within the macrophage parasitophorous vacuole by preventing the fusion of lysosomes with it.

3b Division is by endodyogeny, a process of internal budding.

3c The division cycle produces rosettes of organisms termed tachyzoites.

3d Replication results in the lysis of the host cell. Organisms are phagocytosed by new macrophages or other cell types and repeat the cycle.

3e Host resistance develops, slowing down the rate of reproduction of *T. gondii,* resulting in the pseudocyst. Replication occurs slowly within the pseudocyst, producing hundreds to thousands of bradyzoites. Pseudocysts can remain dormant within host tissues for years. Excystment occurs within the same host if cellular-based defense mechanisms are suppressed or significantly reduced.

4 The developing fetus can become infected via the placenta from the infected mother.

Sexual Cycle

5a The sexual cycle of *T. gondii* occurs only in feline hosts. The intermediate host (e.g., mouse) becomes infected by ingesting either oocysts or pseudocysts.

5b The mouse develops pseudocysts throughout its own tissues.

5c The cat becomes infected when it eats infected meat (e.g., rodent tissues) containing the pseudocysts or ingests oocysts. Bradyzoites or sporozoites penetrate columnar epithelial cells and differentiate into merozoites. Following replication, merozoites rupture infected epithelial cells and infect adjacent ones. Some merozoites differentiate into pre-sex cells termed macrogametocytes (♀) and microgametocytes (♂).

5d The microgametocytes fuse with macrogametocytes, forming zygotes termed oocysts. Oocysts enter the lumen of the small intestine and are defecated. Each oocyst sporulates in the soil, producing eight infectious sporozoites, the infectious stage for the intermediate host. The asexual cycle can also occur in feline hosts.

6 *Toxoplasma gondii* can infect any mammal and all cell types within a given individual. No other parasite, be it virus, bacteria, fungus or helminth can match *T. gondii* for its diversity of host range or its lack of site specificity within the host.

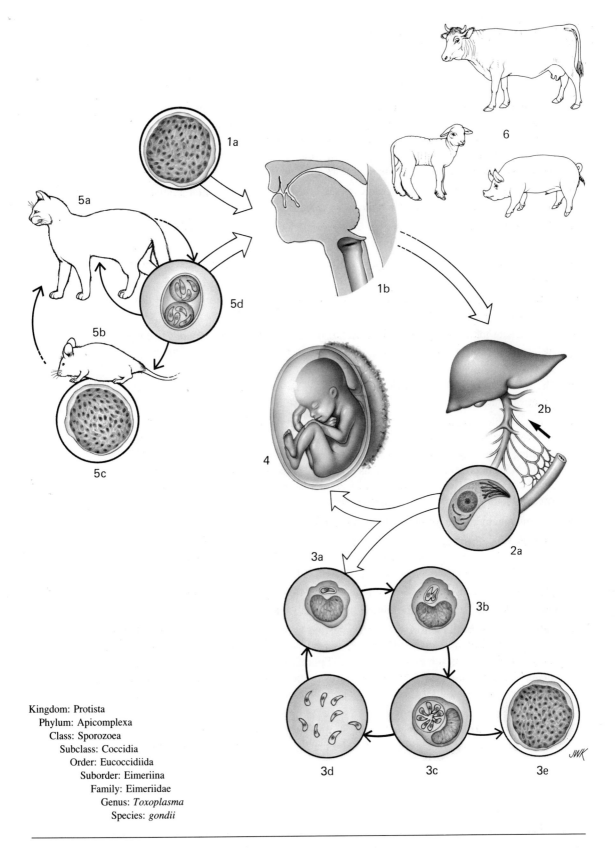

Kingdom: Protista
Phylum: Apicomplexa
Class: Sporozoea
Subclass: Coccidia
Order: Eucoccidiida
Suborder: Eimeriina
Family: Eimeriidae
Genus: *Toxoplasma*
Species: *gondii*

Cryptosporidium Sp.

1a The sporulated oocyst is the infectious stage of *Cryptosporidium* sp. Each oocyst measures 3–5 μm in diameter, and contains four infectious units termed sporozoites and a characteristic refractile residual body. It is not known whether or not there is more than one species of *Cryptosporidium*, since the organism is morphologically indistinguishable regardless of the source of infection.

1b Infection begins when the sporulated oocyst is ingested. Feces-contaminated food and water are the most common sources of infection.

2 The oocyst releases the sporozoites in the small intestine upon contact with host digestive enzymes.

3a Each sporozoite is capable of infecting a columnar epithelial cell, thus beginning the asexual cycle.

3b The sporozoite attaches to the surface of the epithelial cell and embeds itself down to the base of the microvilli.

3c The parasite induces the host cell to extend the microvilli up and around its entire surface, following which the parasite differentiates into the trophozoite. The parasite is now intracellular.

3d The trophozoite transforms into the schizont, resulting in the production of eight organisms termed merozoites.

3e The merozoites burst out of their membrane-bound host cell and are now capable of infecting another epithelial cell. This cycle usually occurs once more, now resulting in the production of only four merozoites. However, in individuals suffering from immunodeficiencies, such as AIDS, the merozoites can reinfect for many cycles. Alternatively, a newly arrived merozoite may differentiate into either a microgametocyte (δ) or a macrogametocyte ($\female$).

4a The microgametocyte produces 12 to 16 microgametes.

4b The microgametes burst out of their infected host cell. Each microgamete is able to fuse with a macrogametocyte (shown on left). The macrogametocyte remains within the host cell cytoplasm until it is fertilized.

5 The resulting zygote, termed the oocyst, differentiates, secretes an impervious outer wall, and then enters the lumen of the small intestine.

6 Before leaving the lumen of the large intestine with the fecal mass, the fertilized oocyst is unsporulated. Upon reaching the external environment, the oocyst immediately sporulates, thus achieving infectivity. Sporulation can also occur if the unsporulated oocyst is ingested. The entire life cycle takes approximately 2 to 4 weeks in healthy individuals. In immunosuppressed persons, the cycle can go on indefinitely.

7 *Cryptosporidium* can initiate infection in a wide variety of mammalian species. Calves and suckling pigs are thought to be the most common reservoir hosts.

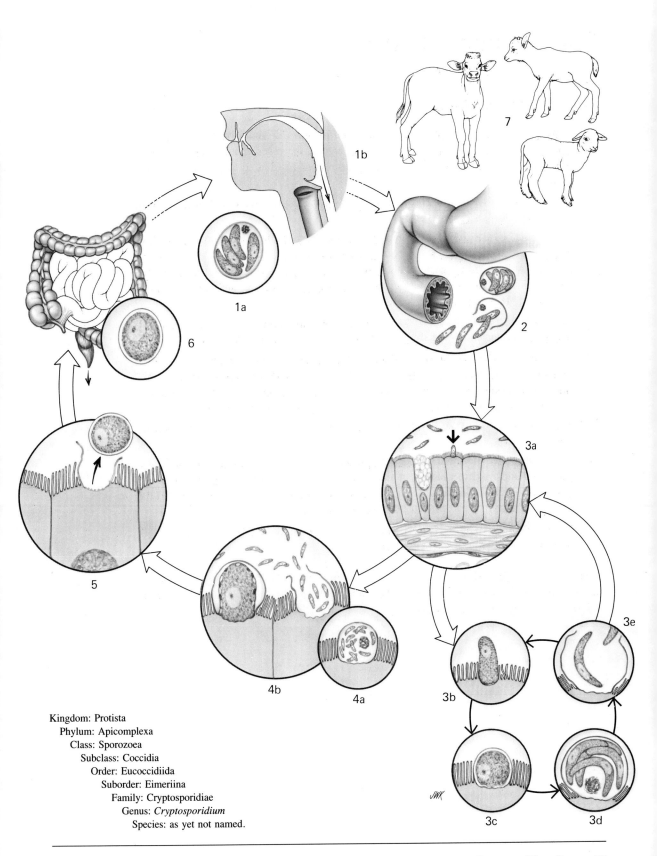

Kingdom: Protista
Phylum: Apicomplexa
Class: Sporozoea
Subclass: Coccidia
Order: Eucoccidiida
Suborder: Eimeriina
Family: Cryptosporidiae
Genus: *Cryptosporidium*
Species: as yet not named.

Cryptosporidium Sp.   27

Plasmodium Vivax

Sexual Cycle (Mosquito)

1 Different species of anopheline mosquitoes transmit different species of malaria. The mosquito becomes infected when she ingests the macrogametocytes (♀) and microgametocytes (♂) present in the peripheral blood of an infected human (intermediate host).

2 The red cell cytoplasm is digested away from the gametocytes within the lumen of the mosquito's stomach.

3 Microgametocytes differentiate and divide into 6 to 8 flagellated microgametes. The process of microgamete formation is termed exflagellation. Each microgamete can fuse with a single macrogamete, thus forming a zygote termed the ookinete. After fusion of the two nuclei, the organism becomes diploid. Ookinete formation takes about 18 hours for completion.

4 The ookinete penetrates between the columnar epithelium and comes to rest just under the connective tissue sheath and further differentiates into the oocyst.

5 Each oocyst undergoes nuclear reduction, then a series of nuclear and cytoplasmic division cycles, resulting in the production of thousands of haploid sporozoites. Sporozoite production is complete within 8–10 days after ingestion of gametocytes. The sporozoites enter the hemocoel by penetrating the wall of the oocyst.

6a Each sporozoite is approximately 2–3 μm long and possesses a single centrally located nucleus.

6b Sporozoites site select within the cytoplasm of the cuboidal epithelium lining the salivary glands and the lumen of the glands themselves. They gain entrance into the human intermediate host when the mosquito injects them, together with salivary secretions, during the taking of her next blood meal.

7 Female mosquitoes in the genus *Anopheles* are the definitive hosts for all species of malaria, including *Plasmodium vixax*.

Note: The same general scheme of sexual development (*1–6b*) applies to *P. ovale, P. falciparum,* and *P. malariae,* as well, although the exact timing for each stage of development varies from species to species.

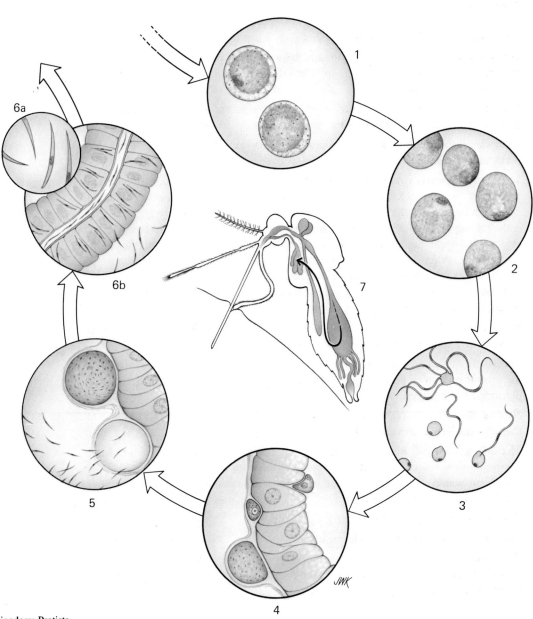

Kingdom: Protista
Phylum: Apicomplexa
Class: Sporozoea
Subclass: Coccidia
Order: Eucoccidiida
Suborder: Haemosporina
Family: Plasmodiidae
Genus: *Plasmodium*
Species: *vivax*

Plasmodium Vivax

Asexual Cycle

1a The sporozoite is the infectious stage and is 2–3 μm long.

1b Sporozoites are injected, along with the salivary secretion of the mosquito, into the human intermediate host when an infected female anopheline mosquito takes a second or third blood meal.

2a The sporozoites travel via the hematogenous route to the liver, where they enter parenchymal cells, thereby initiating the exoerythrocytic cycle.

2b Following differentiation into merozoites, the organisms divide by schizogony into hundreds of infectious units.

3 The exoerythrocytic cycle takes about 6–8 days to complete, culminating in the rupture of the infected parenchymal cell, with the consequent release of about 10,000 parasites into the bloodstream. Merozoites cannot enter new parenchymal cells but can enter red blood cells. Entry into the red cell signals the onset of the erythrocytic cycle. Some merozoites, instead of repeatedly dividing within the parenchymal cell, differentiate into a dormant non-dividing stage termed a hypnozoite (*). This stage can go on to replicate into merozoites at a later time in the infection. Activation of hypnozoites results in a relapse of infection and can occur at any time after initial infection up to 5 years.

4a Replication of *P. vivax* within the red blood cell occurs through an asexual division process, and begins with the trophozoite stage.

4b The single nucleated trophozoite grows within the red cell, feeding mainly upon the protein portion of hemoglobin. During this time, the infected red cell becomes deformed and enlarged.

4c Nuclear division occurs repeatedly, resulting in 16 to 32 nuclei. The cytoplasm then divides, separating each nucleus into a merozoite.

4d The infected red cell ruptures, releasing the parasites into the bloodstream. After entering a new red cell, the division cycle is repeated. One erythrocytic cycle is completed within 41–45 hours. Some early trophozoites (4a), instead of dividing, differentiate into presexual stages.

5a The macrogametocyte is the female presexual stage

5b The microgametocyte is the male presexual stage.

5c These two stages are infective for the definitive host, the female anopheline mosquito, and are acquired by the insect when she takes a blood meal. There are no reservoir hosts for any species of human malaria.

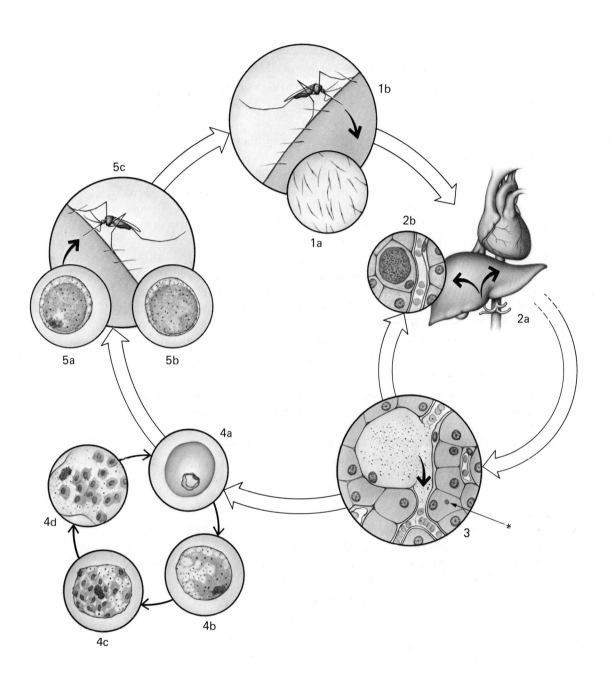

Plasmodium Ovale

Asexual Cycle

1a The sporozoite is the infectious stage and is 2–3 μm long.

1b The sporozoites of *Plasmodium ovale* are injected, along with the salivary secretions of the mosquito, into the host when an infected female anopheline mosquito takes a second or third blood meal.

2a Sporozoites are passively carried by the bloodstream to all organs, but only survive if they reach the liver. In the liver, the sporozoites break out of the capillaries and penetrate parenchymal cells, initiating the exoerythrocytic cycle.

2b The parasites differentiate into merozoites. Some merozoites differentiate further into hypnozoites (*), a nondividing stage, while others undergo multiple divisions, resulting in the formation of mature schizonts. Each schizont gives rise to about 15,000 organisms and takes 9 days to fully mature.

3 Mature schizonts rupture, thereby releasing merozoites into adjacent capillaries. Invasion of red cells by the merozoites then ensues, thus beginning the erythrocytic cycle. Merozoites are unable to invade parenchymal cells. Hypnozoites can mature into schizonts with attendant release of merozoites, thus initiating a new erythrocytic cycle. When this occurs, the infected individual experiences a relapse of the infection. Relapses can apparently occur at anytime up to 5 years after the initial infection.

4a Invasion of a red cell by a merozoite results in the development of the early trophozoite stage, known as the signet ring stage.

4b Growth of the trophozoite culminates in the digestion of most of the hemoglobin of the red cell. A particular waste product of hemoglobin digestion, hemozoin, accumulates in the unoccupied portion of host cell cytoplasm. The overall diameter of the infected red cell increases and its shape becomes irregular.

4c Nuclear division takes place within a syncytium of parasite cytoplasm. Following nuclear division, the cytoplasm divides. Thus 8 to 10 merozoites are formed and are collectively termed the mature schizont. The entire process of nuclear and cytoplasmic division is termed schizogony.

4d The mature schizont ruptures, freeing its complement of merozoites into the bloodstream. Each released merozoite has the opportunity to invade a new red cell. The erythrocytic cycle takes 49–50 hours to complete. Not all merozoites that enter red cells divide. Rather, some differentiate into pre-sex cells.

5a The female pre-sex cell is termed the macrogametocyte.

5b The male pre-sex cell is called the microgametocyte.

5c The mosquito acquires her infection by ingesting macro and microgametocytes along with her blood meal. There are no reservoir hosts for any species of human malaria.

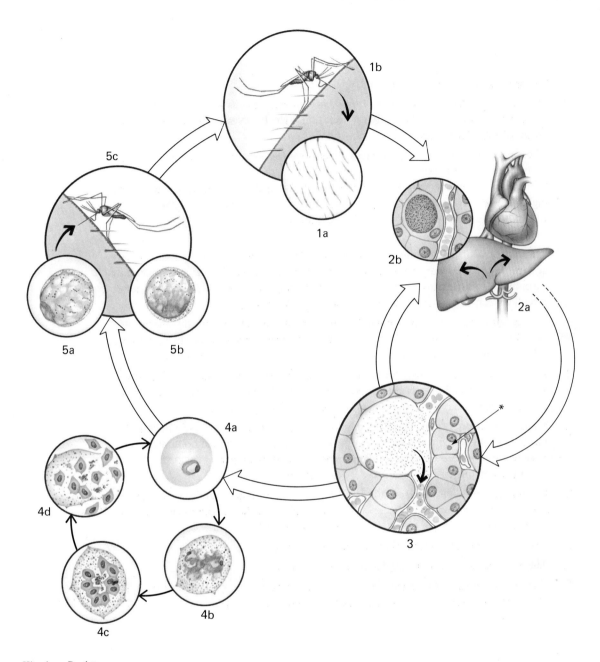

Kingdom: Protista
Phylum: Apicomplexa
Class: Sporozoea
Subclass: Coccidia
Order: Eucoccidiida
Suborder: Haemosporina
Family: Plasmodiidae
Genus: *Plasmodium*
Species: *ovale*

Plasmodium Malariae

Asexual Cycle

1a   The sporozoite is 2–3 μm long and is the infectious stage.

1b   Infection in the human host by *Plasmodium malariae* begins when the sporozoites are injected, along with the salivary secretion, into the blood vessels in the skin by an infected female anopheline mosquito.

2a   The sporozoites are passively carried to the liver as well as to other parts of the body by the bloodstream.

2b   In the liver, the sporozoites enter parenchymal cells and differentiate into merozoites, signaling the beginning of the exoerythrocytic cycle. Division of the merozoites results in the production of about 2,000 parasites, taking about 12–16 days to complete.

3   The mature schizont ruptures the infected cell and the merozoites enter the bloodstream. Merozoites are unable to invade parenchymal cells. *P. malariae* does not form hypnozoites, therefore it is not a cause of relapsing malaria. However, initial infections can last for up to 30 years, even after treatment.

4a   The erythrocytic cycle starts with the invasion of the red cell by the merozoite. As with all other species of malaria, the early trophozoite stage is commonly referred to as the signet ring stage.

4b   The trophozoite feeds upon the protein portion of hemoglobin and enlarges to fill most of the host cell cytoplasm. Unlike *P. vivax* and *P. ovale*, *P. malariae* infection does not alter either the size or shape of the infected erythrocyte.

4c   Nuclear and cytoplasmic division (schizogony) sequentially occur, resulting in the production of merozoites. Hemozoin, a solid waste product of hemoglobin digestion, is sequestered into the center of the infected red cell cytoplasm. The red cell plus the organisms inside it is called the mature schizont.

4d   The infected red cell ruptures, thereby releasing the parasites. Invasion of another red cell by a merozoite initiates another cycle of division. Some merozoites, instead of undergoing schizogony, differentiate into pre-sex cells.

5a   The female pre-sex cell is called the macrogametocyte.

5b   The male pre-sex cell is termed the microgametocyte.

5c   The female mosquito becomes infected by ingesting both types of pre-sex cells. There are no reservoir hosts for any species of human malaria.

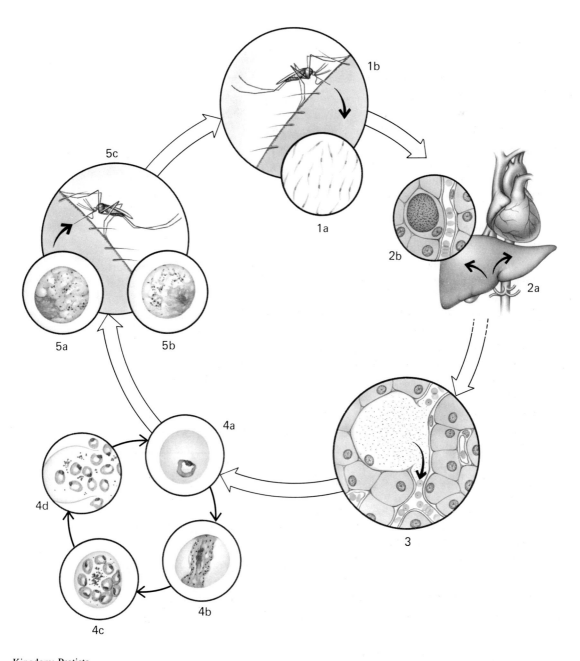

Kingdom: Protista
  Phylum: Apicomplexa
   Class: Sporozoea
    Subclass: Coccidia
     Order: Eucoccidiida
      Suborder: Haemosporina
       Family: Plasmodiidae
        Genus: *Plasmodium*
         Species: *malariae*

Plasmodium Falciparum

Asexual Cycle

1a The sporozoite is the infectious stage and is 2–3 μm in length.

1b Infection begins in the human host when an infected female anopheline mosquito injects sporozoites, along with the salivary secretion, into blood vessels in the skin while she is taking a second or third blood meal.

2a The bloodstream transports the sporozoites to all parts of the body. However, in order to continue the life cycle, sporozoites must reach the liver and penetrate into parenchymal cells.

2b Once in their intracellular niche, each sporozoite differentiates into a merozoite and begins to divide, beginning the exoerythrocytic cycle. Schizogony takes 5–7 days to complete, resulting in the production of approximately 40,000 parasites per infecting sporozoite.

3 The mature tissue schizont ruptures its infected parenchymal cell and the merozoites enter the bloodstream. Merozoites only infect red cells. Hence reinvasion of the liver is not possible. Only a sporozoite transmitted by the bite of another infected mosquito can initiate a new exoerythrocytic cycle of division. No hypnozoites are formed by *P. falciparum*.

4a Merozoites begin the erythrocytic cycle by invading red cells. With *P. facliparum* it is common to have more than one parasite in each red cell. This early stage of development is called the trophozoite and is commonly found in the peripheral circulation.

4b Unlike the other three species of malaria that infect humans, *P. falciparum* develops beyond the trophozoite, inside red cells attached to endothelial cells lining the capillaries of the body, especially those in the deep tissues. The mechanisms by which this takes place apparently involve the parasite-directed elicitation of ''knobs'' on a portion of the infected red cell membrane. The physicochemical properties of these ''knobs'' together with other parasite-derived proteins enable them to bind to endothelial cell membrane. The attachment lasts throughout schizogony. The trophozoite grows within the immobilized infected red cell, feeding upon the protein portion of hemoglobin.

4c Schizogony occurs every 48 hours and results in the production of 8 to 16 merozoites.

4d The mature schizont breaks open, releasing its complement of merozoites.

4e Noninfected red cells often become trapped in capillaries that harbor infected red cells.

4f These trapped red cells are quickly infected by merozoites freed after schizogony. Gametocyte formation occurs in the peripheral circulation.

5a The macrogametocyte is the female pre-sex cell.

5b The microgametocyte is the male pre-sex cell.

5c The female mosquito acquires her infection by ingesting both pre-sex cells along with a blood meal from an infected individual. There are no reservoir hosts for any species of human malaria.

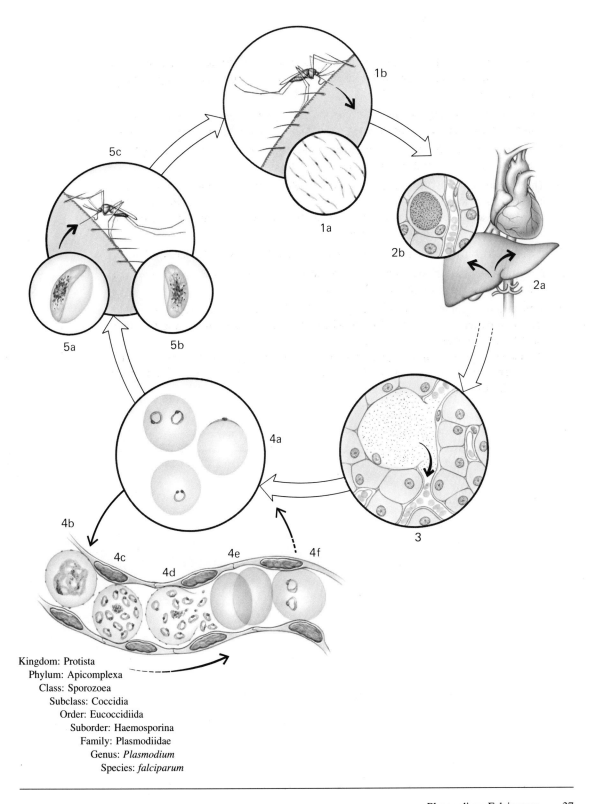

Kingdom: Protista
Phylum: Apicomplexa
Class: Sporozoea
Subclass: Coccidia
Order: Eucoccidiida
Suborder: Haemosporina
Family: Plasmodiidae
Genus: *Plasmodium*
Species: *falciparum*

Balantidium Coli

1a   The infective stage for the human is the cyst. The cyst is 55 μm in diameter and is surrounded by a resistant thickened wall. Its cytoplasm contains a single micro- and macronucleus.

1b   The cyst must be ingested in order for the life cycle to begin. Food and water contaminated with feces from infected individuals serve as the sources of infection.

2   Excystment occurs in the small intestine, while the trophozoites reside in the large intestine. Each cyst produces a single trophozoite.

3a   The trophozoite is 70 μm long by 45 μm in width and is completely surrounded by cilia. Its cytoplasm contains a contractile vacuole, a single micronucleus, and a single cresent-shaped macronucleus. In addition, the trophozoite has a cytostome through which it ingests its food; namely, living host cells.

3b   It divides by binary fission within the walls of the submucosa of the large intestine.

4a   Encystation occurs in the lumen. The process results in the production of a thick wall that surrounds and protects the organism.

4b   Encystation is complete when the cyst wall is fully contiguous. Cysts pass into the environment with the fecal mass where they can remain infective for another host for extended periods of time.

5   Although other mammalian species, such as the Guinea pig and the domestic pig, can become infected with *B. coli,* it is not known if any of them are important reservoir hosts.

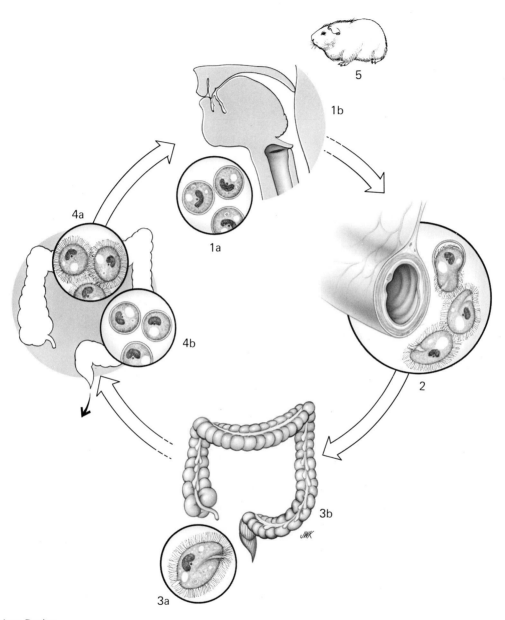

Kingdom: Protista
  Phylum: Ciliophora
    Class: Kinetofragminophorea
      Subclass: Vestibuliferia
        Order: Trichostomatida
          Suborder: Trichostomatina
            Family: Balantidiidae
              Genus: *Balantidium*
                Species: *coli*

2 Cestoidea

General Characteristics of Cestodes

All adult cestodes (tapeworms) are parasitic and live within the digestive tract of their hosts. All vertebrates can harbor tapeworm adults, but only a few species of tapeworms infect the human host. Tapeworms vary greatly in size, with some achieving lengths of over 10 meters, while others grow only centimeters in length. Nearly all cestodes rely on intermediate hosts for transmission, which may in some cases be a mammal (e.g., *Taenia saginata* in the cow and *Taenia solium* in the pig).

The adult worm typically consists of a head (scolex) and a segmented body (strobila), each segment of which is termed a proglottid. None possesses a digestive tract; hence they absorb all nutrients through their outer surface (tegument).

The scolex attaches to the host epithelium by means of suckers, hooks, grooves, or a combination of these holdfast organs, depending upon the species in question. Proglottids are produced near the neck of the strobila and exhibit increasing degrees of maturation the further away from the scolex they are found. Finally, the last segments are those that contain fertilized eggs and usually detach from the colony of proglottids, or disintegrate, releasing their eggs into the lumen of the intestine. Eggs can either be eaten by an intermediate host and undergo further development, or hatch, infect an intermediate host, and then undergo morphogenesis to the next stage. Ultimately, the definitive host must ingest the infective larval tapeworm to acquire the infection.

The entire surface of the tegument is covered with small fingerlike projections (microtriches), which are thought to both aid in adherence of the worm to the intestinal surface, and to increase its own absorption surface. As already mentioned, all nutrients must be absorbed, either passively or actively through the tegument.

Below the tegument lies a complex arrangement of muscle, nerve, excretory, and reproductive tissues. The musculature runs both longitudinally and circularly. Their muscle cells lack T-tubules and are nonstriated. The excretory tubules run on either lateral side of each segment and transport wastes to the host intestinal lumen. Specialized ciliated cells called flame cells aid in fluid movement. The tegument and excretory system have been implicated in osmoregulation. The scolex possesses ganglia from which emanate various branches of nerves running the length of the strobila. The head may contain sensory nerves ending in specialized regions that aid the worm in seeking nutrient gradients. The nerves communicate via lateral commissures.

Each segment usually contains a complete set of male and female reproductive organs. As already mentioned the farther away from the scolex the segment is, the more sexually mature it is. Each proglottid makes a full complement of sperm and eggs. Often, the sperm are stored and self-fertilization in each proglottid occurs. However, segments can also exchange sperm. If two worms of the same species are present in the same host, they can mate with each other. Sperm are produced in the testes, which are connected to the vas efferens. Sperm are stored in the external seminal receptacle. The female system reproductive system consists of the ovary, vitelline glands, oviduct, and Mehlis' gland. Egg yolk is formed by the vitelline cells which join with the ovum to produce the unfertilized egg. Fertilization occurs when the egg passes through the oviduct. Meiosis is complete after fertilization. The vitelline membrane is then laid down and the zygote and/or vitelline cells secrete the eggshell, itself depending on the species. Embryonation then ensues, resulting in gravid proglottids, which may contain hundreds to thousands of infectious eggs.

Classification

Bold type indicates orders represented in book by parasites

Kingdom: Animal
  Phylum: Platyhelminthes
    Class: Turbellaria
    Class: Monogenea
    Class: Trematoda
    Class: Cestoidea
      Subclass: Cestodaria
        Family: Amphilinidae
        Family: Austramphilinidae
        Family: Gyrocotylidae
      Subclass: Eucestoda
      Order: Caryophyllidea
        Family: Caryophyllaeidae
      Order: Spathebothriidea
        Family: Cyathocephalidae
        Family: Spathebothriidae
      Order: Trypanorhyncha
        Family: Dasyrhynchidae
        Family: Eutetrarhynchidae
        Family: Gilquiniidae
        Family: Gymnorhynchidae
        Family: Hepatoxylidae
        Family: Hornelliellidae
        Family: Lacistorhynchidae
        Family: Mustelicolidae
        Family: Otobothriidae
        Family: Paranybeliniidae
        Family: Pterobothriidae
        Family: Sphyriocephalidae
        Family: Tentaculariidae
      Order: Pseudophyllidea
        Family: Amphicotylidae
        Family: Bothriocephalidae
        Family: Cephalochlamydidae
        Family: Diphyllobothriidae
        Family: Echinophallidae
        Family: Haplobothriidae
        Family: Parabothriocephalidae

        Family: Ptychobothriidae
        Family: Triaenophoridae
      Order: Lecanicephalidea
        Family: Adelobothriidae
        Family: Balanobothriidae
        Family: Disculicepitidae
        Family: Lecanicephalidae
      Order: Aporidea
        Family: Nematoparataeniidae
      Order: Tetraphyllidea
        Family: Dioecotaeniidae
        Family: Onchobothriidae
        Family: Phyllobothriidae
        Family: Triloculariidae
      Order: Diphyllidea
        Family: Ditrachybathridiidae
        Family: Echinobothriidae
      Order: Litobothridea
        Family: Litobothridae
      Order: Proteocephalata
        Family: Proteocephalidae
      Order: Cyclophyllidea
        Family: Amabiliidae
        Family: Anoplocephalidae
        Family: Catenotaeniidae
        Family: Davaineidae
        Family: Dilepididae
        Family: Dioecocestidae
        Family: Diploposthidae
        Family: Hymenolepididae
        Family: Mesocestoididae
        Family: Nematotaeniidae
        Family: Progynotaeniidae
        Family: Taeniidae
        Family: Tetrabothriidae
        Family: Triplotaeniidae
      Order: Nippotaeniidea
        Family: Nippotaeniidae

Diphyllobothrium Latum

1a The infective stage for the human host of *D. latum* is the pleroceroid, which lives between the myomeres in muscle tissue of freshwater fish.

1b The mode of infection is by oral ingestion of undercooked or raw unfrozen infected freshwater fish.

2a Following ingestion, the pleurocercoid develops to the immature adult. The scolex of the adult worm attaches to the wall of the small intestine by means of two bilateral grooves called bothria.

2b Differentiation, growth, and maturation occurs within the lumen of the small intestine.

3a Hundreds of immature, mature, and gravid segments are produced within 20 days after ingestion of the pleurocercoid. Adult worms can achieve lengths exceeding 14 meters.

3b The mature proglottid can be distinguished from other adult tapeworms infecting the human host by the fact that its birth pore exits from the center of the dorsal surface, rather than laterally.

4a Gravid proglottids periodically release eggs into the lumen.

4b The eggs become included within the fecal mass prior to being passed outside the host during defecation. It has been estimated that a large adult worm can produce some 10^6 eggs each day.

4c The unembryonated eggs have a single operculum and must be deposited in fresh water for continuation of the life cycle.

5a After an incubation period of approximately 18–20 days, the operculated end of the egg opens, and the free-swimming coracidium emerges into the aquatic environment. This stage moves about aided by extremely long cilia covering its entire outer surface. The coracidium can survive for 12–14 hours as a free-swimming larva before it exhausts its stored energy supply and dies.

5b The coracidium is able to develop to the next stage only after being ingested by crustaceans in the genus *Diaptomus*. After the coracidium is eaten, it penetrates the hemocoel of *Diaptomus* and transforms into the procercoid stage over a 2- to 3-week period.

5c Minnows and other small fish feed upon both infected and noninfected Diaptomus. If an infected *Diaptomus* is eaten, then the procercoid is released from the crustacean, penetrates the fish's small intestine, and finally migrates to between the myomeres. There it develops to the plerocercoid, the infective stage for the human host.

5d Humans do not usually eat raw or undercooked minnows, and therefore these infected smaller fish do not serve as important vectors for the infection. However, if an infected minnow is eaten by a larger predator species of fish (e.g., trout, walleyed pike, Northern pike, or perch), then the pleurocercoid can relocate between the myomeres of the musculature of the larger fish. Hence transmission of the infection is through the ingestion of these latter intermediate hosts.

6   Bears can serve as reservoir hosts for *Diphyllobothrium latum*.

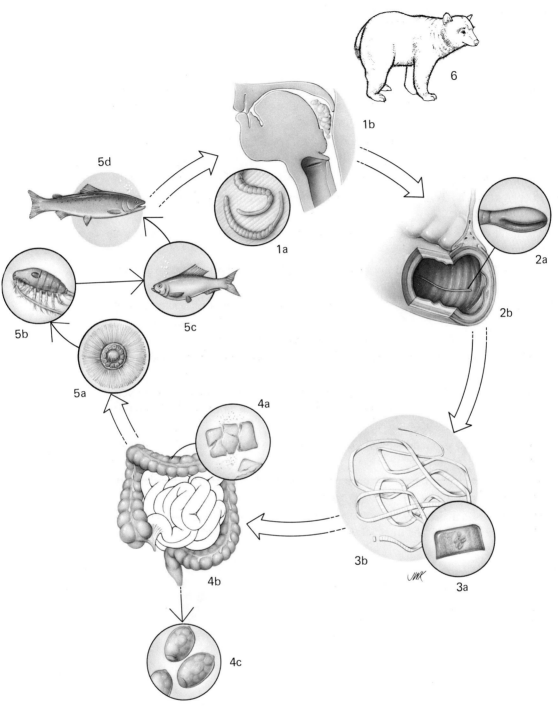

Kingdom: Animal
 Phylum: Platyhelminthes
  Class: Cestoidea
   Order: Pseudophyllidea
    Family: Diphyllobothriidae
     Genus: *Diphyllobothrium*
      Species: *latum*

Dipylidium Caninum

1   The infective stage of *Dipylidium caninum* is the cysticercoid (6b) and lives within the haemocoel of the dog flea, *Ctenocephalides canis*. The infected flea must be ingested to initiate infection in the human host.

2   The flea's tissues are digested away from the cysticercoid in the stomach and small intestine.

3a   The hook-studded scolex of *D. caninum* attaches to the wall of the small intestine.

3b   In approximately 20–25 days, the worm matures to adulthood within the lumen of the small intestine.

4a   The adult of *D. caninum* is 30–40 cm in length, but can achieve a length of over 70 cm.

4b   The characteristic proglottid has two genital pores, each of which opens laterally on either side of the segment.

5a   Gravid proglottids break off from the parent colony and pass out, *intact,* in the feces.

5b   The packets of eggs contained within each proglottid are held together by an outer embryonic membrane. The proglottids disintegrate in the soil, releasing the packets of eggs.

6a   The eggs must then be ingested by the larvae of fleas to continue the life cycle. The eggs hatch within the flea's midgut, and the hexacanth tapeworm larva migrates into the hemocoel, where it transforms into the cysticercoid.

6b   The cysticercoid is retained by the flea during its own morphogenesis to an adult insect.

6c   The adult flea, harboring the cysticercoid, must now be ingested by the definitive mammalian host for the life cycle to become complete.

7   Dog is the usual definitive host for this tapeworm. The cysticercoid is usually ingested together with the infected flea (i.e., the intermediate host).

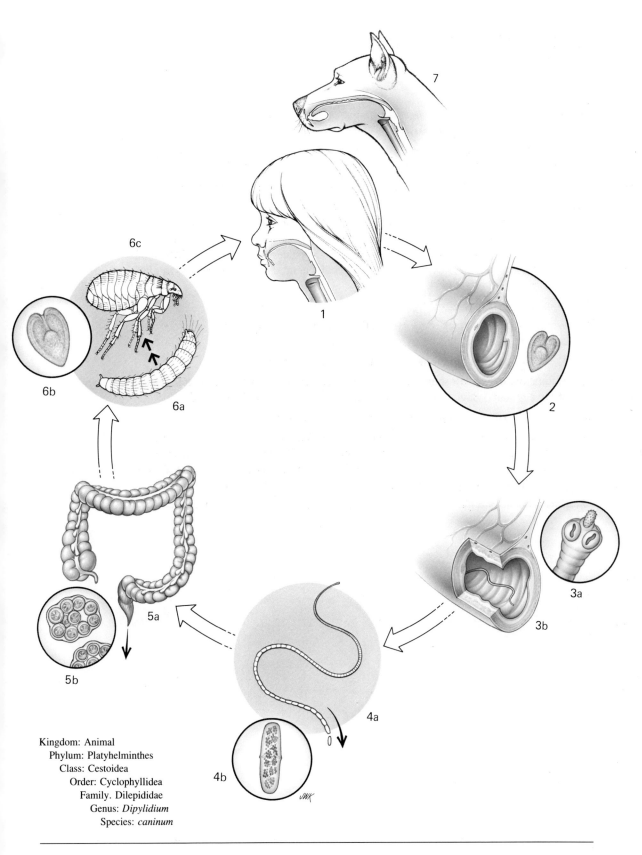

Kingdom: Animal
Phylum: Platyhelminthes
Class: Cestoidea
Order: Cyclophyllidea
Family. Dilepididae
Genus: *Dipylidium*
Species: *caninum*

Hymenolepis Nana

1a The embryonated egg of *Hymenolepis nana* contains polar filaments, thereby distinguishing it from that of *Hymenolepis diminuta*.

1b The egg can be ingested directly by the definitive host. Feces containing eggs is the source of infection.

2   The eggs hatch within the lumen of the small intestine releasing the hexacanth embryo.

3   The hexacanth embryo penetrates the villus tissue of the small intestine and develops into the cysticeroid. Alternatively, eggs can be ingested by the intermediate host, various beetles species, and proceed to develop to cysticercoids within the hemocoel, as with *H. diminuta*. Thus, *H. nana* can infect its definitive host directly or through an intermediate insect host.

4a In the direct life cycle, the cysticercoid exits from the villus.

4b Within 6 days it attaches to the wall of the lumen of the small intestine after everting the scolex.

5a The scolex of *H. nana* possesses both hooks and suckers.

5b Maturation to the adult stage takes approximately 30 days from the time of ingestion of the egg and 5 days less than that if an infected arthropod is ingested.

6a The proglottid of *H. nana* has a single lateral genital pore.

6b The adult worm measures about 30–40 cm in length. Eggs are passed into the lumen of the small intestine either through the genital atrium of gravid segments or are released after such proglottids break off from the parent colony and disintegrate. The eggs are passed into the outside environment by defecation.

7   Small rodents are the most common reservoir hosts.

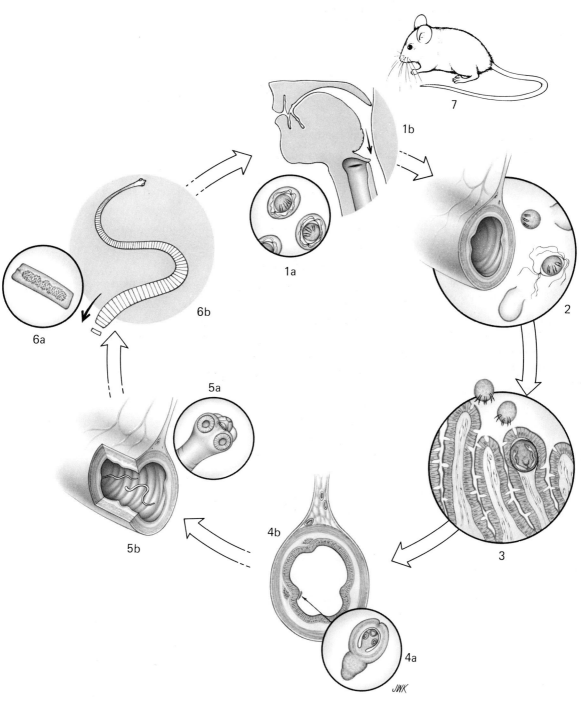

7

1b

1a

2

6a

6b

3

5a

5b

4b

4a

JWK

Kingdom: Animal
  Phylum: Platyhelminthes
    Class: Cestoidea
      Order: Cyclophyllidea
        Family: Hymenolepididae
          Genus: *Hymenolepis*
            Species: *nana*

Hymenolepis Diminuta

1a The intermediate host is usually a coleopteran in the genus *Tribolium*. However, various other genera of beetles can also serve this function in the life cycle.

1b The beetle, infected with the cysticerocid larva of *H. diminuta,* must be ingested in order to initiate infection with this cestode.

2 The tissues of the infected beetle are digested away from the cysticercoids in the stomach and small intestine.

3a The scolex, which possesses four suckers, everts from the cysticercoid shortly after being released from the beetle.

3b The scolex then attaches to the wall of the lumen of the small intestine where it matures within 20 days.

4a The gravid proglottid has a single lateral genital pore.

4b The adult worm is small in length compared to the *Taenia* spp. or *D. latum,* achieving an average length of 30 cm.

5a The eggs are passed out the genital atrium of gravid segments, or are released into the lumen of the small intestine when egg-laden segments break off from the parent colony and disintegrate.

5b Eggs thus released are included into the fecal mass and are passed out of the host during defecation.

6a The eggs become ingested by the larvae of *Tribolium* spp. beetles and other Coleoptera. In the insect's small intestine, the egg hatches, releasing the hexacanth embryo. The embryo then penetrates the intestinal tract and eventually transforms into the cysticercoid (i.e., the infective stage for the definitive host) in the hemocoel.

6b The cysticercoid survives the insect's morphogenesis to an adult arthropod.

7 While humans often become infected with *H. diminuta,* it is more commonly a parasite of rodents, such as rats and mice.

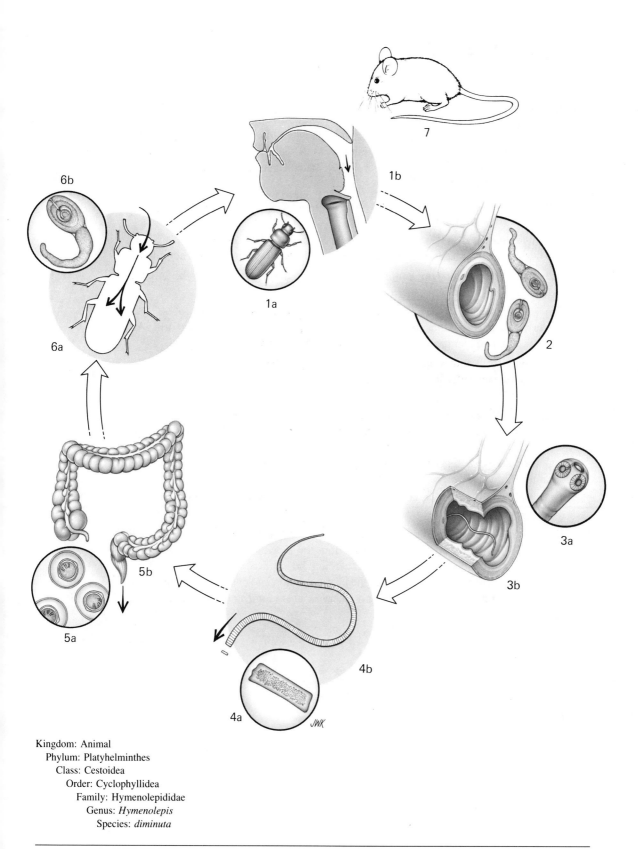

Kingdom: Animal
  Phylum: Platyhelminthes
    Class: Cestoidea
      Order: Cyclophyllidea
        Family: Hymenolepididae
          Genus: *Hymenolepis*
            Species: *diminuta*

Hymenolepis Diminuta   53

Taenia Saginata

1a The infective stage for the human (i.e., definitive) host is the juvenile worm termed the cysticercus. No other mammal can serve as the definitive host for this tapeworm. The cysticercus lives encysted within the tissues of the intermediate host, the cow. All bovine tissues may harbor cysticerci, but skeletal muscle is the most common source of infection.

1b The cysticercus must be ingested in raw or undercooked unfrozen beef for the life cycle to begin within the human host.

2 The cysticerci are digested away from the tissues of the cow in the stomach. The freed cysticerci enter the small intestine and initiate development toward adulthood.

3a In the small intestine, the immature tapeworm evaginates its scolex (note the absence of hooks).

3b The scolex attaches to the inner wall of the small intestine by means of its four suckers, and in approximately 8–12 weeks develops into a fully mature worm. An adult *T. saginata* can grow to as long as 10 meters, but 6 meters is typical.

4a The gravid proglottid contains some 100,000 eggs. The uterus has more than 12 branches on each side, thereby distinguishing it from that of *T. solium* (see Figure 4a, page 57).

4b Gravid proglottids break off from the parent colony and pass live through the anus to the external environment. During its passage through the anal sphincter, some eggs may be expressed from the proglottid and come to rest on the perianal region of the host. Eggs may be expelled from the *intact* parent colony, but this is an uncommon mode of egg dispersal.

5a The embryonated eggs become liberated from the proglottids when the segments disintegrate in the soil.

5b Ingestion of embryonated eggs by cattle results in their hatching within the small intestine. The hexacanth larvae then penetrate the bloodstream and are carried to various organs throughout the body, including brain, eye, skeletal musculature, and the heart. There, within 2 months, the larvae develop into cysticerci, the infective stage for the human host. There are no reservoir hosts for *Taenia saginata*.

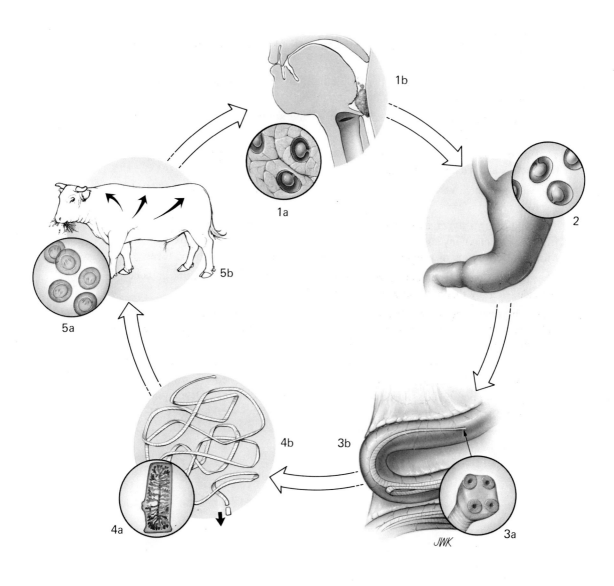

Kingdom: Animal
Phylum: Platyhelminthes
Class: Cestoidea
Order: Cyclophyllidea
Family: Taeniidae
Genus: *Taenia*
Species: *saginata*

Taenia Solium

1a The stage leading to adult tapeworm infection for the human host is the cysticercus (i.e., juvenile tapeworm).

1b The cysticercus, together with a portion of infected undercooked or raw unfrozen pork must be ingested in order to begin the cycle.

2 Cysticerci are liberated from muscle tissue in the stomach. The freed cysticerci then enter the small intestine by peristalsis.

3a The scolex evaginates and attaches to the wall of the small intestine. It utilizes both hooks and suckers to remain there.

3b The worm matures within the lumen of the small intestine over a period of 10–12 weeks.

4a The adult worm averages 4 meters in length. The gravid proglottids break off from the parent colony and actively migrate out the anus to the external environment. More rarely, groups of proglottids break off and are passed out with the feces.

4b The gravid proglottid, containing thousands of eggs, has less than 10 uterine branches per side, thereby distinguishing it from that of *T. saginata* (see page 54).

5a The embryonated eggs are infectious for the pig (i.e., the intermediate host) upon being passed from the human host in feces. Humans can also become infected with the larval form.

5b After the pig ingests the eggs, they hatch in the small intestine; the hexacanth larvae penetrate the gut and enter the bloodstream and are carried to various organs throughout the body where they encyst and develop to cysticerci. Development to this stage after penetrating a given organ takes about 3–5 weeks. The cysticerci are then infectious for the definitive host.

6 No other mammal can harbor the adult of *T. solium*.

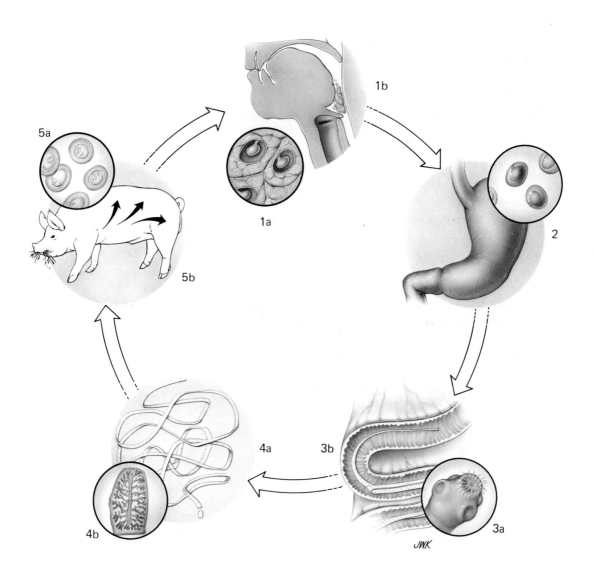

Kingdom: Animal
  Phylum: Platyhelminthes
    Class: Cestoidea
      Order: Cyclophyllidea
      Family: Taeniidae
        Genus: *Taenia*
          Species: *solium*

Taenia Solium (Cysticercosis)

1a The infectious stage for the intermediate host is the egg. The pig is the usual intermediate host (see life cycle for the adult stage of *Taenia solium*). However, humans can also harbor the juvenile stage of *T. solium* if they ingest eggs rather than cysticerci (i.e., the juvenile stage).

1b Ingestion of eggs initiates the infection. Food and inanimate objects contaminated with feces from humans harboring the adult tapeworm are the usual sources of infection.

2a The eggs hatch in the small intestine.

2b The oncosphere (hexacanth larva) is stimulated to hatch when the egg encounters bile salts in the small intestine.

3 The oncospheres penetrate into the bloodstream and are carried to a variety of organs. There, they undergo extensive growth and development, transforming into cysticerci.

4a-d The cysticercus is ovoid in shape and measures approximately 10 mm at its widest point (4a). A variety of organs can become infected with cysticerci, but subcutaneous tissue is the most common site invaded. The cysticerci lodge between the muscle bundles (4b). The eye (4c) and brain (4d) are other common sites of larval *T. solium* infection.

5a The adult worm in the human host is the source of infectious eggs.

5b The eggs are found within gravid proglottids of the adult worm and pass into the environment when defecated proglottids disintegrate.

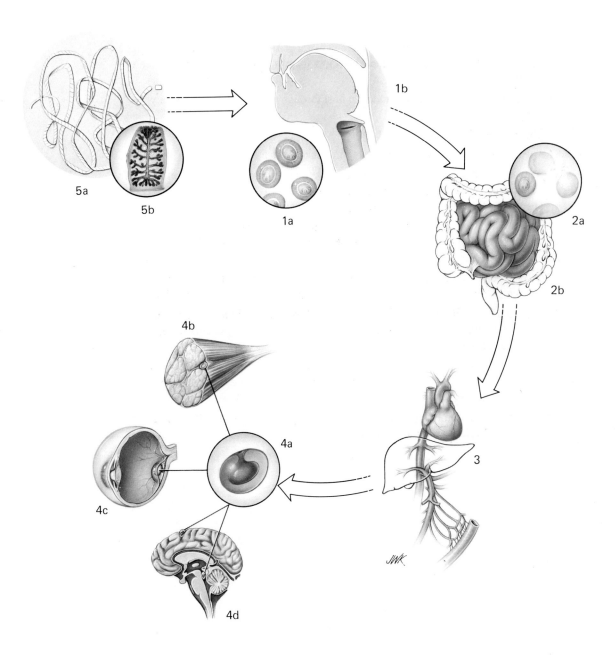

Taenia Multiceps

1a   The embryonated eggs are infectious for a wide variety of mammals, including sheep (5c) and humans. Feces containing eggs from infected dogs is the source of infection.

1b   The eggs are ingested by the intermediate host through contamination of the environment by dog feces.

2   Hatching occurs in the small intestine.

3a   The hexacanth larva is morphologically similar to all taeniid tapeworm species.

3b   The hexacanth larva (35 μm in diameter) penetrates the small intestine and enters the bloodstream via the portal system and is carried to any one of a variety of organs within the body. There it develops to the next stage, the coenurus.

4a   The brain (shown in coronal section) is a common site for the coenurus to develop. The coenurus is a large fluid-filled cyst that grows to an average diameter of 35 mm.

4b   Inside the coenurus, the germinal layer gives rise to infectious units termed protoscolices, each of which is capable of developing to an adult in the definitive host.

5a   The dog and other carnivores serve as definitive hosts of *T. multiceps*. They acquire their infection through the ingestion of coenuri. This usually occurs when dogs are fed infected organs of slaughtered sheep.

5b   Adult worms develop within the dog's small intestine. After the worms mature, embryonated eggs are passed in the feces and become ingested by sheep and, occasionally, humans.

5c   The sheep is a common intermediate host for *T. multiceps*. In the human the parasite's life cycle is considered aberrant.

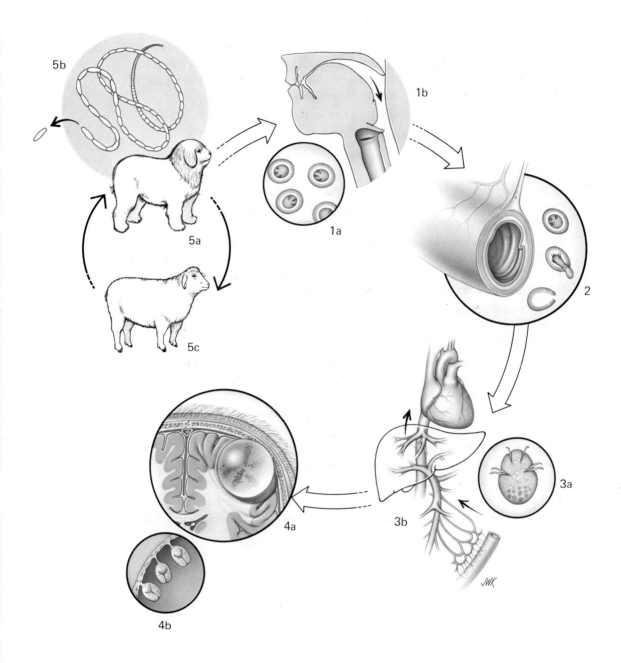

Kingdom: Animal
Phylum: Platyhelminthes
Class: Cestoidea
Order: Cyclophyllidea
Family: Taeniidae
Genus: *Taenia*
Species: *multiceps*

Echinococcus Granulosus

1a The embryonated eggs are infectious for the intermediate hosts, which include various ruminants and humans. Food and inanimate objects contaminated with dog feces containing eggs are the most common source of infection. In many parts of the world, sheep are the most common intermediate host.

1b The eggs must be ingested to begin infection in the human host.

2 Hatching occurs in the small intestine.

3a The hexacanth larva, referred to as the oncosphere, is typical of all tapeworm larvae, possessing six hookletes.

3b Through the use of its hookletes, the oncosphere penetrates the wall of the intestinal tract and enters the portal system. Usually, the oncosphere penetrates the liver where it transforms into the cyst stage. More rarely, other organs are infected.

4a The cyst takes several months to mature, becoming thin-walled and filled with fluid, hence the term "hydatid cyst." Its average diameter at maturity can be as much as 30 cm. In the brain the size of the cyst is much less, since the space limitations of the cranium do not permit further expansion.

4b The wall of the hydatid cyst consists of an outer acellular laminate membrane and an inner cellular germinal layer. The protoscolices are produced by budding from the inner surface of the germinal layer.

4c Small packets of protoscolices, referred to as brood capsules, may contain as many as 6 to 12 protoscolices. Each protoscolex, if ingested, can develop into an adult worm in the definitive host.

5a Canines, particularly domestic dogs, serve as definitive hosts for *E. granulosus*. They usually acquire their infection by ingesting organs of slaughtered sheep or reindeer which harbor the hydatid cyst.

5b Thousands of adult worms may develop in the intestinal tract of the dog after the ingestion of a single large, mature hydatid cyst.

5c Sheep acquire their cysts from ingestion of eggs passed in the feces of infected dogs. The eggs are passed in an embryonated state and are immediately infectious.

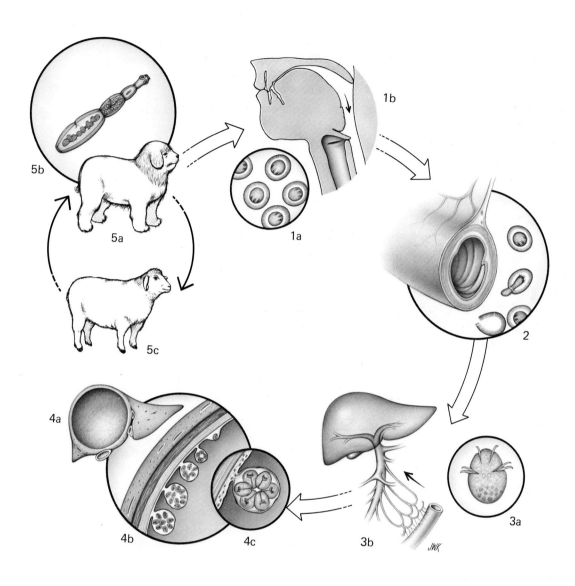

Kingdom: Animal
Phylum: Platyhelminthes
Class: Cestoidea
Order: Cyclophyllidea
Family: Taeniidae
Genus: *Echinococcus*
Species: *granulosus*

Echinococcus Multilocularis

1a The embryonated egg is the infectious stage for the intermediate host, usually small rodents. Feces containing eggs from the definitive host (e.g., fox) is the source of infection. Humans who become infected resemble intermediate hosts in regard to the stage of the life cycle which develops after infection.

1b Ingestion of the eggs is necessary for the initiation of infection in the intermediate host.

2 The oncosphere hatches from the egg in the small intestine.

3a The hexacanth larva (oncosphere) is similar in morphology to all other cestode oncospheres.

3b The oncosphere penetrates the small intestine, enters the bloodstream and is carried to the liver.

4a In the vole and human hosts, the multilocular cyst develops in the liver.

4b In the human, no protoscolices develop. Rather, only the laminate acellular outer membrane and the inner germinal layer can be demonstrated.

4c Viable protoscolices are produced within each compartment of the cyst. Protoscolex development only occurs in the vole and related rodent species.

4d Each protoscolex is produced from the inner surface of the germinal layer within each compartment.

5a The definitive host is the fox (and related carnivores in the family Caniidae), acquiring its worms through the ingestion of the infected intermediate host.

5b The adult worm, similar in morphology to that of *Echinococcus granulosus*, lives attached to the luminal surface of the small intestine of the definitive host.

5c The vole serves as the most important intermediate host for *E. multilocularis*, and acquires its infection through ingesting the eggs passed in the feces of infected foxes.

6 Dogs are the definitive hosts for *Echinococcus granulosus*.

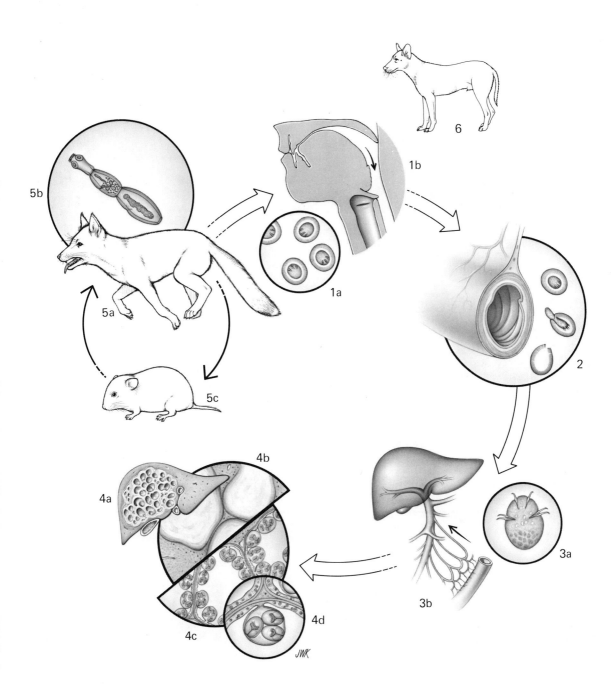

Kingdom: Animal
Phylum: Platyhelminthes
Class: Cestoidea
Order: Cyclophyllidea
Family: Taeniidae
Genus: *Echinococcus*
Species: *multilocularis*

3 Trematoda

General Characteristics of Trematodes

All adult trematodes in the subclass Digenea, commonly referred to as flukes, are parasitic, occupying a wide variety of sites within the human host. Some live within the lumen of organs, while others infect solid tissue, such as liver and lung.

The nonsegmented adult worms vary greatly in morphology, depending upon the species. There are two distinct types: one in which the sexes are separate (e.g., Family Schistosomatidae), and the other in which both sets of reproductive organs are found within the same individual. In the latter group (i.e., the majority of Families within the Subclass Digenea), self- or cross-fertilization may occur, while the schistosomes require both sexes for egg production. Both groups of flukes are surrounded by a tegument whose surface contains various projections and spines. Nutrients are obtained by active transport of small molecular weight substances across the tegument and by ingestion and digestion of host tissues. The products of digestion are absorbed across the gut wall and enter the parenchymal tissues of the worm. The source of nutrients varies greatly for each worm species, and is largely determined by the worms' location within each host. Each adult worm has two suckers, one anterior and one ventral. The suckers are multipurposed, serving functions related to attachment and movement.

Below the level of the tegument lie the parenchymal, muscle, nerve, excretory, and reproductive systems.

Eggs may be produced either embryonated or nonembryonated, depending upon the species in question. In all cases, eggs must eventually exit from the host. The male reproductive organs typically consist of the testes, vas deferens and the external seminal vesicle and cirrus. The female reproductive system includes the ovary, vitelline cells, Mehlis' gland, oviduct, uterus and metraterm. Eggs, in an advanced state of embryogenesis, leave the ovary, pass down the oviduct, acquire yolk, and are fertilized. The eggshell is produced by the vitelline cells. Eventually, the eggs exit from the genital pore and must pass out of the host into an aquatic environment for the life cycle to continue. All trematodes utilize snails as their first intermediate host. Within the snail, the worm undergoes remarkable changes, both in morphology and in numbers, resulting in infectious larvae, which exit from the snail and either encyst or penetrate the human host to complete their life cycle. Those species that encyst usually do so on plants or on invertebrates or vertebrates. Often, the second intermediate host is an amphibian. Thus, these flukes must be eaten in order to carry out their life cycles.

Classification

Bold type indicates superfamilies represented in book by parasites

Kingdom: Animal
 Phylum: Platyhelminthes
  Class: Cestoidea
  Class: Turbellaria
  Class: Monogenea
  Class: Trematoda
   Subclass: Digenea
    Superorder: Anepitheliocystidia
     Order: Strigeata
      Superfamily: Strigeoidea
      Superfamily: Clinostomatoidea
      Superfamily: Schistosomatoidea
      Superfamily: Azygioidea
      Superfamily: Transversotrematoidea
      Superfamily: Cyclocoeloidea
      Superfamily: Brachylaemoidea
      Superfamily: Fellodistomatoidea
      Superfamily: Bucephaloidea
     Order: Echinostomata
      Superfamily: Echinostomatoidea
      Superfamily: Paramphistomoidea
      Superfamily: Notocotyloidea
    Superorder: Epitheliocystidia
     Order: Plagiorchiata
      Superfamily: Plagiorchioidea
      Superfamily: Allocreadioidea
     Order: Opisthorchiata
      Superfamily: Isoparorchioidea
      Superfamily: Opisthorchioidea
      Superfamily: Hemiuroidea

Schistosoma Mansoni

1   The cercaria penetrates the skin at the level of the hair follicle thereby initiating infection. The forked tail is lost during penetration, and the worm is now referred to as a schistosomula. The schistosomula penetrates the dermis, where it undergoes further development over the next several days. The schistosomule then migrates to the lungs, undergoing morphogenic changes there, as well.

2a   It is not known how schistosomules reach the liver, but the hematogenous route is the most likely one.

2b   Following maturity within the capillaries of the liver, mating ensues. The surface of the adult male is covered with small knoblike protuberances. Adults are 12 mm in length and 2 mm in diameter. Each worm has an anterior and ventral sucker with which it attaches to endothelial cells.

3   Pairs of worms migrate within the portal circulation, finally residing in the mesenteric venules of the small intestine. The female begins to lay eggs shortly after arriving there. Eggs exit from the genital pore, which is applied to the surface of the venule. Each female produces about 300 eggs per day.

4a   The egg contains the larval stage termed the miracidium. The miracidium secretes proteases which facilitates its penetration through venule endothelial cells, the connective tissue and the wall of the small intestine. Nearly 50% of the eggs reach the lumen of the small intestine. The other 50% are swept back into the presinusoidal capillaries of the liver where they no longer participate in the life cycle.

4b   Eggs are 110 μm long by 60 μm wide and possess a unique lateral spine.

5   Eggs reaching the lumen of the small intestine are passed from the host during defecation, and must be deposited in fresh water in which the appropriate snail host lives if the life cycle is to continue.

6a   The miracidium hatches from the egg in fresh water. This ciliated stage swims about seeking its snail host.

6b   The miracidium penetrates the snail. The most common vector snail species throughout tropical Central and South America is *Biomphalaria glabrata*. Other susceptible species of *Biomphalaria* occur in Africa. The trematode reaches the snail's hepatopancreas where it undergoes a series of morphogenic changes and then multiplies, transforming first into larvae termed sporocysts, then multiplying further into second-generation sporocysts. Secondary sporocysts give rise to many cercariae, the infectious stage for the human host.

6c   The phototropic cercariae exit from the snail and swim toward the surface of the water, aided by their forked tails. Cercariae live for about a day, then die if a host is not found.

7   Monkeys of various species can serve as reservoir hosts.

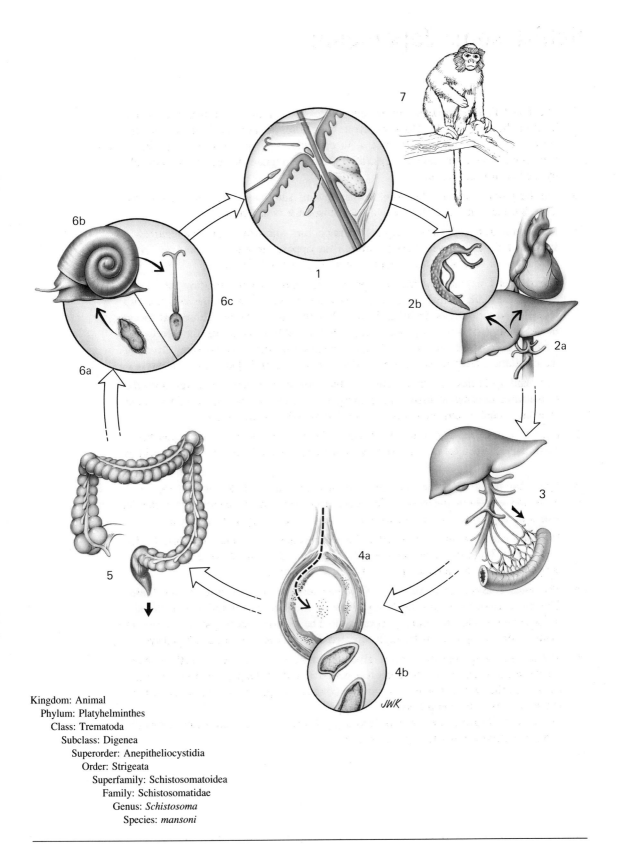

Kingdom: Animal
  Phylum: Platyhelminthes
    Class: Trematoda
      Subclass: Digenea
        Superorder: Anepitheliocystidia
          Order: Strigeata
            Superfamily: Schistosomatoidea
            Family: Schistosomatidae
              Genus: *Schistosoma*
                Species: *mansoni*

Schistosoma Japonicum

1   The fork-tailed cercaria penetrates the unbroken skin of the human host at the level of the hair follicle. Upon penetration, it loses its tail and burrows into the dermis. It is now referred to as a schistosomula. The schistosomula undergoes development there for several days, after which it migrates to the lungs, probably by the hematogenous route.

2a The lung schistosomule develops further toward adulthood, then migrates to the liver, but the route taken by the lung schistosomule is not known.

2b Maturation to an adult and subsequent mating occurs within the liver. The tegumental surface of *S. japonicum* adults is smooth, as opposed to either *S. mansoni* or *S. haematobium*. The adults are about 15 mm long and 0.5 mm wide.

3   Paired adults migrate out into the portal circulation against the flow of blood. Most of the adult worms locate in the mesenteric venules, but some may take up residence in the venules draining the spinal column or the brain. Those that locate in the mesenteric venules produce eggs that are able to continue the life cycle, while eggs produced in the other above-mentioned sites become sequestered in the capillaries. Each female worm produces about 2,000–3,000 eggs each day.

4a Eggs laid up against the endothelium of the mesenteric venules penetrate into the surrounding connective tissue and eventually migrate into the lumen of the small intestine, aided by enzymes produced by the miracidia within them.

4b Each *S. japonicum* egg is about 90 μm by 70 μm, is ovoid in shape, and has a small curved spine on its outer surface. Each egg has a ciliated miracidium within it.

5   Eggs that reach the lumen of the small intestine are included within the fecal mass and exit from the host during defecation. Eggs must reach fresh water in which an appropriate snail host lives in order for the life cycle to continue.

6a Hatching occurs within 1 hour after the embryonated egg comes in contact with fresh water. The miracidium emerges and swims rapidly about seeking its intermediate snail host. Each miracidium is either male or female.

6b The most common snail hosts for *S. japonicum* are in the genus *Oncomelania*. The miracidium penetrates the fleshy tissue of the snail and transforms at the site of penetration into the primary sporocyst. The primary sporocyst gives rise to many secondary sporocysts through repeated division cycles termed polyembryony.

6c The secondary sporocysts in turn, give rise to the cercariae, the infectious stage for the mammalian host. The cercariae penetrate out of the snail and swim to the surface of the water, where they must encounter an appropriate mammalian host if the cycle is to be completed.

7   Primates of all species are susceptible to *S. japonicum* and many nonhuman primates serve as reservoir hosts for human infection.

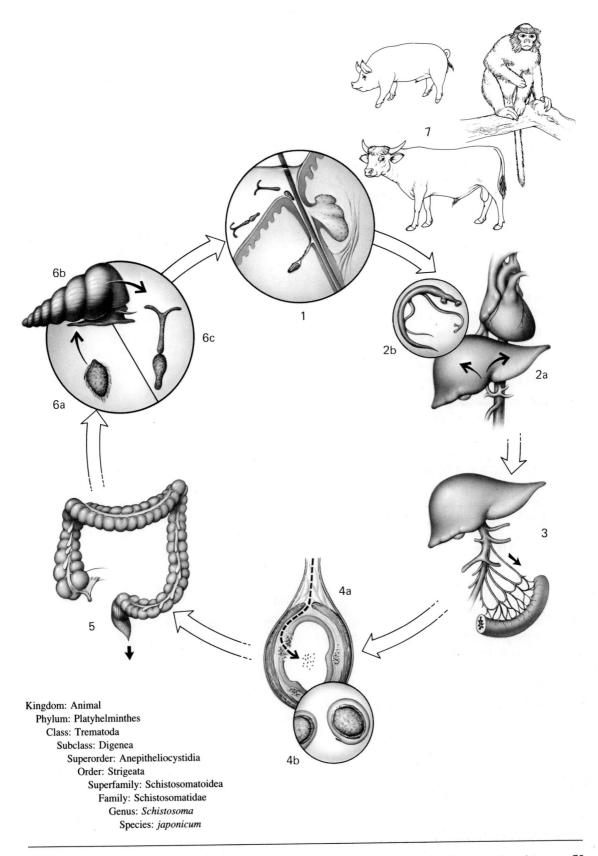

Kingdom: Animal
  Phylum: Platyhelminthes
    Class: Trematoda
      Subclass: Digenea
        Superorder: Anepitheliocystidia
          Order: Strigeata
            Superfamily: Schistosomatoidea
              Family: Schistosomatidae
                Genus: *Schistosoma*
                  Species: *japonicum*

Schistosoma Haematobium

1   The cercaria initiates the infection in the human host by penetrating the unbroken skin at the level of the hair follicle. Usually the area of skin most frequently penetrated is that which is at the surface of the water. The forked tail is lost upon entering the follicle; thus the cercaria transforms into the schistosomula. This stage penetrates into the dermis and, during the next several days, undergoes development toward adulthood. Subsequently, the skin schistosomule migrates to the lungs, probably via the hematogenous route, and undergoes further morphogenesis.

2a   From the lungs, the immature blood fluke migrates to the liver, where it completes its development into an adult trematode. The sexes are separate. Mating occurs within the blood vessels of the liver.

2b   The adults remain *in copula* for life. The adult of *S. haematobium* measures about 12 mm long and 1 mm wide. The protuberances on the male of *S. haematobium* are not as prominent as those found on the tegumental surface of *S. mansoni*.

3   The mature flukes migrate, as mated pairs, from the liver to the venous plexus surrounding the bladder, where the female worm begins her production of eggs. Eggs are produced in an embryonated state. It is not known how many eggs are produced each day by each female worm.

4a   The eggs of *Schistosoma haematobium* measure 140 μm by 60 μm and are characterized by an external terminal spine. The miracidium (i.e., the ciliated larva) lies within the egg.

4b   The adult female lays her eggs up against the endothelial cells of the venule. The miracidium within the egg secretes lytic enzymes which allows the egg to penetrate through the vessel wall and eventually through the smooth muscle wall of the bladder itself. Eggs reaching the lumen of the bladder are voided with the urine. About 50% of all eggs laid reach the lumen of the bladder. The rest wash back into the venous return and are trapped in the liver and, to a lesser extent, the lungs. These eggs do not exit from the host, and hence do not participate in the life cycle.

5a   Hatching occurs in fresh water. The ciliated miracidium swims about seeking its appropriate snail intermediate host. Various species of *Bulinus* serve in this capacity.

5b   The miracidium, upon finding a *Bulinus* snail, penetrates it and migrates to the hepatopancreas where the worm undergoes further development. Each miracidum is either male or female. This stage develops further, via division, into many sporocysts, then into secondary sporocysts. Each secondary sporocyst gives rise to many cercariae, the infectious stage for the human host.

5c   The forked tail cercariae penetrate out of the snail and immediately begin seeking out their human host. As with all other species of schistosomes, the cercaria of *S. haematobium* is positively phototactic and negatively geotropic, thus ensuring that it will quickly rise to the water's surface. If it does not find a host within 2 days, it loses its infectivity and dies shortly thereafter.

6   Non-human primates serve as reservoir hosts for *S. haematobium*.

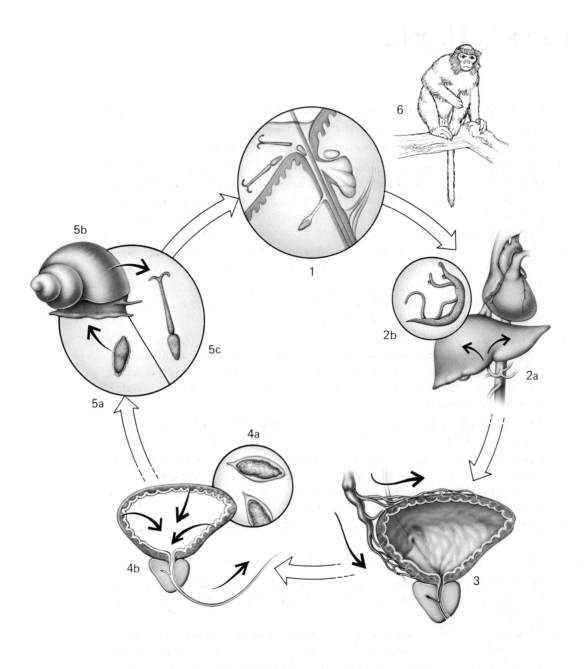

Kingdom: Animal
 Phylum: Platyhelminthes
  Class: Trematoda
   Subclass: Digenea
    Superorder: Anepitheliocystidia
     Order: Strigeata
      Superfamily: Schistosomatoidea
       Family: Schistosomatidae
        Genus: *Schistosoma*
         Species: *haematobium*

Fasciola Hepatica

1 Infection in the human host is initiated by swallowing the metacercaria (encysted larva) together with contaminated watercress or other littoral plants.

2 The metacercaria excysts within the lumen of the small intestine.

3 The immature fluke burrows through the wall of the small intestine, enters the peritoneal cavity, and penetrates the liver, where it then begins to feed upon the parenchymal cells. *Fasciola hepatica* grows slowly, achieving sexual maturity after 2 months in the liver. Fasciola is hermaphroditic, and self-mating may occur. Eggs are produced by each worm after another month of development.

4a The adult flukes are among the largest that infect the human host. Each adult measure 25–30 mm in length and about 10–15 mm in width.

4b Eggs are laid unembryonated within the tunnels created by the feeding worms in the liver tissue. The eggs reach the lumen of the small intestine by way of the hepatic ducts and, eventually, the common bile duct.

4c Each egg measures approximately 115–120 μm in length by 55–60 μm in width and has an operculum at one end. The egg contains a single cell surrounded by yolk material. The egg exits from the host in the feces and must be deposited in fresh water to embryonate. Hatching takes place within 10–15 days after entering its aquatic environment.

5a The ciliated miracidium swims about seeking its appropriate snail host. Upon encountering it, the miracidium penetrates the snail and develops within snail tissue.

5b Snails in the genera *Lymnaea, Stagnicola,* and *Fossaria* serve as intermediate hosts for *Fasciola hepatica*. Morphogenesis within the snail proceeds sequentially from the miracidium to the sporocyst, then the redia stage. Each new stage signals an increase in the number of individual immature flukes.

5c Each redia gives rise to many cercariae, which then penetrate out of the snail and into the water.

6a The cercariae encyst upon watercress and other littoral plants.

6b The encysted cercariae, now termed metacercariae, are resistant to mild changes in temperature and some chemicals. The metacercaria is the infective stage of the infection.

7 Sheep are the most commonly infected mammalian hosts in nature, and serve as reservoirs for the human infection. Other herbivores, such as cattle, can also become infected in endemic areas. Experimentally, *F. hepatica* will infect a wide variety of mammals, including the rat and rabbit.

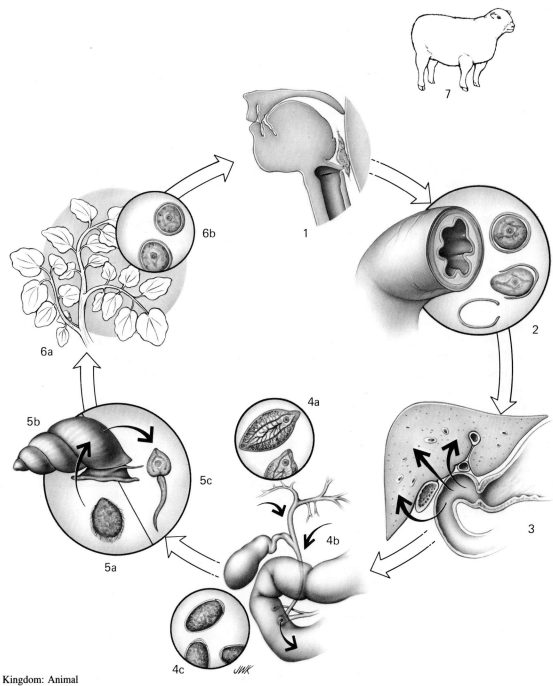

Kingdom: Animal
  Phylum: Platyhelminthes
    Class: Trematoda
      Subclass: Digenea
        Superorder: Anepitheliocystidia
          Order: Echinostomata
            Superfamily: Echinostomatoidea
              Family: Fasciolidae
                Genus: *Fasciola*
                  Species: *hepatica*

Fasciolopsis Buski

1a The metacercaria is the infective stage for the human host.

1b Infection is acquired by swallowing the metacercariae, which have encysted upon freshwater aquatic plants.

2 Excystation occurs in the lumen of the small intestine.

3a The immature fluke attaches to the luminal surface of the small intestine and begins grazing upon the columnar epithelium of the villus tissue. Maturation to a reproductive adult takes place within 3 months after hatching.

3b The adult worm measures 25–80 mm in length and 10–20 mm in width.

4 Unembryonated eggs are passed into the lumen of the small intestine and must reach fresh water to continue the life cycle. Each egg measures about 130 μm in length by 75 μm in width, and possesses a terminal operculum. The egg contains the yolk material and a single embryonic cell.

5a Embryonation proceeds slowly, with the miracidium taking up to 6–8 weeks to fully develop. Hatching ensues, and the ciliated miracidium then seeks out its appropriate intermediate snail host. Upon contact, the miracidium penetrates the snail tissue, develops to the sporocyst stage and migrates to the hepatopancreas. Each sporocyst produces many primary rediae, each of which in turn gives rise to secondary rediae.

5b The most common genus of snail that serves as the first intermediate host is *Segmentina*.

5c The secondary rediae give rise to many cercariae, which leave the snail and enter the water.

6 Cercariae of *F. buski* encyst upon a variety of aquatic plants, many of which serve as food for human consumption. Water caltrop (illustrated), water chestnut, and bamboo shoots are among the most common sources of plants upon which encystment occurs.

7 Many mammals besides the human host can also become infected with *Fasciolopsis buski*. Farm animals such as the pig, cat, and dog serve as reservoir hosts.

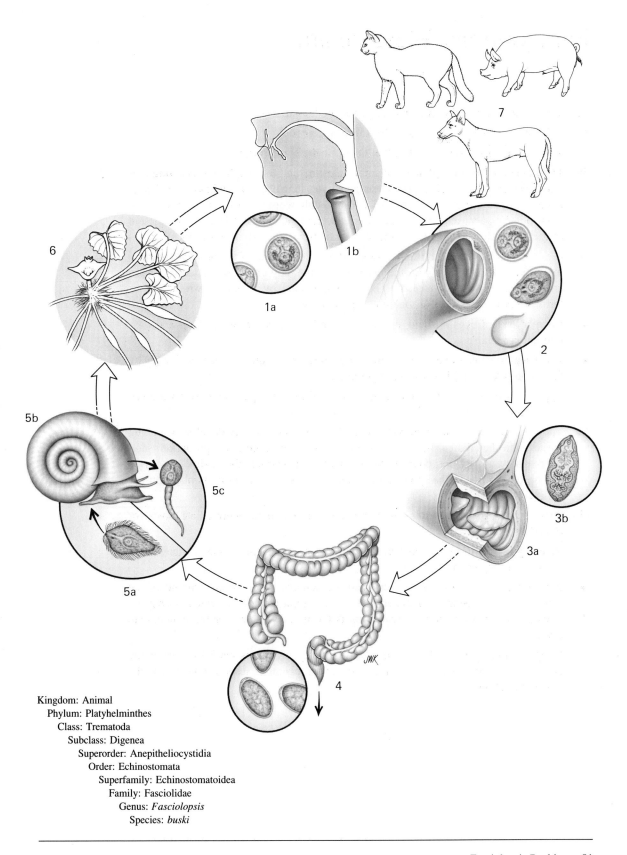

Kingdom: Animal
  Phylum: Platyhelminthes
    Class: Trematoda
      Subclass: Digenea
        Superorder: Anepitheliocystidia
          Order: Echinostomata
            Superfamily: Echinostomatoidea
              Family: Fasciolidae
                Genus: *Fasciolopsis*
                  Species: *buski*

Paragonimus Westermani

1a   The metacercaria is the infective stage for the human host.

1b   Infection is acquired by ingestion of the metacercaria.

2   The metacercaria excysts within the lumen of the small intestine.

3a   The immature fluke penetrates the small intestine and the diaphragm and migrates into the pleural cavity. There, the worm penetrates lung tissue and takes up residence. Other tissues of the body can also harbor adult worms, such as brain or even striated skeletal muscle. However, these aberrant sites do not lead to completion of the life cycle, since eggs are unable to exit from the body in these locations.

3b   *P. westermani* matures in 8 to 12 weeks after entering the host. The adults usually live as pairs of worms within the necrotic capsule they create while feeding upon lung tissue. Each adult measures 8 to 15 mm long by 5 mm in width. Cross-fertilization is necessary for viable egg production.

4a   Unembryonated eggs are laid in the worm-induced capsule of the lung and pass into the bronchioles.

4b   The unembryonated egg of *P. westermani* measures about 100 μm in length by 55 μm in width, and has a single operculum.

5   Eggs reach fresh water by either being coughed up and expectorated or swallowed and defecated.

6a   The eggs embryonate in fresh water and take 2–3 weeks to fully develop. Hatching ensues, and the ciliated miracidium then swims about seeking its appropriate snail intermediate host. Upon contact, the miracidium penetrates the snail's soft tissue and develops through the sporocyst and redia stages, increasing in numbers during the process.

6b   Snails of the genus *Semisulcospira* are the most common intermediate hosts for *P. westermani*.

6c   Rediae give rise to many cercariae, which, upon leaving the infected snail, swim about until they encounter crustacea.

6d   Freshwater crabs (illustrated) or crayfish are suitable hosts for encystment of the cercariae. The crustacean is penetrated by the cercaria, then the cercaria encysts, transforming into the metacercaria. This is the infective stage for the mammalian host.

7   Besides humans, pigs, dogs, and a wide variety of felines can also harbor the adult of *P. westermani*. Hence there are many potential reservoir hosts for the human infection.

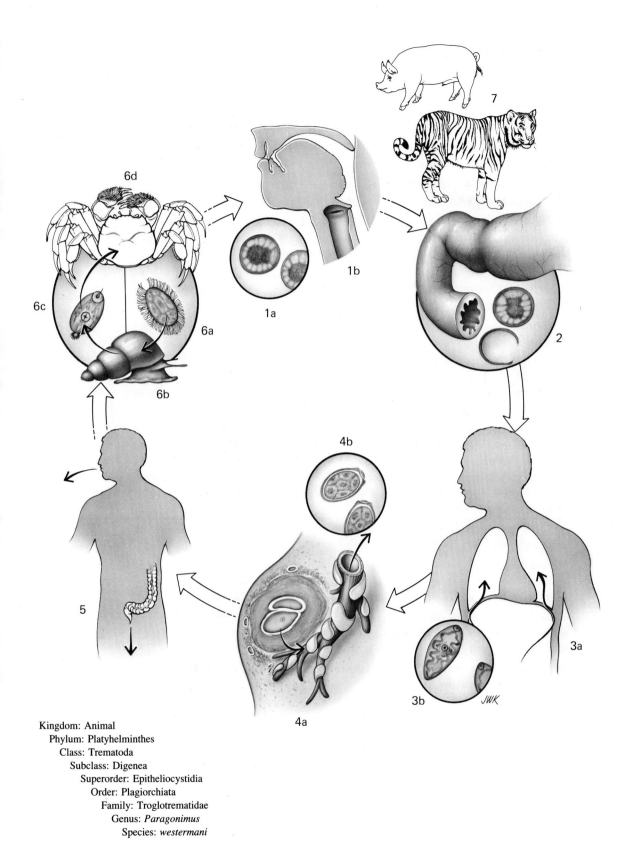

Kingdom: Animal
Phylum: Platyhelminthes
Class: Trematoda
Subclass: Digenea
Superorder: Epitheliocystidia
Order: Plagiorchiata
Family: Troglotrematidae
Genus: *Paragonimus*
Species: *westermani*

Clonorchis Sinensis

1a The metacercaria of *Clonorchis sinensis* is the infective stage for the human host.

1b The metacercaria initiates infection upon ingestion. This occurs when raw or under-cooked infected fish is eaten.

2 The metacercaria excysts in the lumen of the small intestine.

3a The immature fluke then seeks out its niche in the host.

3b The immature fluke migrates into the common bile duct and up the biliary tract, completing its growth and development within one of the bile ducts or the gall bladder. Egg production begins about 1 month after infection.

4a The adult of *Clonorchis sinensis* measures 10–20 mm in length by 2–5 mm in width, and is hermaphroditic. Its food consists of epithelial cells that line the common duct and gallbladder.

4b The worm releases embryonated eggs which must pass into the lumen of the small intestine if the life cycle is to continue.

4c The egg of *Clonorchis sinensis* is small compared to the eggs of most other flukes that infect the human host, measuring only 25–30 μm in length by 15 μm in width. It possesses an operculum at one end and a small knoblike protuberance at the other end. Each egg contains a well-developed miracidium.

5a The egg exits from the host in the feces during defecation and must be deposited in fresh water. Hatching occurs when an appropriate intermediate snail host ingests the eggs. The miracidium then penetrates the wall of the snail's intestine and begins its development within the hepatopancreas. The sporocyst stage is produced first, which, in turn, gives rise to rediae. Each redia produces about 25 cercariae. The entire process takes about 30 days.

5b Snails in the genus *Parafossarulus* are the most commonly occurring intermediate hosts for *Clonorchis sinensis*.

5c The cercariae leave the snail and swim about, encysting upon any of a wide variety of freshwater fishes in the family Cyprinidae. Crustaceans can also be infected with the metacercaria of this fluke, but this occurs more rarely than in fish.

5d When a fish is encountered by a cercaria, the cercaria penetrates beneath the scales of the fish and encysts, transforming into the metacercaria, the infectious stage for the mammalian host.

6 Dogs and cats can also be infected with this fluke, and serve as reservoir hosts for the human infection.

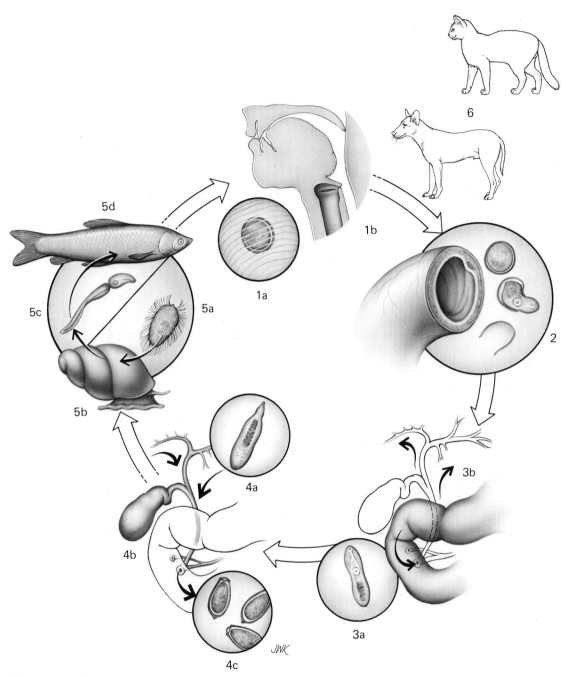

Kingdom: Animal
Phylum: Platyhelminthes
Class: Trematoda
Subclass: Digenea
Superorder: Epitheliocystidia
Order: Opisthorchiata
Superfamily: Opisthorchioidea
Family: Opisthorchiidae
Genus: *Clonorchis*
Species: *sinensis*

Opisthorchis Viverrini

1a Infection in the human host is initiated by the metacercaria.

1b The metacercaria must be ingested; this occurs when raw or undercooked infected fish is eaten.

2   The metacercaria excysts within the lumen of the small intestine.

3a The immature fluke seeks out its niche.

3b After migrating up the biliary tract, the worm feeds upon the epithelium of the bile ducts and develops to an adult worm there.

4a The adult worm is very similar in morphology and size to that of *Clonorchis sinensis*.

4b Eggs must pass out of the bile duct into the lumen of the small intestine in order to continue the life cycle.

4c The egg resembles that of *C. sinensis*.

5a Eggs eventually pass from the host in the feces during defecation. They must then be eaten by an appropriate intermediate snail host. Hatching occurs within the gut tract of the snail. The miracidium burrows into the hepatopancreas and develops into a sporocyst, which produces rediae, which in turn give rise to cercariae.

5b Snails in the genus *Bulinus* are common intermediate hosts for this parasite.

5c The cercariae leave the snail and swim about, seeking a freshwater fish. The cercaria penetrates the fleshy part of the scale and encysts, transforming into the metacercaria.

5d Fish in the family Cyprinidae (e.g., grass carp) serve as important paratenic (i.e., transport) hosts for *O. viverrini*.

6   Dogs, cats, and pigs serve as reservoir hosts for *O. viverrini*.

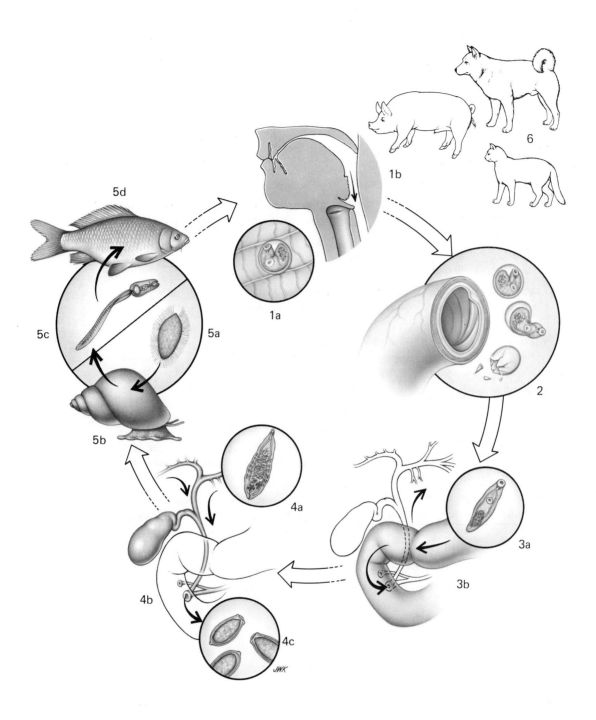

Kingdom: Animal
Class: Trematoda
Subclass: Digenea
Superorder: Epitheliocystidia
Order: Opisthorchiata
Superfamily: Opistohorchioidea
Family: Opisthorchiidae
Genus: *Opisthorchis*
Species: *viverrini*

Heterophyes Heterophyes

1a   The metacercaria is the infective stage for the mammalian host.

1b   Infection occurs by the oral route when the metacercaria is eaten together with infected raw or undercooked fish.

2   Excystation occurs in the lumen of the small intestine.

3a   The immature fluke attaches to the intestinal villus tissue and proceeds to feed upon epithelial cells. The worm develops to an adult within 8 days after beginning its life in the small intestine.

3b   Each adult worm is 1–2 mm in length by 0.4 mm in width, making it one of the smallest trematodes to infect the human host.

4a   Embryonated eggs are passed directly into the lumen of the small intestine and leave the host during defecation. They must be deposited in fresh water if the life cycle is to continue.

4b   The egg measures 30 μm long by 15 μm wide, and possesses an operculum at one end. Each egg contains a single fully-developed miracidium.

5a   The egg must be ingested by an appropriate intermediate snail host in order to continue the life cycle.

5b   Snails in the genus *Cerithidia* (illustrated) are common hosts in Asia, while those in the genus *Pironella* are important hosts in the Middle East. The miracidium hatches from the egg and penetrates the gut tract of the snail. Development to the sporocyst stage occurs within the hepatopancreas. The sporocyst gives rise to rediae. Many cercariae are produced by each redia.

5c   The cercaria leaves the snail and swims about seeking to encyst upon a fresh- or brackish-water fish. The cercaria, upon coming into contact with the fish, encysts beneath the scales and transforms into the metacercaria, the infectious stage for the mammalian host.

5d   Mullet are the dominant fish upon which *H. heterophyes* encysts.

6   The cat and dog can serve as reservoir hosts for *H. heterophyes*.

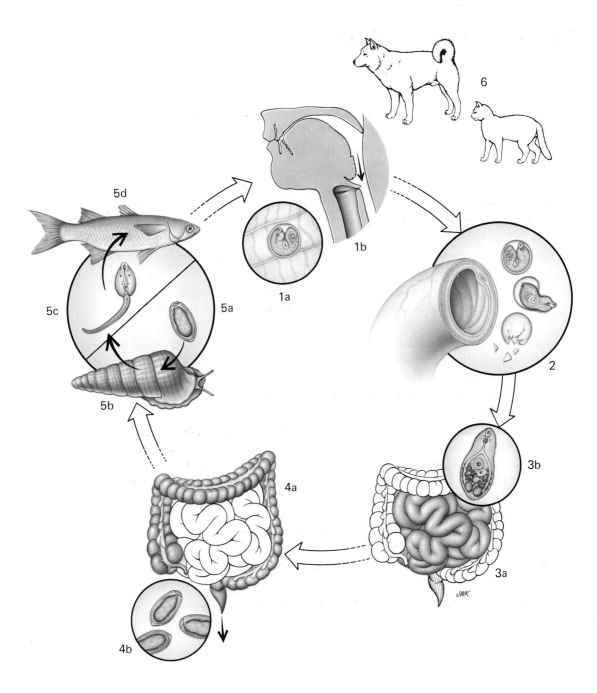

Kingdom: Animal
Phylum: Platyhelminthes
Class: Trematoda
Subclass: Digenea
Superorder: Epitheliocystidia
Order: Opisthorchiata
Superfamily: Opisthorchioidea
Family: Heterophyidae
Genus: *Heterophyes*
Species: *heterophyes*

Metagonimus Yokogawai

1a The infective stage for the mammalian host is the metacercaria. Many fish-eating mammals, in addition to humans, can be infected with *M. yokogawai*.

1b Infection occurs through the oral route by ingestion of raw or undercooked fish harboring the metacercarial stage.

2 Excystation occurs in the small intestine.

3a The immature fluke attaches to the villus surface of the small intestine and begins feeding upon epithelium. Development to the adult stage occurs within 10 days after being ingested.

3b The adult worm measures 1.5 mm long by 0.7 mm wide and lives attached to the wall of the small intestine.

4a Embryonated eggs are passed into the lumen of the small intestine where they become included within the fecal mass and eventually pass from the host during defecation.

4b Each egg measures 25 μm long by 15 μm wide and has an operculum. The opposite end is smooth. This egg closely resembles that of *H. heterophyes*. Each egg contains a fully developed miracidium.

5a Eggs must reach fresh water, where they become ingested by an appropriate intermediate snail host.

5b Snails in the genus *Semisulcospira* are most frequently infected with *M. yokogawai*. After ingestion, hatching ensues, and the miracidium penetrates the gut tract and begins its development in the hepatopancreas. The miracidium transforms into the sporocyst stage, which, in turn, gives rise to the redia stage. Numerous cercariae are produced by each redia.

5c The cercaria penetrates out of the snail and swims about, seeking a freshwater fish. When a cercaria encounters a fish, it penetrates beneath scale and encysts, transforming into the metacercaria, the infectious stage for the mammalian host.

5d Fish in the genus *Plecoglossus* are commonly infected with metacercaria of *M. yokogawai*.

6 The dog and cat are the most common reservoir hosts for *M. yokogawai*.

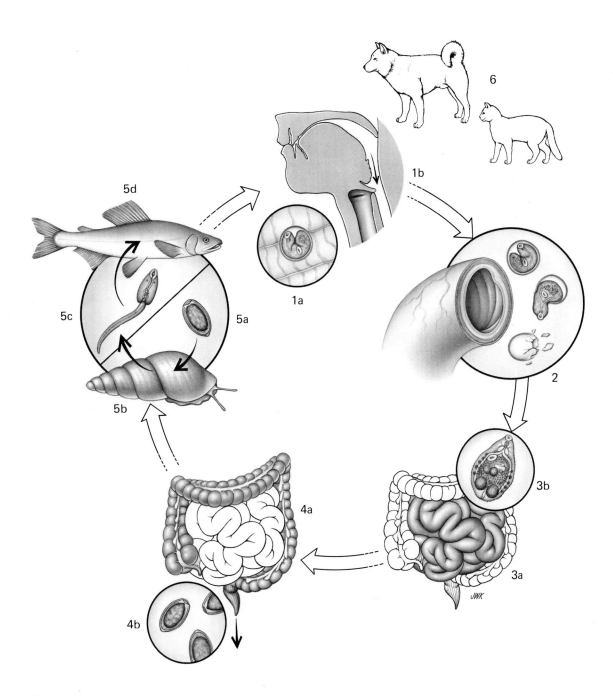

Kingdom: Animal
　Phylum: Platyhelminthes
　　Class: Trematoda
　　　Subclass: Digenea
　　　　Superorder: Epitheliocystidia
　　　　　Order: Opisthorchiata
　　　　　　Superfamily: Opisthorchioidea
　　　　　　　Family: Heterophyidae
　　　　　　　　Genus: *Metagonimus*
　　　　　　　　　Species: *yokogawai*

4 Nematoda

General Characteristics of Nematodes

Nematodes comprise a large group of organisms, the majority of which are free-living. Characteristically, they are nonsegmented round worms, and the sexes are separate and usually morphologically distinct. The life cycles of parasitic nematodes can be rather simple. For example, some species of nematodes lay eggs that leave the host in feces and embryonate in soil. In these cases, the eggs enter the host by the oral route and the worms develop to adults in the intestinal tract. Other species of nematodes have more complex cycles, involving intermediate invertebrate or vertebrate hosts, often with complex migration routes, once inside the host. The route of entry into the host can also vary, with some species being capable of penetrating directly into the host through the unbroken skin. Nematode parasites have been selected for life in a broad spectrum of niches within the mammalian host, including intracellular and intramulticellular environments.

Structurally, all nematodes are similar, being covered by a thick, acellular collagen-rich cuticle. A hypodermal region directly beneath the cuticle synthesizes new cuticula before each molt, and also serves as a point of attachment for muscles. All nematodes molt four times as larvae before developing to adulthood. With each molt, the worm achieves a more advanced stage of development. All muscle cells contain both thick and thin filaments and, uniquely, insert processes into the lateral, dorsal, and ventral nerve branches, which run the length of the worm. Adult worms possess a complete gut tract, typically subdivided into three regions; namely, foregut (pharynx and esophagus), midgut, and hindgut. The foregut and hindgut are lined with an extension of the outer cuticle, while the epithelium of the midgut is covered with microvilli and usually serves as the absorption surface through which nutrients enter the pseudocoelom. For many species, the source of food is known. For example, *Ascaris lumbricoides* adults ingest whatever food the host has eaten, while hookworm adults feed directly on villous tissue and, in addition, suck blood. In contrast, for *Trichinella spiralis* and *Trichuris trichiura,* the food sources remain unknown.

Metabolically, parasitic nematodes possess both aerobic and anaerobic energy pathways, and complete metabolic pathways for synthesizing all classes of macromolecules.

The nervous system consists of an anterior nerve ring from which emanate the dorsal, ventral, and lateral branches. A number of sensory nerve endings are found clustered near the anterior and/or posterior ends of the adult stage of most species of round worms. These aid the nematode in navigating through the many microenvironments of the host, and also enable male and female worms to find each other in the milieu of the host prior to mating.

The excretory system consists of two lateral tubes and associated anterior pores. A large portion of worm biomass is devoted to reproduction. The female reproductive tract is tubelike and consists of the ovary, seminal receptacle, uterus, oviduct, and vulva. Many species lay eggs, while others give birth to live larvae. The male reproductive tract consists of the testis, seminal vesicle, vas deferens, and cloaca. Sperm are nonflagellated amoeboidlike cells, which are deposited into the vulval opening during copulation.

Classification

Bold type indicates families represented in book by parasites

Phylum: Nematoda
  Class: Aphasmida
    Order: Trichurata
      Family: Anatrichosomatidae
      Family: Capillariidae
      Family: Cystoopsidae
      Family: Trichinellidae
      Family: Trichosomoididae
      Family: Trichuridae
    Order: Dioctophymata
      Family: Dioctophymatidae
      Family: Eustrongylidae
      Family: Soboliphymatidae
  Class: Phasmidea
    Order: Rhabditata
      Family: Rhabdiasidae
      Family: Strongyloididae
    Order: Strongylata
      Family: Amidostomatidae
      Family: Ancylostomatidae
      Family: Angiostrongylidae
      Family: Cloacinidae
      Family: Cyathostomidae
      Family: Deletrocephalidae
      Family: Diaphanocephalidae
      Family: Dictyocaulidae
      Family: Filaroididae
      Family: Heligmosomatidae
      Family: Ichthyostrongylidae
      Family: Metastrongylidae
      Family: Oesophagostomatidae
      Family: Ollulanidae
      Family: Pharyngostrongylidae
      Family: Protostrongylidae
      Family: Pseudaliidae
      Family: Stephanuridae
      Family: Strongylacanthidae
      Family: Strongylidae
      Family: Syngamidae
      Family: Trichostrongylidae
    Order: Ascaridata
      Family: Acanthocheilidae

Family: Angusticaecidae
Family: Anisakidae
Family: Ascaridae
Family: Ascaridiidae
Family: Crossophoridae
Family: Goeziidae
Family: Heterocheilidae
Family: Inglisonematidae
Family: Oxyascarididae
Family: Toxocaridae
Order: Oxyurata
  Superfamily: Oxyuroidea
    Family: Heteroxynematidae
    Family: Oxyuridae
    Family: Ozolamidae
    Family: Pharyngodonidae
    Family: Syphaciidae
  Superfamily: Atractoidea
    Family: Atractidae
    Family: Crossocephalidae
    Family: Cruziidae
    Family: Hoplodontophoridae
    Family: Labiduridae
    Family: Schrankianidae
    Family: Travnematidae
  Superfamily: Cosmocercoidea
    Family: Cosmocercidae
    Family: Gyrinicolidae
    Family: Lauroiidae
  Superfamily: Heterakoidea
    Family: Aspidoderidae
    Family: Heterakidae
    Family: Spinicaudidae
    Family: Strongyluridae
  Superfamily: Kathlaniodea
    Family: Kathlaniidae
  Superfamily: Subuluroidea
    Family: Maupasinidae
    Family: Parasubuluridae
    Family: Subuluridae
Order: Spirurata
  Family: Acuariidae

Family: Ascaropsidae
Family: Cobboldinidae
Family: Crassicaudidae
Family: Desmidocercidae
Family: Gnathostomatidae
Family: Gongylonematidae
Family: Habronematidae
Family: Haplonematidae
Family: Hedruidae
Family: Physalopteridae
Family: Pneumospiruridae
Family: Rhabdochonidae
Family: Rictulariidae
Family: Salobrellidae
Family: Schistorophidae
Family: Seuratidae
Family: Spinitectidae
Family: Spirocercidae
Family: Spiruridae
Family: Streptocaridae
Family: Tetrameridae
Family: Thelaziidae
Order: Camallanata
  Family: Anguillicodidae
  Family: Camallanidae
  Family: Dracunculidae
  Family: Oceanicucullanidae
  Family: Philometridae
  Family: Phlyctainophoridae
  Family: Skrjabillanidae
  Family: Tetanonematidae
Order: Filariata
  Family: Aproctidae
  Family: Desmidocercidae
  Family: Diplotriaenidae
  Family: Filariidae
  Family: Onchocercidae
  Family: Setariidae

Capillaria Philippinensis

1a   The third stage larva is the infectious stage of *Capillaria philippinensis*.

1b   Infection is initiated by ingestion of certain species of uncooked fresh or brackish water fish and crustaceans which are infected with third-stage larvae.

2   Larvae are released from the intermediate host tissue in the stomach. They then are carried to the small intestine where they penetrate into the villous tissue and develop into adults. The adult female measures 3–5 mm in length and 30 μm in diameter, while the male measures 1–2 mm in length and 30 μm in diameter.

3a   Adult females begin their reproductive cycle by shedding first-stage larvae.

3b   These larvae are capable of infecting the same host by penetrating adjacent villous tissue, molting four times, and developing into adults. Thus large numbers of worms can accumulate in the small intestinal tissue in a few weeks.

3c   Within weeks after infection, adult females switch to egg production. What factors control this change in reproductive strategy are not yet known.

3d   The eggs reach the lumen of the small intestine.

4   Fertilized eggs exit from the host in the feces.

5a-c   In order for the cycle to continue, eggs (5a) must reach fresh or brackish water where they complete their embryonation. They are ingested by small fish (5b) and crustaceans (5c). Little is known about the infection in the intermediate host. Experimental infection in various water birds has been successfully carried out. Thus, birds may be capable of serving as reservoir hosts.

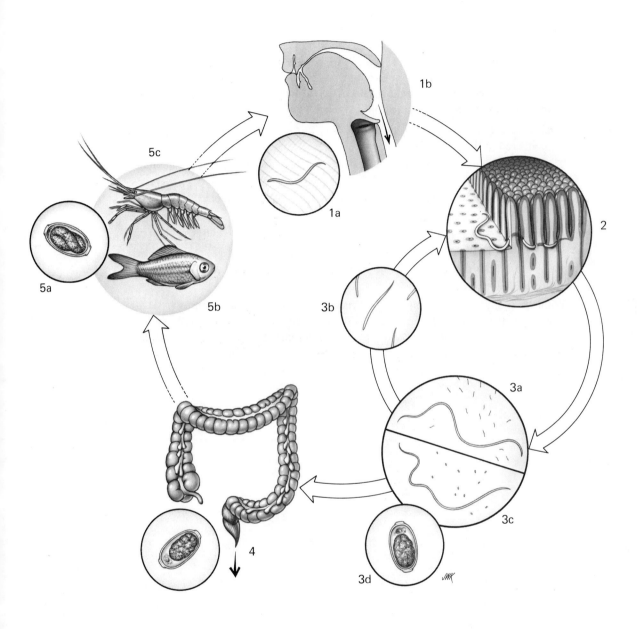

Kingdom: Animal
Phylum: Nematoda
Class: Aphasmida
Order: Trichurata
Family: Capillariidae
Genus: *Capillaria*
Species: *philippinensis*

Trichinella Spiralis

Enteral Phase

1   *Trichinella spiralis* is not host specific. All mammals are susceptible. Infection begins by the ingestion of infected raw or undercooked unfrozen meat containing the infectious first-stage larvae in striated skeletal muscle tissue. At this point the worm is 1 mm in length by 35 μm in diameter.

2   Parasites are freed of host tissue by digestive enzymes in the stomach and then are delivered to the small intestine.

3   Within the small intestine the larva quickly penetrates a row of columnar epithelium. It is now considered an intramulticellular parasite. There, the worm undergoes four molts within 28 hours, developing into an adult male or female.

4   Mating occurs within 30 hours after infection. The precise location in the gut where mating takes place is still undetermined. After mating (shown here in cross section) adult worms reside within the intramulticellular niche.

5a   Males are 1.5 mm by 36 μm, while females (shown here) are 3 mm in length by 36 μm in diameter.

5b   Within 5–6 days following infection, females begin shedding newborn (first-stage) larvae into the intracellular milieu. Newborn larvae are 80 μm in length by 6–7 μm in diameter. The newborn larva penetrates through the villous tissue into the lamina propria by using a spearlike stylet within its esophagus. They then enter either a draining lymph or blood vessel.

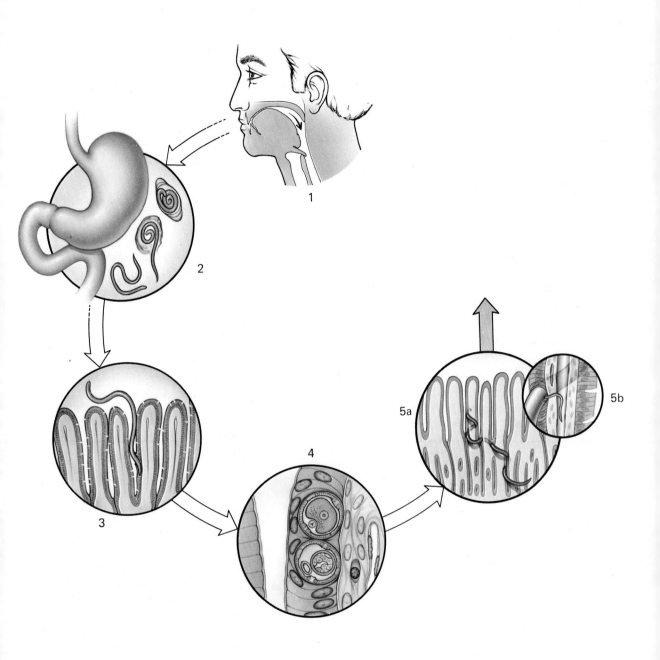

1

2

3

4

5a

5b

Kingdom: Animal
Phylum: Nematoda
Class: Aphasmida
Order: Trichurata
Family: Trichinellidae
Genus: *Trichinella*
Species: *spiralis*

Trichinella Spiralis

Parenteral Phase

6 Larvae eventually enter the general circulation and become distributed throughout the body.

7a Penetration of tissue by newborn larvae appears to occur solely by use of its esophageal stylet.

7b Migrating newborns penetrate out of capillaries into whatever tissue happens to be adjacent to the vessel, but will only remain within striated skeletal muscle cells. Larvae in tissues other than muscle reenter the general circulation.

8 The larvae grow and differentiate within the intracellular matrix of the infected muscle cell. During the process, the larva induces dramatic changes in the muscle cell, resulting in a totally new arrangement of host cytoplasm. Most of the cellular changes are complete by day 9 after intracellular infection.

9 Further host cell modifications at day 10–12 result in a nearly mature unit now referred to as the Nurse cell. The name describes the activity of this cell, the purpose of which is to facilitate nutrient acquisition by the larva and export of its metabolic wastes.

10 The larva-Nurse cell complex is fully grown at day 20 after infection. The first-stage larva has now achieved its maximum growth.

11 Any species of mammal can serve as a reservoir host for the infection, but transmission from animal to animal is largely by carnivorism and scavenging. In most of Europe, Asia and North America the pig is the usual source of infection. Polar bears, wart hogs and bush pigs are reservoirs commonly responsible for infections in arctic and tropical environments.

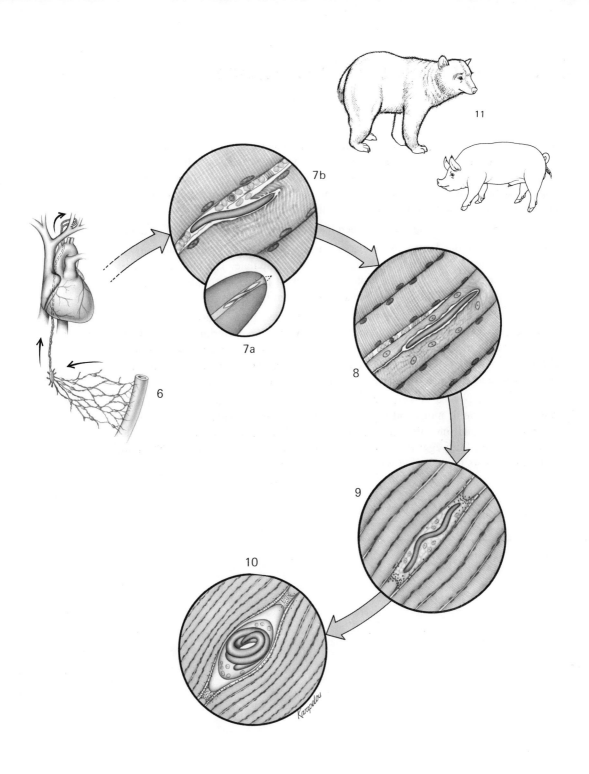

Trichuris Trichiura (Whipworm)

1 Infection with *Trichuris trichiura* is initiated by ingestion of embryonated eggs. Feces-contaminated soil and various uncooked vegetables that have been fertilized with human feces are the two most common sources of such eggs. Because of their impervious outer shell, embryonated eggs can survive in warm, moist soil for many months to years without losing their infectivity.

2 The egg contains a first-stage larva, which hatches upon reaching the small intestine.

3 Peristalsis carries the larvae to the large intestine, where they penetrate into the epithelium. After four molts, the worms, now adults, copulate. The female measures 4–6 cm in length and 1–2 mm in width at its thickest point. The male is somewhat smaller, measuring 2–3 cm in length and 0.6–0.8 mm in width.

4 The anterior portion of each worm remains embedded in a parasite-induced host syncytium composed of fused epithelial cells, while the posterior portion of the worm protrudes into the lumen of the large intestine. Worms begin producing eggs about 1 to 1½ months after infection. Female worms shed about 3,000–5,000 fertilized unembryonated eggs each day, and may continue to do so for up to 2 years.

5 Eggs must be deposited in a suitable external environment for development to continue. Loamy, warm, moist soil represents an ideal niche for embryonation. Larvae are fully developed into first-stage worms within 2–3 weeks after deposition. The entire life cycle, from egg to adult to egg takes approximately 2 months. There are no reservoir hosts for infection with *Trichuris trichiura*.

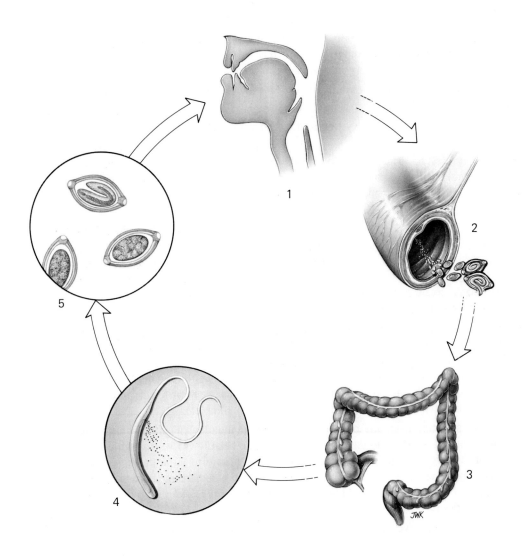

Kingdom: Animal
    Phylum: Nematoda
    Class: Aphasmida
    Order: Trichurata
    Family: Trichuridae
    Genus: *Trichuris*
    Species: *trichiura*

Strongyloides Stercoralis

1　The third-stage (filariform) infectious larva enters the host by penetrating the unbroken skin. Infection can also occur by ingestion of this stage. The larva penetrates into a capillary and is carried passively into the general circulation.

2　Larvae reach the pulmonary circulation where they penetrate out of the alveolar capillaries into the alveolar spaces.

3　Larvae migrate up the respiratory tree into the pharynx and are then swallowed.

4　*S. stercoralis* parasitic larvae develop only to adult females within the villus tissue of the small intestine. Male worms only exist in the free-living cycle. Reproduction in the parasitic female is by a process involving sequential production of sperm, then eggs. She is a protanderous hermaphrodite, measuring 2 mm in length by 0.04 mm in width.

5　Within several weeks after developing to adulthood, the worms begin to shed fully embryonated eggs into the surrounding tissue. There, the embryos develop to first-, then to second-stage larvae, after which they hatch. Once free of the eggshell, the second-stage larvae migrate out into the lumen of the small intestine. The worms are carried passively to the large intestine, where they are included within the fecal mass, and are defecated into the external environment.

6　If feces containing larvae are deposited in warm, moist, loamy or sandy soil, then the larvae feed, grow, and molt twice more, developing into free-living males and females. Several reproductive cycles can occur in this situation, provided that moisture, temperature, and food remain optimal. Many infectious third-stage larvae can result from the free-living cycle. Thus, the soil serves as a reservoir for the infection. The entire free-living life cycle takes several weeks to complete.

7　Individuals suffering from any one of a number of immunological difficiencies may permit second-stage larvae to develop into third-stage (filariform) worms within the lumen of the large intestine. When this occurs, the filariform larva can infect the same host by penetrating the large intestine, entering the bloodstream and completing the migration as described here in steps 1–3. Hence, *Strongyloides stercoralis* can be autoinfectious.

8　Many animals can serve as reservoir hosts, including dogs and monkeys.

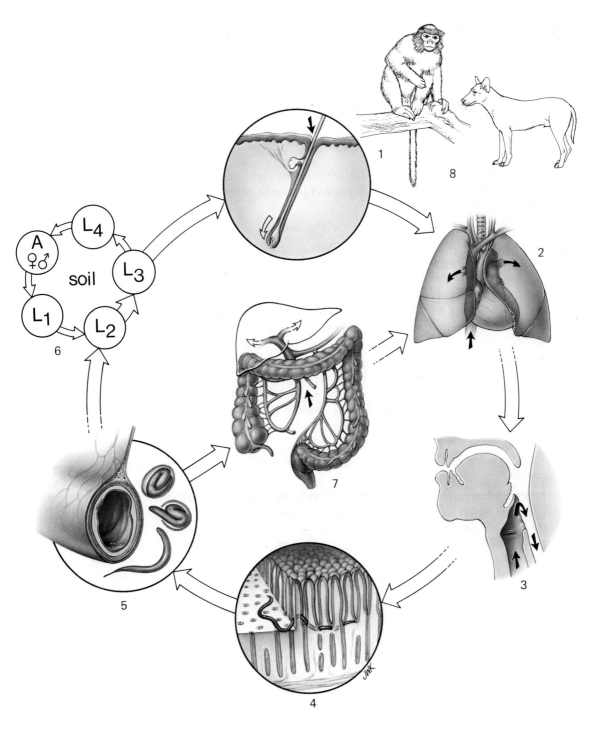

Kingdom: Animal
 Phylum: Nematoda
  Class: Phasmida
   Order: Rhabditata
    Family: Strongyloididae
     Genus: *Strongyloides*
      Species: *stercoralis*

Necator Americanus (Hookworm)

1a   The infectious filariform (third-stage) larva enters the host by either penetrating the unbroken skin or by being ingested.

1b   Larvae penetrating skin usually enter the circulation through a capillary at the base of a hair shaft.

2   Worms are passively carried through the bloodstream to the heart, where they are pumped into the pulmonary circulation and penetrate out of an alveolar capillary into the alveolar space.

3   After crawling up the respiratory tract to the pharynx, larvae are swallowed.

4   Upon arrival in the lumen of the small intestine, larvae attach to the villous tissue, molt twice, and develop to adults. The female is 10 mm in length by 0.35 mm in width, while the male is 7 mm in length by 0.30 mm in width. Mating ensues with male and female worms living *in copula*. Each female produces about 10,000 eggs each day. Worms live for about 2–4 years. Adult worms feed directly on villous tissue and suck blood. It is not known whether worms use blood as a food source.

5   Eggs are passed fertilized and begin to embryonate immediately. Feces containing eggs must be deposited in warm, moist, sandy or loamy soil if the life cycle is to continue. Embryogenesis is rapid, taking only 3–5 days. The larvae hatch in feces and consume bacteria, developing to rhabditiform (second-stage) larvae, then molt again into filariform (third-stage) worms.

6a   The filariform larvae do not feed, and, as already mentioned, are the infectious stage. The life cycle from larva to adult to filariform larva takes about 1 to 1½ months.

6b   Infectious larvae seek out the highest object in their immediate environment and remain there during periods of maximum moisture. This usually correlates with the early daylight hours. When moisture levels drop, they retreat into the soil and remain there until conditions favor migration. There are no reservoir hosts for *Necator americanus*.

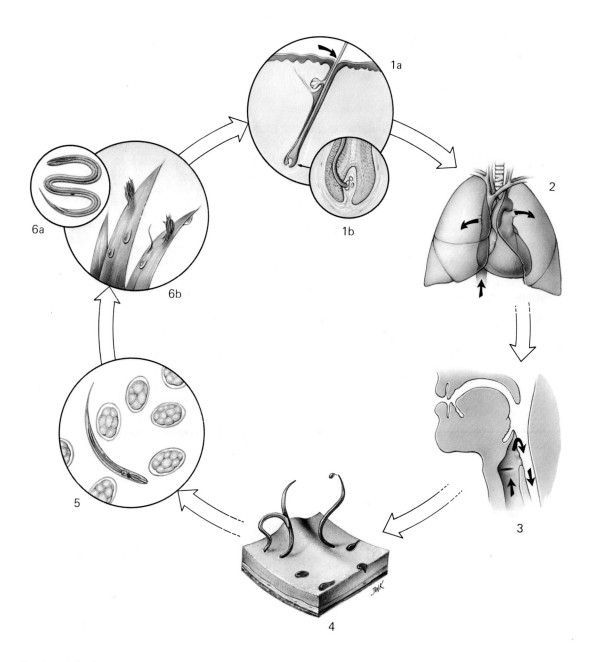

Kingdom: Animal
Phylum: Nematoda
Class: Phasmida
Order: Strongylata
Family: Ancylostomatidae
Genus: *Necator*
Species: *americanus*

Ascaris Lumbricoides (Giant Intestinal Worm)

1a The embryonated egg is the infectious stage of *Ascaris lumbricoides*. Feces-contaminated raw vegetables are the most common sources of eggs. Like *Trichuris*, the eggs of *A. lumbricoides* can survive in warm, moist, sandy or loamy soil for months or even years.

1b Eggs are swallowed in order to initiate infection.

2 Upon reaching the small intestine, the second-stage larva is stimulated to hatch. It then rapidly penetrates the small intestinal villus and enters the portal circulation. It arrives in the liver, and then penetrates out of the capillary into the parenchyma. The larva develops to a third-stage worm during this brief (1–2 weeks) migratory period.

3 The third-stage larva is now larger in diameter than a capillary. The worm reenters the returning circulation to the heart and is pumped into the pulmonary artery.

4 Worms become stuck in the small vessels of the alveolus, where they penetrate out into the alveolar spaces.

5 *A. lumbricoides* larvae migrate up the respiratory tract to the pharynx, and become swallowed.

6 After two more molts in the small intestinal lumen, worms grow to their full length; a process that takes 3 months. The adult female is 20–35 cm in length, by 0.5 cm in diameter, while the male is smaller, measuring 15–20 cm in length by 0.3–0.8 cm in diameter. Ascaris adults ingest and utilize intestinal luminal contents. After mating, the female begins to produce fertilized unembryonated eggs at the rate of about 200,000 per day. *Ascaris* adults can live up to 5 years, but average 2½ to 3 years. Eggs embryonate in soil, and take 2–4 weeks to do so. The entire life cycle from egg to adult to egg takes from 3½ to 4 months to complete. There are no reservoir hosts for Ascaris.

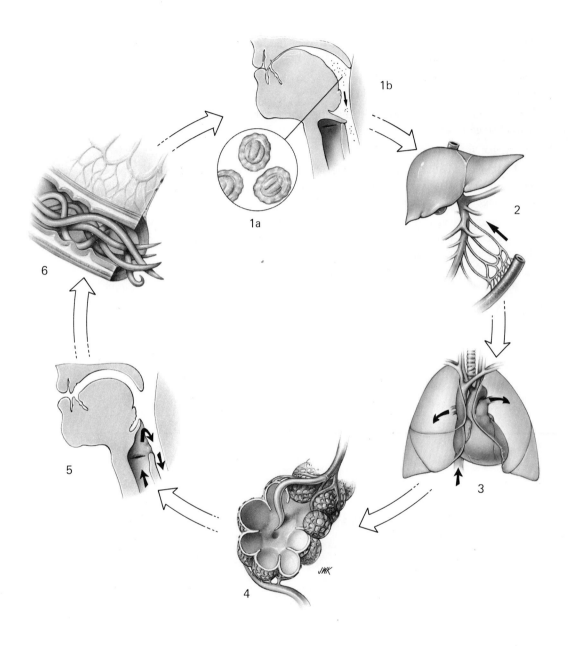

1a

1b

2

3

4

5

6

Kingdom: Animal
Phylum: Nematoda
Class: Phasmida
Order: Ascaridata
Family: Ascaridae
Genus: *Ascaris*
Species: *lumbricoides*

Ascaris Lumbricoides (Giant Intestinal Worm)

Toxocara Canis and Cati

1a   The adults of *Toxocara canis* and *cati* live in the lumen of the small intestine of dogs and cats, respectively.

1b   The life cycle in dogs and cats is similar to that of *Ascaris lumbricoides* in the human host (see pages 110 and 111).

2   In all hosts, infection begins by ingestion of embryonated eggs containing the second stage larva.

3   Larvae hatch in the small intestine.

4   In the human host larvae penetrate the small intestine, enter the portal circulation and wander aimlessly from organ to organ. Parasites develop only to the third larval stage in the human host.

5   Organs most frequently infected include the liver (5a), the brain (5b) and the eye (5c). In contrast its cycle continues in dogs and cats resulting in adult worms in the small intestinal lumen.

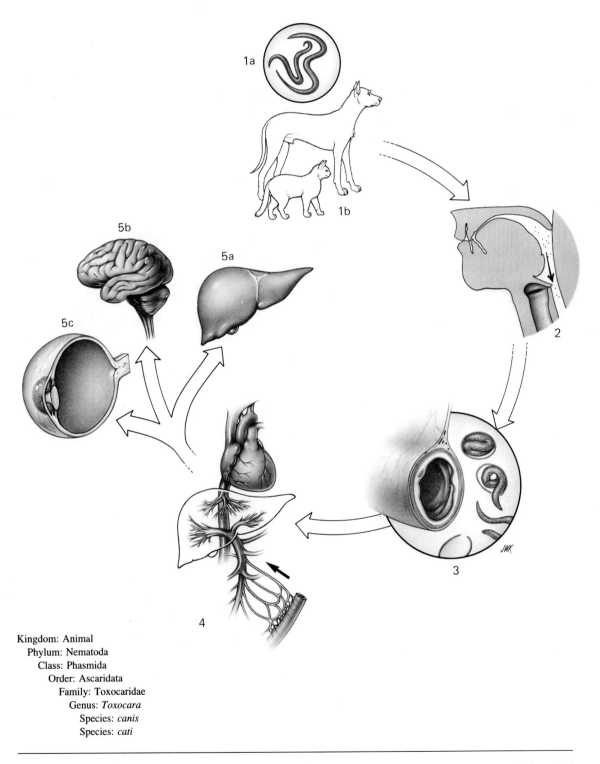

Kingdom: Animal
Phylum: Nematoda
Class: Phasmida
Order: Ascaridata
Family: Toxocaridae
Genus: *Toxocara*
Species: *canis*
Species: *cati*

Enterobius Vermicularis (Pinworm)

1 Infection with *Enterobius vermicularis* is usually initiated by ingestion of embryonated eggs. Eggs can also hatch on the perianal region and infect via the anus. Aberrant infections result from larvae migrating into the vaginal tract instead of the anus.

2 The embryonated egg contains the larva. As it is carried down the small intestine, it develops further and comes to reside in the lumen of the transverse and descending colon as an adult. Male worms measure 0.2 mm in width by 2.5 mm in length, while females measure 0.5 mm in width by 8–13 mm in length.

3 Mating occurs in the colon. Gravid females each contain from 10,000 to 11,000 eggs. The gravid females, in response to lower body temperature, reduced oxygen tension, or both, migrate out of the body, usually while the person is asleep.

4 The female worms come to rest on the area surrounding the anus.

5a There they either experience prolapse of their uterus, or simply die and disintegrate.

5b The embryonated eggs develop within 6 hours to first-, then second-stage worms. The larvae are now infectious. The outer egg shell is thin and susceptible to drying. Pinworm larvae die within 2 to 3 days in a low-humidity environment. The entire cycle from egg to adult to egg takes approximately 6 weeks.

6 Repeated infections eventually sensitize the host to worm antigens. The resulting itching and scratching cycle facilitates the contamination of fingers with embryonated eggs, which in turn ensures the reinfection of the same host. There are no reservoir hosts for this parasite. Furthermore, the human host is not susceptible to infection from any other species of pinworm.

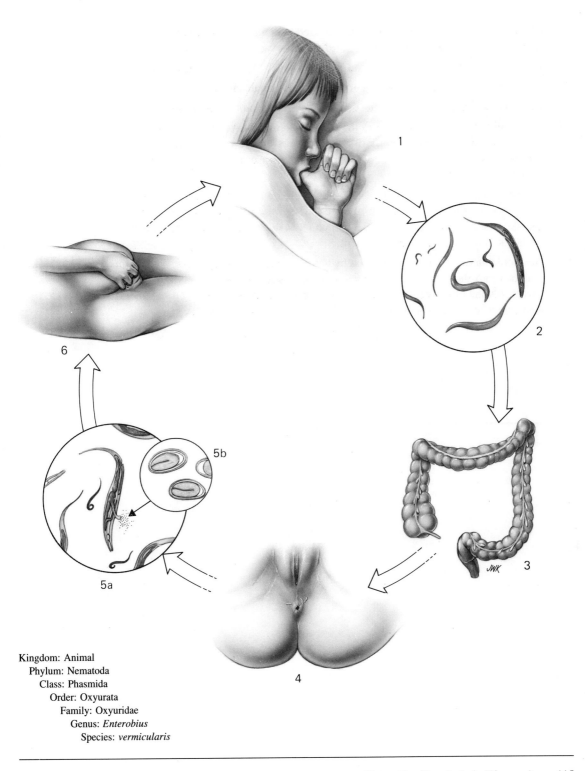

Kingdom: Animal
Phylum: Nematoda
Class: Phasmida
Order: Oxyurata
Family: Oxyuridae
Genus: *Enterobius*
Species: *vermicularis*

Enterobius Vermicularis (Pinworm)   115

Dracunculus Medinensis

1   Infection begins by drinking water contaminated with microscopic crustaceans (e.g., cyclops) which are infected with the third-stage larvae of *D. medinensis*.

2a The infected crustaceans are digested in the stomach, freeing the infectious larva.

2b The worm is carried passively by peristalsis to the small intestine.

3   The larva penetrates the small intestine and enters the subcutaneous tissues.

4   Larvae migrate within this tissue to the lower extremities. Adult males and females develop within the subcutaneous tissues. Females are 100 mm in length by 1.5 mm in width, while the males are much smaller, measuring only 40 mm in length by 0.4 mm in width.

5a Following mating, the female induces a fluid-filled blister at her anteriormost end. Upon encountering water, the worm experiences a uterine prolapse, releasing live first-stage larvae into the blister fluid. Simultaneously, the blister ruptures, releasing the larvae into the aquatic environment.

5b The motile larvae are quickly ingested by various species of crustaceans. The worms penetrate into the hemocoel and develop to third-stage infectious larvae within 2–3 weeks. None of the various mammals susceptible to infection with *D. medinensis* are thought to serve as reservoirs of infections for the human host.

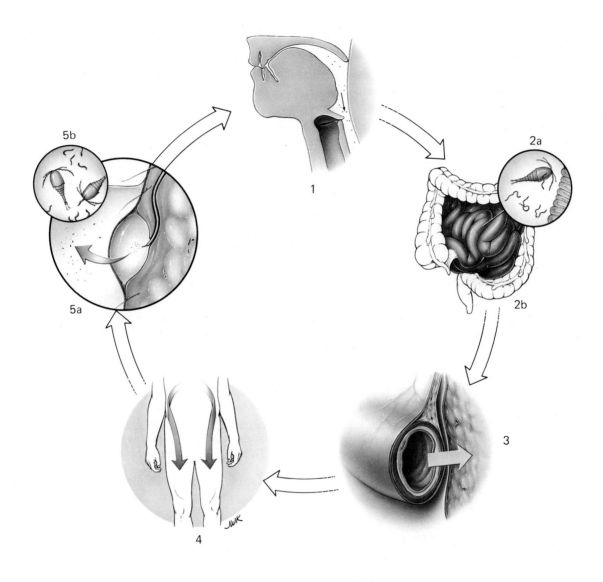

Kingdom: Animal
  Phylum: Nematoda
    Class: Phasmida
      Order: Camallanata
        Family: Dracunculidae
          Genus: *Dracunculus*
            Species: *medinensis*

Wuchereria Bancrofti

1a   *Wuchereria bancrofti* is transmitted from person to person by culicine and anopheline mosquitoes.

1b   When an infected mosquito bites, the infectious third-stage larva crawls out of the biting mouthparts of the mosquito onto the skin. When she withdraws her mouthparts after taking a blood meal, the larva crawls into the bite wound.

2   Worms migrate by the lymph to the draining lymph nodes.

3   Adult males and females develop to sexual maturity in the afferent lymph vessels adjacent to the lymph nodes. Females are 8 cm long by 300 μm in diameter, and males are 4 cm long by 100 μm in diameter. Development in the mammalian host is slow, taking approximately 1 year to complete.

4   Females give birth to living larvae called microfilariae. These larvae migrate through the lymph node, and eventually enter the general circulation of the blood. Microfilariae are 270 μm in length by 9 μm in diameter and live for about 1½ years.

5a   *W. bancrofti,* in most places in the world, exhibits periodic behavior. Microfilariae are found in peripheral blood of those individuals experiencing periods of extended rest (i.e., sleep).

5b   Microfilariae are not found in peripheral blood during periods of physical activity. In some geographic regions, *W. bancrofti* exhibits non-periodic behavior (i.e., they are found in peripheral blood at all times).

6   When a mosquito ingests blood containing microfilariae, the blood is digested, and the worms penetrate the intestine, enter the hemocoel, then migrate to the flight wing muscles in the thorax. There, they penetrate single muscle fibers and grow and develop to third-stage infectious larvae. Following maturation, they migrate into the hemocoel and take up residence in the biting mouthparts. Infectious larvae develop within 2 weeks after being ingested. There are no reservoir hosts for *Wuchereria bancrofti*.

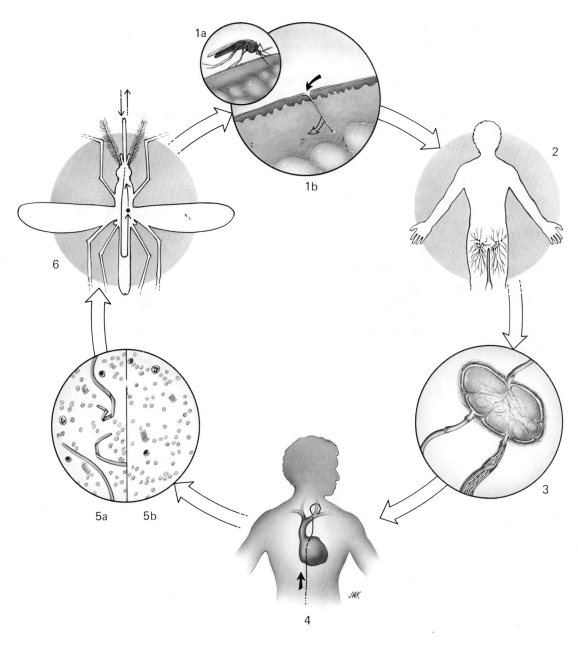

Kingdom: Animal
Phylum: Nematoda
Class: Phasmida
Order: Filariata
Family: Onchocercidae
Genus: *Wuchereria*
Species: *bancrofti*

Loa Loa

1a Dipteran flies in the genus *Chrysops* are the vectors for *Loa loa*.

1b Infection occurs when an infected fly takes a blood meal. The third-stage larvae crawl out of the biting mouthparts onto the skin adjacent to the bite site. When the fly leaves the host, the larvae enter the bite wound and migrate to the subcutaneous tissues.

2 Larvae grow to adulthood in the subcutaneous tissues. Adult male and female *L. loa* develop to sexual maturity within 1–4 years after initial infection. Females are 60 mm long by 0.5 mm wide. Males are 32 mm long by 0.4 mm wide. Females give birth to live larvae (microfilariae), which find their way into the general circulation of the blood.

3 Microfilariae exhibit diurnal periodicity, appearing in peripheral blood during daylight hours, and remaining sequestered in the deep vascular beds of the lungs at night.

4 *Chrysops* spp. feed during daylight hours, acquiring their infection by taking a blood meal from an infected individual.

5 The microfilariae penetrate the intestine, enter the hemocoel, and then migrate to the flight wing muscles where they each penetrate a single muscle fiber. After two molts, they are fully infectious. The larvae then migrate out of the muscle tissue into the hemocoel, then into the biting mouthparts. There are no reservoir hosts for this parasite.

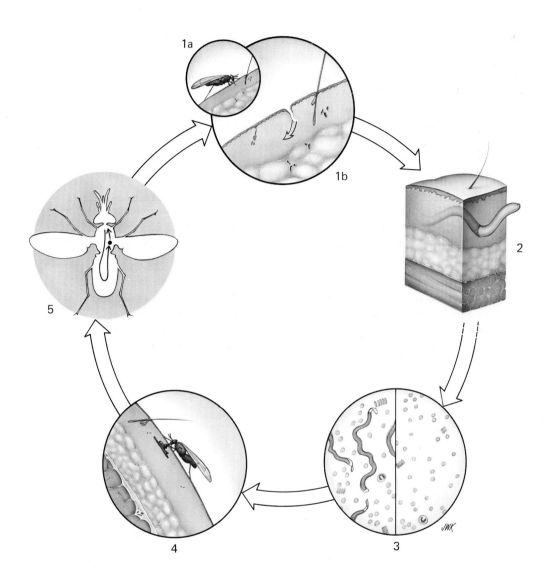

Kingdom: Animal
 Phylum: Nematoda
  Class: Phasmida
   Order: Filariata
    Family: Onchocercidae
     Genus: *Loa*
      Species: *loa*

Onchocerca Volvulus

1a The female blackfly (*Simulium* sp.) is the vector of *Onchocerca volvulus*.

1b The infective larva crawls out of the blackfly mouthparts onto the bite site while the infected insect feeds. When it withdraws its mouthparts, the larva crawls into the wound and enters the subcutaneous tissues.

2 Larvae molt and develop to adults in the subcutaneous tissue within a parasite-induced nodule, and take one year to do so. Adult females are 45–50 cm in length by 300 μm in diameter, while the smaller males are 20–40 mm in length by 200 μm in diameter. After mating, each female begins to shed live larvae (microfilariae). Adult worms can live for 8–10 years and produce hundreds of thousands of offspring during that time.

3 Microfilariae migrate away from the adult worm, remaining within the confines of the subcutaneous tissue. Microfilariae can live for up to 6 months.

4 The larvae are ingested by female blackflies when they take a blood meal from an infected person.

5 Once within the blackfly, the larvae penetrate the intestine, enter the hemocoel, and migrate to the flight wing muscles, where they penetrate into single muscle fibers. Two molts ensue within 6 days, resulting in an infectious (third-stage) larva. The worms then migrate to the mouthparts and are introduced onto the host during the next blood meal that the insect takes. No reservoir hosts exist for *Onchocerca volvulus*.

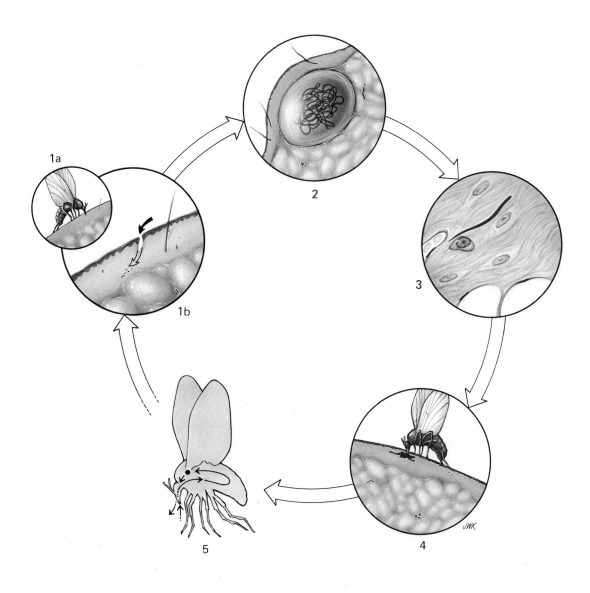

Kingdom: Animal
Phylum: Nematoda
Class: Phasmida
Order: Filariata
Family: Onchocercidae
Genus: *Onchocerca*
Species: *volvulus*

Selected Readings

General

Ash L, Oriel T: Atlas of Human Parasitology. Chicago, American Society of Clinical Pathologists, 1987

Ash L, Oriel T: Parasites: A Guide to Laboratory Procedures and Identification. Chicago, American Society of Clinical Pathologists, 1987

August JT (ed): Molecular Parasitology. New York and London, Academic Press, 1984

Bailey WS (ed): Cues That Influence Behavior of Internal Parasites. New Orleans, Agricultural Research Service, USDA, 1982

Campbell WC, Rew R (eds): Chemotherapy of Parasitic Diseases. New York and London, Plenum, 1986

Cox FEG (ed): Modern Parasitology. Oxford and London, Blackwell Scientific Publications, 1982

Evered D, Collins GM (eds): Cytopathology of Parasitic Diseases. London, Pitman, 1983

Howell MJ (ed): Parasitology—Quo Vadit. Canberra, Australian Academy of Science, 1986

Katz M, Despommier DD, Gwadz R: Parasitic Diseases. New York and Heidelberg, Springer-Verlag, 1982

Kennedy CR (ed): Ecological Aspects of Parasitology. Amsterdam and Oxford, North-Holland Publishing, 1976

Newton BN, Michal F (eds): New Approaches to the Identification of Parasites and Their Vectors. Basel, Schwabe, 1984

Nicoli RM, Penaud A (eds): 50 Cycles Epidemiologique. Paris, Médicine et Sciences Internationale, 1983

Price PW (ed): Evolutionary Biology of Parasites. Princeton NJ, Princeton University Press, 1980

Rogers WP (ed): The Nature of Parasitism. New York and London, Academic Press, 1962

Peters W, Gilles HM: Color Atlas of Tropical Medicine and Parasitology. Chicago IL, Year Book Medical Publishers, 1977

Schmidt G, Roberts L (eds): Foundations of Parasitology. St. Louis MO, Mosby, 1981

Strickland GT (ed): Hunters' Tropical Medicine. Philadelphia and London, Saunders, 1984

Trager W (ed): Living Together: The Biology of Animal Parasitism. New York, Plenum, 1986,

Wakelin D (ed): Immunity to Parasites: How Animals Control Parasite Infections. London, Edward Arnold, 1984

Warren KS, Bowers JZ (eds): Parasitology: A Global Perspective. New York, Springer-Verlag, 1983

Whitfield PJ (ed): The Biology of Parasitism. Baltimore, University Park Press, 1979

Protozoa

Baker JR: The Biology of Parasitic Protozoa. London, Edward Arnold, 1982

Bruce-Chwatt LJ: Essentials of Malariology. New York, Wiley, 1985

Erlandsen SL, Myer EA (eds): Giardia and Giardiasis. New York, Plenum, 1984

Hudson L (ed): The biology of trypanosomes. Curr Topics Microbioal Immunol 117:183, 1985

Jensen JB (ed): In Vitro Cultivation of Protozoan Parasites. Boca Raton FL, CRC Press, 1983

Lee JJ, Hunter SH, Bovee EC (eds): An Illustrated Guide to the Protozoa. Lawrence KS, Allen Press, 1985

Levine ND, et al: A newly revised classification of the Protozoa. J Protozool, 27:37–58, 1980

Martinez-Paloma A: The Biology of Entamoeba histolytica. Chichester, England, Wiley, 1982

Molyneux DH, Ashford RW (eds): The Biology of Trypanosomes and Leishmania Parasites of Man and Animals. New York, Taylor and Francis, 1983

Cestodes

Arai MP (ed): Biology of the Tapeworm Hymenolepis Diminuta. New York and London, Academic Press, 1983

Arme C, Pappas PW (eds): Biology of the Eucestoda, Vol 1, 2. New York and London, Academic Press, 1983

Flisser A, Williams K, Laclette C, et al (eds): Cysticercosis: Present State of Knowledge and Perspectives. New York and London, Academic Press, 1982

Schmidt G: Key to the Identification of Tapeworms. Boca Raton, FL, CRC Press, 1986

Thompson RSA, Allen G: Biology of Echinococcus and Hydatid Disease. London, Allen and Unwin, 1986

Trematodes

Bruce JJ, Sornmani S (eds): The Mekong Schistosome. Whitmore Lake MI, Malacological Review, 1980

Jordan P: Schistosomiasis. The St. Lucia Project. Cambridge, England, Cambridge University Press, 1985

Smyth JD, Halton DW (eds): The Physiology of Trematodes. Cambridge, England, Cambridge University Press, 1983

Nematodes

Campbell WC (ed): Trichinella and Trichinosis. New York, Plenum, 1983

Croll NA (ed): The Organization of Nematodes. London and New York, Academic Press, 1976

Crompton DWI, Nesheim MC, Pawlowski ZF (eds): Ascariasis and Its Public Health Significance. London and Philadelphia, Taylor and Francis, 1985

Kim CW (ed): Trichinellosis. Albany NY, New York State University Press, 1985

Zuckerman BM (ed): Nematodes as Biological Models, Vol 1, 2. London and New York, Academic Press, 1980

Alphabetical Listing of Parasites

Learning
AIDS

An Information Resources Directory

SECOND EDITION
1989

EDITORS	Trish Halleron, MPH, Director of Education
	Janet Pisaneschi, PhD, Program Consultant
	Margi Trapani, Project Director
PROJECT STAFF	Alan Clore, Assistant Project Director
	Anthony Ranieri, Project Librarian
	Rita Kirsonis, Data Entry
	Jose Cenac
	Peter Muller
ABSTRACT WRITERS	Barbara Davis
	Barbara Nathenson
	Louise Northcut
	Johanna Van Wert
DATA PRODUCTION CONSULTANT	Michael Smith
	Village Consulting, Inc.
DESIGN	Brian Crede
	Paula Wiech
SPECIAL TECHNICAL ASSISTANCE	Dennis Diamond
	Video D
PROJECT VOLUNTEERS	Steve Jones
	Bob O'Shaughnessy
	Kristen B. Schleifer
	Jim Selfe

Please direct all inquiries to

Trish A. Halleron, MPH
American Foundation for AIDS Research
1515 Broadway, Suite 3601
New York, New York 10036
212-719-0033

Distributed by

R.R. Bowker
245 West 17th Street
New York, NY 10011
212-337-6934
1-800-521-8110

TABLE OF CONTENTS

**From the Surgeon General
of the United States:**

*I must salute the members of the
American Foundation for AIDS
Research for the work they have
done in assembling the second
edition of this information
resources directory, a much
needed and useful tool for both
assessing and accessing AIDS information and education resources. This work is much more than
a simple compilation or bibliography.*

*Learning AIDS is a unique,
qualitative assessment of available educational materials. The
careful, indepth evaluation is
typical of the "extra step" AmFAR
has taken over the years to better
educate our youth and the
American public at large about
AIDS.*

*C. Everett Koop, M.D., Sc.D
Surgeon General
U.S. Public Health Service
May 1989*

PREFACE

This directory is intended as a reference tool for educators, service providers, program managers, policy makers and other individuals interested in or affected by the AIDS/HIV epidemic. In order to meet the information needs of diverse groups, every attempt was made to solicit material nationwide. However, since the development of new material is continuous, some products will become available after this book is produced. Some local information is beyond the scope of this directory and so is not listed here.

In order to make this book as useful to readers as possible, materials described in Chapter 1 were reviewed by AIDS and education experts. Their qualitative assessments are intended to provide readers with a guide to material appropriate for their needs; however, evaluations by the expert panel do not necessarily reflect the opinion of AmFAR.

The information in the Directory should serve as only the first step in identifying qualitative and suitable materials. The editors recommend that the user obtain a sample or preview copy of the products selected from the Directory and carefully assess each item in terms of ones specific program goals and special needs and characteristics of the intended audience.

ABOUT THIS DIRECTORY

HOW THE DIRECTORY WAS DEVELOPED

AmFAR solicited submissions for the directory through a national survey distributed to over 12,000 organizations. Not all the information gathered is contained in this directory since some of it, such as services information, is beyond the scope of this work and is contained in other publications.

Over thirty AIDS, health, and education experts representing diverse constituencies assisted in the review of materials submitted for this second edition.

REVIEW AND SELECTION PROCESS

Over 900 items were collected for possible inclusion in the directory. Each item was screened initially to determine if it:
1) pertained to AIDS/HIV;
2) was intended for use as an educational tool in formal or informal instructional settings (e.g., videotapes, curricula, etc.) or for general public information (eg., public service announcements, posters, etc.)
3) was a periodical, a reference book, a statement of policy or guidelines, or a source book for supplemental or more indepth information.

Items that were not AIDS/HIV-specific were not reviewed and do not appear in this directory. Items that are formal or informal educational tools, or are for general public information were reviewed and appear in Chapter 1. And, those items that are "references," were not reviewed, but appear in Chapter 2 listings.

MATERIAL REVIEW

Members of the Expert Review Panel met over a three day period to provide qualitative evaluation of materials collected. Each item selected for review was evaluated by a team of three experts. Material assignment for each team was based on target audience, knowledge, and preferences of individual reviewers, as well as appropriate distribution and balance of expertise within the team. Teams were instructed to provide, if possible, a consensus rating and comments for each product. If a consensus was not possible, the majority opinion was adopted.

In some cases, when a specific expertise was not available at the review conference (e.g., translations for certain languages, a unique target audience, etc.), materials were sent to experts around the country for review. All materials were reviewed by at least three experts.

RATING AND COMMENTS

The basic criteria used in the evaluation of the materials were: medical accuracy, appropriateness for target audience, and production quality. Reviewers were given more detailed evaluation criteria guidelines for each type of product reviewed (see appendix). These criteria guidelines were used not only to rate products but also to assist reviewers in developing statements for their review comments. All of the reviewed materials are presented in Chapter 1. Those that were rated average or above are fully described, including abstract and reviewers' comments. Those that were rated below average are simply listed by title and producer.

EXPERT REVIEW PANEL

Abdul Rahim Ali
Project Director, BEBASHI
Blacks Educating Blacks
About Sexual Health Issues
Philadephia, PA

William A. Bogan
Executive Vice President
National Coalition of Hispanic
Health and Human Services
Organizations (COSSMHO)
Washington, D.C.

**Steve L. Buckinghham,
LCSW, ACSW**
Director of Psychosocial
Services
Pacific Oaks Medical Group
Sherman Oaks, California

Dagmaris Cabezas, M.S.
Associate Director Community
Affairs & Special Projects
HIV Center for Clinical &
Behavioral Studies, Columbia
University
New York, NY

Maribel Clements, RN, MA
Puget Sound Blood Center
Hemophilia Program
Seattle, WA

Douglas J. Conway, JD
San Francisco, CA

Joan L. Cooney, MA
Health Education Coordinator
AIDS Project American
College Health Association
Rockville, MD

**Frances J. Dunston, MD,
MPH FAAP**
Director, Richmond City
Health Department
President, US Conference
of Local Health Officials
Richmond, VA

Gilberto Garica, LPN
National Association of People
with AIDS
Tucson, AZ

Aida L. Giachello, Ph.D.
Jane Addams College
of Social Work
University of Illinois at Chicago
Chicago, IL

Joel Gray , BSN, RN
National Association of People
with AIDS
Tucson, AZ

Christopher S. Hall
Coordinator, Clearinghouse
and Resource Development
National AIDS Network
Washington, D.C.

John L.S. Holloman, Jr., MD
The William F. Ryan Health
Center
New York, NY

Trish Houtteman
AIDS Education Task Force
UAW-GM Human Resource
Health and Safety Center
Madison Heights, MI

Lynelle T. Johnson
Volunteer Program Coordinator
National Minority AIDS
Council
Washington, D.C.

Dianne Kerr, MA, MEd
AIDS Education Project
Coordinator
American School Health
Association
Kent, OH

Iris W. Lee, MPH
Director, Division of AIDS
Education
DC Commission of Public
Health
Washington, DC

James L. Mckittrick, Ed.D
Director, Media Services
School of Medicine
University of Alabama
Birmingham, AL

Alison Moed, RN, BSN
Head Nurse
San Francisco General Hospital
Medical Center
San Francisco, CA

Patricia Nichols, BSN, MS
Health Education Consultant
Michigan Department of
Education
Lansing, MI

Lyn Paleo
Education Director
San Francisco AIDS Foundation
San Francisco, CA

Patricia M. Parrish, MSW
Program Specialist
Atlanta Area Health Education
Center, Inc.
Atlanta, GA

Margaret R. Reinfeld
Director of Education
Gay Men's Health Crisis
New York, NY

Gloria Rodriguez
New Jersey State Department
of Health
Division of AIDS Prevention
and Control
East Orange, NJ

Rev. John H. Vaughn, M.Div.
Executive Director
East Harlem Interfaith
New York, NY

Armin D. Weinberg, Ph.D
Director
Center for Cancer Control
Research
Baylor College of Medicine
The Methodist Hospital
Houston, TX

James A. Wells, Ph.D
Senior Policy Analyst
Project HOPE Center
for Health Affairs
Chevy Chase, MD

James Williams, MEd
Director
National Education Association
Health Information Network
Atlanta, GA

**REVIEWERS FOR
SPECIAL PRODUCTS AND
TRANSLATIONS**

Lori K. Beaulieu
Program Specialist
National Native American
AIDS Prevention Center
Minneapolis Branch
Minneapolis, Minnesota

Jocelyne Daniel
Women and AIDS Resource
Network (WARN)
Brooklyn, NY

Sharon Day
Special Assistant Director
Chemical Dependency Division
Minnesota Department of
Human Services
St. Paul, Minnesota

Michael Fleming
Chinese American Planning
Council
New York, NY

Pete Flores
Health Director
Pascua Yaqui Health
Department
Tuscan, AZ

Gloria Garica
AIDS Coordinator
Pascua Yaqui Health
Department
Tuscan, AZ

Marie Gaspard, MA
WARN
Brooklyn, NY

Janet Gilman
Director, Public Relations
The Asian Society
New York, NY

Mr. Kim Huot Kiet
Project Director
Cambodian American Society
Humanitarian Association
Brooklyn, NY

**Marie-Lucie-Brutus MA,
MPH**
WARN
Brooklyn, NY

Jean Paul, MA
WARN
Brooklyn, NY

Josefine Petit-Frere, BA
WARN
Brooklyn, NY

Marie Saint Cyr
Executive Director, Women
and AIDS Resource Network
Brooklyn, NY

David Sam
Resource Specialist
Alaska Native Health Board
Anchorage, Alaska

Lois Steele, MD
Clinical Director
Pascua Yaqui Health
Department
Tuscan, AZ

EVALUATION CRITERIA

CONTENT

The content is accurate and current.

Medical/scientific information is stated and interpreted factually and without bias.

The content is appropriate to the level of the learner and to the objectives.

The content is adequate in detail relative to the objectives and the target audience.

Pertinent variant views are clearly acknowledged.

INSTRUCTIONAL DESIGN

Objectives are clearly stated or obviously implied and address the needs of the target audience.

Objectives address: enhancing knowledge, changing attitudes or beliefs, modifying behavior, and building skills.

Product achieves (or is suitably designed to achieve) its stated or implied objectives.

Principles of good communication and instruction are applied.

Language level and vocabulary used are appropriate for the target audience.

The length of the product is suited to the attention span of the targeted audience.

Material is organized and presented in a logical, understandable manner.

The product stimulates the user's interest.

It is appropriately concise and to the point.

Product can be used for or by audiences other than the one specifically targeted.

Appropriate support materials are provided.

TECHNICAL PRODUCTION

The format is appropriate for the product's objectives.

Visual elements are used as appropriate or needed.

Visual/audio elements are clear, sharp, and well integrated.

The print/graphics/artwork are readable and consistent.

Visuals are used to highlight all educationally significant details.

Performances, sets, and graphic design contribute to effectiveness.

Noticeable technical flaws do not impede learning.

Overall, technical production enhances instructional effectiveness.

The concept or execution is innovative.

The designated user will find the product easy to use.

The overall design is appealing.

Overall, the product is effective.

Additional Criteria

For Instructional Programs:

INSTRUCTIONAL METHODS

The methods suit the objectives.

The methods are appropriate to the audience.

The methods selected are consistent with current, accepted learning theory.

SUPPORT MATERIALS

The variety of support materials is suitable to the target audience and objectives.

The support materials implement the strategies.

ASSESSMENT/ ADMINISTRATION

There are provisions for measuring learning or achievement.

The cost of the curriculum is reasonable.

The program is part of a larger health curriculum.

The program provides for or stipulates the need for thorough training of the instructor.

A Guide To Selected AIDS Educational Materials

This chapter contains the listing of all products that were reviewed by either the 1988 (first edition) or the 1989 (second edition) expert review panel. These Products are categorized first by target audience (e.g., Children And Adolescents) and then, within each target audience, by type of product (e.g., Brochure). Items that were rated as average or above (i.e., recommended for use), as well as those that were rated below average (i.e., not recommended) are listed. The items that are recommended for use are displayed differently from those not recommended.

Products Recommended by the Expert Review Panel

The following information is provided for all recommended products: symbol indicating both recommended status and the edition of item's first appearance, title, producers name, physical description, publication date, original and other available languages, an abstract, and reference to ordering information. For all types of products except brochures, reviewers' comments are also provided. In the case of brochures reccomended in the first edition, both abstracts and reviewers' comments have been omitted. Below is a sample item.

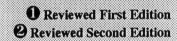

❶ AIDS Is Killing Blacks, Too

Minority AIDS Project
11 x 17; color; 1988; $1.50; English.

This tri-color-print poster informs blacks that AIDS/HIV crosses sexual, racial, and socio-economic lines. Using direct language, it specifies ways to avoid AIDS/HIV.

Reviewers' Comments: This poster gets right to the point; its strong language conveys the message.

▲ For Ordering Information, see p. 223

Products Not Recommended by the Expert Review Panel

The following information is provided for all not-recommended products: Symbol indicating not-recommended status, title, and producers name. Below is a sample.

◯ Safer Sex

**Division of Health,
AIDS/HIV Program**

❶ Reviewed First Edition
❷ Reviewed Second Edition

◯ Not Recommended

BLACK COMMUNITY

BROCHURES

❶ AIDS And People Of Color

Massachusetts Department of Public Health
3 panels; charts; free, limited copies; Dec 1987; English.

▲ For Ordering Information, see p. 222

◯ AIDS And The Black Community

Massachusetts Department of Public Health

◯ AIDS And The Black Community

Texas Department of Health Bureau of AIDS and STD Control

❷ AIDS Can Tear You Apart

Blacks Against AIDS
3 panels; illustrations; free; 1988; English.

This brochure asserts that protecting yourself and your family from AIDS/HIV is your responsibility, without giving specific information for doing so. It does explain that the virus is transmitted through body fluids and that it does not discriminate on any basis. Individuals are encouraged to contact Blacks Against AIDS for more information and one panel is a call for volunteers.

▲ For Ordering Information, see p. 215

❷ AIDS: Concerns For People Of Color

NO/AIDS Task Force
3 panels; $.10; special rates / discounts; 1988; English.

This brochure provides readers with basic AIDS/HIV information including transmission, a description of AIDS/HIV and how it affects the immune system, and the fact that the virus does not discriminate according to gender, sexuality, race, age, or drug use habits. It includes a list of "warning signs" of AIDS/HIV infection and a list of "things to remember" such as "You can't tell if a person has the AIDS virus by looking at them," and "Drugs and alcohol can trick you into doing something that might put you at increased risk for getting AIDS." It encourages people of color to become informed about AIDS/HIV. New Orleans and Louisiana hotline numbers are included.

▲ For Ordering Information, see p. 225

❶ AIDS - Facts About AIDS Young Black Men Need To Know
AIDS - Facts About AIDS Young Black Women Need To Know

Bebashi, Inc.
2 panels; illustrations; English.

▲ For Ordering Information, see p. 215

❷ AIDS In The Black Community

Ohio Department of Health - AIDS Unit
3 panels; free, limited copies; Apr 1988; English.

This brochure confronts the myth that AIDS/HIV is not a problem in the black community. It states that although 12 percent of the US population is black, 25 percent of those with AIDS/HIV, including 50 percent of women and 60 percent of children with AIDS/HIV, are black. It mentions what AIDS is, its symptoms, and how it is and is not transmitted. No specific prevention information is provided.

▲ For Ordering Information, see p. 225

❷ AIDS In The Black Community

People of Color Against AIDS Network
3 panels; illustrations; free, limited copies; 1988; English.

This brochure describes what AIDS/HIV is, how it is spread, who gets AIDS/HIV, and how to prevent transmission of the virus. It lists the percentages of black American men, women, and children who have the virus and encourages testing for anyone planning to have a child. Ways HIV is not transmitted are also listed. Various Seattle area information numbers are given.

▲ For Ordering Information, see p. 226

❷ AIDS In The Black Community

Virginia Department of Health - AIDS Program
3 panels; free; 1988; English.

In this brochure, statistics are given to demonstrate that AIDS/HIV is affecting minority communities. HIV is described, prevention methods are listed, and risky and dangerous behaviors are outlined, as are types of casual contact that cannot spread the virus. Symptoms are listed and Virginia hotline numbers are given.

▲ For Ordering Information, see p. 231

❶ 1ST EDITION RECOMMENDED   ❷ 2ND EDITION RECOMMENDED   ◯ NOT RECOMMENDED

❶ AIDS In The Black Community - The Facts

National Coalition of Black Lesbians and Gays
2 panels; illustrations; Sep 1987; English.

▲ For Ordering Information, see p. 224

❷ AIDS In The Black Community - The Facts

North Carolina AIDS Control Program
2 panels; free; 1988; English.

This brochure emphasizes that AIDS/HIV does not discriminate, offering statistics on the prevalence of AIDS/HIV among blacks in the United States. It lists symptoms, identifies high-risk behaviors, and suggests steps for HIV transmission prevention to those engaging in high risk behaviors. Symptoms of HIV infection are listed and National hotline numbers are given.

▲ For Ordering Information, see p. 225

❶ AIDS In The Black Community - When In Doubt...Pull The Condom Out

The Kupona Network
4 panels; illustrations; free; 1987; English.

▲ For Ordering Information, see p. 229

❷ AIDS Is A White Man's Disease

People of Color Against AIDS Network
3 panels; photographs; free, limited copies; 1988; English.

The message in this brochure is that anyone can contract AIDS/HIV and the percentage of people with AIDS/HIV in the U.S. who are black, Hispanic, Asian and Native American is given. Readers are encouraged to use condoms and never share intravenous drug works. The People of Color AIDS Network number is given.

▲ For Ordering Information, see p. 226

◯ AIDS - It's A Black Problem, Too

AIDS Foundation Houston, Inc.

❷ AIDS Knows No Color Or Language

Health Issues Taskforce of Cleveland
3 panels; $.10; 1988; English/Spanish.

This brochure provides information on HIV, its symptoms, transmission, and infection. It also discusses the ways in which the virus is not transmitted. Statistics are presented on the high incidence of AIDS/HIV among black and Hispanic communities in the U.S. The Spanish translation fails to meet the minimum acceptance criteria.

▲ For Ordering Information, see p. 220

◯ AIDS The Equal Opportunity Syndrome

AIDS Prevention Project Dallas County Health Department

◯ Any Color, Any Sex, Any Age, Anybody

Madison AIDS Support Network

◯ Avoiding AIDS

Unique Community Women's Club, Inc.

❷ Black IV Drug Users: Enlightening News On A Crisis In Our Community

D.C. Commission of Public Health
2 panels; illustrations; special rates / discounts; 1987; English.

This brochure clarifies some of the facts about IV drug use and AIDS/HIV, and dispels common misconceptions such as "only gays get AIDS." It explains basic IV drug use-related transmission and urges readers not to share needles and to use condoms. Local telephone numbers are provided for more information.

▲ For Ordering Information, see p. 218

❷ Black People Get AIDS Too!

Black Women's Health Council, Inc.
1 panel; illustrations; free; 1988; English.

Depicting various nationalities in cartooned faces, this leaflet gives statistics about AIDS among Blacks in the United States and in the state of Maryland. It also offers a hopeful message, "Together We Can Learn How to Stop the Spread of AIDS," and phone numbers to call for information in Maryland, as well as the National AIDS Hotline number.

▲ For Ordering Information, see p. 215

○ **Black People Get AIDS Too!**

Sacramento AIDS Foundation

❷ **Black Women: Enlightening News On A Crisis In Our Community**

D.C. Commission of Public Health
2 panels; illustrations; special rates / discounts; 1987; English.

This brochure addresses questions regarding AIDS/HIV; how women become infected with the disease; how they can avoid infection; and how and whether women can deduce that someone has the virus.

▲ For Ordering Information, see p. 218

❷ **Black Youth: Enlightening News On A Crisis In Our Community**

D.C. Commission of Public Health
2 panels; illustrations; special rates / discounts; 1987; English.

This brochure addresses black youth. It explains what AIDS/HIV is and that teens do get it. Basic transmission modes are given with information on transmission prevention. Local telephone numbers for more AIDS/HIV information are provided.

▲ For Ordering Information, see p. 218

❷ **Blacks: Enlightening News On A Crisis In Our Community**

D.C. Commission of Public Health
3 panels; illustrations; special rates / discounts; 1987; English.

This brochure stresses prevention through wearing condoms and not sharing needles. It outlines the warning signs of the disease and offers facts about AIDS/HIV in Washington's black community.

▲ For Ordering Information, see p. 218

❷ **Brothers Loving Brothers Safely**

Gay Men's Health Crisis, Inc.
1 page; photographs; $.30; special rates / discounts; 1988; English.

This brochure teaches gay men about safer sex. It provides a frank, detailed description of safer sex behaviors and risk behaviors. It also details why particular behaviors are safer or risky. The brochure encourages readers to protect themselves from HIV transmission because, "Safe sex is better sex!" The GMHC hotline number is included.

▲ For Ordering Information, see p. 219

❶ **Disease Does Not Discriminate - You Don't Have To Be White Or Gay To Get AIDS**

Good Samaritan Project
3 panels; illustrations; free; Jun 1987; English.

▲ For Ordering Information, see p. 220

❷ **If I Had Known**

African Americans Taking Action Against AIDS Council c/o American Red Cross Hawkeye Chapter
3 panels; 1988; special rates / discounts; English.

This pamphlet was developed to provide AIDS/HIV information to black church communities and families. It includes information on AIDS/HIV and expresses the need for community awareness and concern as well as compassion for people with AIDS/HIV. Transmission and prevention tips on the virus are provided.

▲ For Ordering Information, see p. 213

○ **People Of Color - AIDS Is Preventable - Contracting AIDS Is A Matter Of Choice**

Black Community AIDS Program

❶ **Seven Out Of Ten Women With AIDS Are Women Of Color**

Maryland Department of Health and Mental Hygiene AIDS Administration
3 panels; photographs; free; 1987; English.

▲ For Ordering Information, see p. 222

❷ **Understanding AIDS**

Inglewood Physicians Association
1 page; free; 1988; English.

This leaflet provides a definition of AIDS, information on transmission and infection, basic AIDS/HIV vocabulary, and suggestions for what to do if you are HIV antibody positive. Common concerns such as casual contact transmission and the difference between being infected with HIV and having AIDS are addressed. Phone numbers for more information are listed for the 213 area code only.

▲ For Ordering Information, see p. 221

❶ 1ST EDITION RECOMMENDED   ❷ 2ND EDITION RECOMMENDED   ○ NOT RECOMMENDED

❶ You Don't Have To Be White Or Gay To Get AIDS

Bebashi, Inc.
   3 panels; illustrations; English.

▲ For Ordering Information, see p. 215

❶ You Don't Have To Be White Or Gay To Get AIDS

Health Education Resource Organization (HERO)
   3 panels; photographs; $.30; 1987; English.

▲ For Ordering Information, see p. 220

PAMPHLETS

○ Black People Do Get AIDS, But Not By...

Minority AIDS Project

○ A Message From The Ambassador Of Health

Minority AIDS Project

○ People Of Color - Because We Care - Let's Talk

Minority AIDS Project

❶ Respect Yourself

Los Angeles County Dept. of Health Services AIDS Program Office
   32 pages; illustrations & photographs; 1987; $.25; special rates / discounts; English.

This comic-book, using photographs rather than cartoons, warns sexually active young black men and women that practicing unprotected sex is dangerous. Through the "rappin" of "Master Blaster," the pamphlet educates teenagers about the facts of AIDS/HIV and urges them to respect themselves and practice safe sex.

Reviewers' Comments: The pamphlet gets down to the language and feelings of teenagers. It makes good use of photos and captions. Although targeted for inner city adolescents, it does not discuss drugs and alcohol.

▲ For Ordering Information, see p. 222

POSTERS

❷ AIDS Can Tear You Apart

Blacks Against AIDS
   11 x 17; illustrations; black & white; 1988; free; English.

This poster shows a high contrast collage of black faces that has been torn through the middle. Between the halves are the words, "AIDS can tear YOU apart." The address and phone number of Blacks Against AIDS are included.

Reviewers' Comments: This is a basic poster for an AIDS service organization. The graphics are not effective.

▲ For Ordering Information, see p. 215

○ AIDS Does Not Discriminate

Brooklyn AIDS Task Force

❶ AIDS Is An Equal Opportunity Disease / SIDA Es Una Enfermedad Que Ataca A Toda La Gente

Minority AIDS Project
   1988; $1.50; English/Spanish.

This poster calls attention to the fact that AIDS/HIV strikes men, women, and infants of the black community. It highlights transmission modes and summarizes risk reduction methods, including safer sex and not sharing needles. It gives both English and Spanish hotline numbers.

Reviewers' Comments: This poster succeeds in making the point that AIDS can affect anyone.

▲ For Ordering Information, see p. 223

❶ AIDS Is Color Blind

Massachusetts Department of Public Health
   11 1/2 x 15; illustrations; color; Jan 1988; free, limited copies; English.

This white and red on black poster lists general risk reduction information and offers an AIDS hotline number for English and Spanish speaking people and an alcohol and drug hotline number. The entire caption reads: "AIDS is color blind. AIDS doesn't care what color you are...it just kills!"

Reviewers' Comments: The poster's caption attracts the viewer's attention.

▲ For Ordering Information, see p. 222

❶ AIDS Is Killing Blacks, Too

Minority AIDS Project
11 x 17; color; 1988; $1.50; English.

This tri-color-print poster informs blacks that AIDS/HIV crosses sexual, racial, and socio-economic lines. Using direct language, it specifies ways to avoid AIDS/HIV.

Reviewers' Comments: This poster gets right to the point; its strong language conveys the message.

▲ For Ordering Information, see p. 223

❶ Always The Last To Know And What You Don't Know Can Kill You / Siempre El Ultimo En Saber Y Lo Que No Sabe Lo Puede Matar

Minority AIDS Project
11 x 17; color; 1988; $1.50; English/Spanish.

This black-and-red-on-white poster encourages AIDS/HIV education in the black community. It carries line art illustrations of two young black children. It lists statistics that show how blacks and other minorities make up a significant number of AIDS/HIV cases. It includes three hotline numbers.

Reviewers' Comments: Although not a compelling piece, the poster conveys the message effectively to a multi-cultural audience.

▲ For Ordering Information, see p. 223

❷ Every Two Hours A Black American Dies Of AIDS

D.C. Commission of Public Health
28 x 11; illustrations; black & white; 1987; special rates / discounts; English.

This poster urges black Americans to get the facts about AIDS/HIV, and offers a local phone number. Beneath a drawing of black citizens of various ages and background, the headline states that every two hours a black American dies of AIDS.

Reviewers' Comments: This poster reflects the diversity of the black community and is educational as well as attractive.

▲ For Ordering Information, see p. 218

○ He Can Only Strike You Out If You Let Him

New York City Department of Health AIDS Education Training Unit

❷ Love Is For Everyone, Including People With AIDS

Minority AIDS Project
11 x 17; photographs; color; 1988; $1.50; English.

This poster contains a photograph of a minister and two young men and asks, "Is your church doing its part?" The Minority AIDS Project phone number is listed as a source of information about church support for AIDS in the black community.

Reviewers' Comments: This poster has appeal for both the black community and the church, and it is easily duplicated. It contains space for inserting a local AIDS/HIV information number. Some may be concerned that the poster shows men only.

▲ For Ordering Information, see p. 223

❷ Please Put It On Before You Get It On

Teschuba
14 x 20; illustrations; color; 1988; $3.00; English.

Illustrations of the biological symbols for female and male are at the center of this poster. The poster advocates transmission prevention through safer sex practices, specifically condom use; the arrow protruding from the male circle is sheathed. The organization's local phone number is provided for more information.

Reviewers' Comments: This gives a good basic message about condom use for heterosexual sex. The message is clear, but may be confusing to anyone who is unfamiliar with the biological symbols for male and female.

▲ For Ordering Information, see p. 229

❶ 1ST EDITION RECOMMENDED   ❷ 2ND EDITION RECOMMENDED   ○ NOT RECOMMENDED

❷ Time

Teschuba
14 x 20; illustrations; black & white; 1988; $3.00; English.

This poster declares that time "can be an ally or an enemy" and urges viewers to take the time to use condoms during sex and to sterilize needles used for injecting drugs. An illustration of a clock separates two sections of text. The organization's local phone number is provided for more information.

Reviewers' Comments: This is a basic informational poster which can be used in other communities and in various settings (schools, buses, offices).

▲ For Ordering Information, see p. 229

❷ We Are Not Afraid Of Uncle George

Minority AIDS Project
11 x 17; photographs; color; 1988; $1.50; English.

This poster shows a picture of a black man with AIDS/HIV who embraces two young girls sitting on either side of him. The caption is the girls' exclamation: "We're not afraid of Uncle George. He has AIDS. We love him." The poster encourages understanding of people with AIDS and HIV infection. The Minority AIDS Project phone number is listed.

Reviewers' Comments: This is a good poster which "puts a black face" on the AIDS/HIV epidemic. It speaks to the importance of compassion and models youth/family involvement. It is also easily duplicated.

▲ For Ordering Information, see p. 223

❶ We Didn't Think We Could Get AIDS!

Health Education Resource Organization (HERO)
28 x 11; photographs; color; 1987; $1.50; English.

This poster shows a photograph of a young black couple. The banner text states, "We didn't think we could get AIDS!" The remaining text suggests that 50 percent of all individuals diagnosed with AIDS/HIV are black, and the best defense against AIDS/HIV is information. The size and shape makes the poster suitable for display on public transportation vehicles.

Reviewers' Comments: The poster is most suitable for use in Maryland.

▲ For Ordering Information, see p. 220

PUBLIC SERVICE ADS (TV, RADIO, PRINT)

❷ If You Cheat On Your Partner You Could Wind Up With More Than Just A Broken Heart

CDC National AIDS Information and Education Program
Multimedia; Oct 1988; free; English.

In this America Responds To AIDS print ad, the reader is encouraged to remain monogamous as a means of preventing transmission of HIV. The ad provides the number for the National AIDS Hotline and is available in a variety of sizes. Government agencies and AIDS organizations are free to localize it according to need.

Reviewers' Comments: This ad piques the reader's interest. However, the headline is long and the information it contains is inaccurate. Monogamy is not safer sex, and for people with previous sexual experience, it is not an effective way of preventing transmission.

▲ For Ordering Information, see p. 216

VIDEOS / FILMS

❷ Another View: AIDS In The Minority Community

New Jersey Network
20:30 min.; VHS; Jan 1988; $75.00; rental fee: $50.00/2 weeks; special rates / discounts; English.

In this edition of the program "Another View," the AIDS/HIV problem in New Jersey is discussed. The first segment includes interviews with people with AIDS, physicians, the chairman of Newark's Advisory Committee on AIDS, and an AIDS coordinator at a drug clinic. It offers reports on how the disease is transmitted and how to avoid infection. The second segment presents a taped studio discussion with a panel of three health professionals.

Reviewers' Comments: This video is appropriate for black communities around the country. It provides good basic AIDS/HIV information and shows an appropriate representation of blacks across socio-economic levels. It addresses the problem of IV drug use in the black community; however, it suffers by not showing "mainstream" blacks who practice risky behaviors.

▲ For Ordering Information, see p. 225

❶ Black People Get AIDS, Too

Multicultural Prevention Resource Center (MPRC)
22:30 min.; 1987; $350.00; English.

This videotape emphasizes the AIDS/HIV epidemic among blacks. It presents facts orally, illustrates them in vignettes, and enumerates them in a chart format. Subjects covered include high-risk behaviors, HIV antibody testing, symptoms, protective methods, and the need for education in schools, drug treatment centers, and churches. It recommends the use of condoms and spermicides, provides instuctions on cleaning needles, and discusses the need for confidentiality in antibody testing.

Reviewers' Comments: This motivational and upbeat video provides a good AIDS/HIV-awareness overview. It is suitable for well-educated members of the Black community, especially for policy makers. It devotes too much time to the scientific aspects of AIDS and frequently uses one-on-one interview segments. Some of the statistical information presented needs to be updated.

▲ For Ordering Information, see p. 223

◯ Respect Yourself

Los Angeles County Dept. of Health Services AIDS Program Office

❶ 'Til Death Do Us Part

Durrin Films / New Day Films
16 min.; 1988; $355.00; English.

This video captures a 20-minute play produced by the Everyday Theatre Youth Ensemble in Washington, D.C. It presents basic facts about AIDS/HIV, women-at-risk, and IV drug use. It stresses the importance of taking responsibility for one's actions. The film delivers these messages primarily to adolescent black youth through music, poetry, rap, and dance. The video comes with a discussion guide.

Reviewers' Comments: This video is dramatic and vivid and would serve as a powerful consciousness-raising program, especially for black youth. However, it uses fear as a motivational device, and does not provide specific AIDS/HIV prevention information. A discussion of basic AIDS/HIV facts should follow the viewing of this video.

▲ For Ordering Information, see p. 218

❶ 1ST EDITION RECOMMENDED   ❷ 2ND EDITION RECOMMENDED   ◯ NOT RECOMMENDED

BLOOD AND TISSUE RECIPIENTS

BROCHURES

○ **Fact Sheet No. 10 - The Blood Supply And AIDS**

Gay Community AIDS Project

○ **Patients Who Need Transfusions May Have Questions About AIDS And The Blood Supply. Here Are Some Answers.**

American Association of Blood Banks National Office

❷ **The Safety Of Giving And Receiving Blood**

American Red Cross National Headquarters
3 panels; free; 1989; English.

Attempting to mitigate fears regarding donating and receiving blood, this brochure describes basic facts about HIV transmission and blood screening. The focus is that it is impossible to become HIV infected by donating blood, and that the chances of becoming infected by receiving blood have been greatly reduced.

▲ For Ordering Information, see p. 215

❶ **When You Need A Transfusion You May Have Questions About AIDS And The Blood Supply. Here Are Some Answers.**

American Association of Blood Banks National Office
2 panels; illustrations; special rates / discounts; Jan 1986; English.

▲ For Ordering Information, see p. 214

PAMPHLETS

❶ **Jeffrey Wants To Know**

Florida Association of Pediatric Tumor Programs, Inc.
illustrations; 1987; $1.75; English.

This coloring book provides opportunities for hemophiliac children and their parents to discuss their concerns, questions, and fears about AIDS/HIV. It broaches the issue of safety of blood products and casual contact, the AIDS antibody test, and specific precautions for children with hemophilia.

Reviewers' Comments: The coloring book concept is an excellent device for stimulating communication about AIDS/HIV. In the case of children with chronic illnesses such as hemophilia, the roles of parent and physician are often times just the reverse of how they are presented in this booklet.

▲ For Ordering Information, see p. 219

VIDEOS / FILMS

❶ **Blood Banks In The Age Of AIDS**

American Association of Blood Banks National Office
9:39 min.; VHS 3/4; Feb 1986; $99.00; rental fee: $25.00/day; English.

This documentary-style video presents information for potential blood donors. It discusses "risk groups" for AIDS and why they should not donate blood. It describes the testing of blood for HIV and other agents and emphasizes the safety of the blood supply as well as the safely of donating blood. It stresses the critical need for life-saving blood. There is no discussion guide available.

Reviewers' Comments: This video is a good promotional piece for blood donors.

▲ For Ordering Information, see p. 214

❶ Blood Transfusion Risks And Benefits

American Association of Blood Banks National Office
9 min.; VHS 3/4; Dec 1987; $119.00; rental fee: $25.00/day; English.

Scenes of patients, blood donor centers, testing laboratories, and operating rooms illustrate this documentary as narrators discuss the risks and benefits of blood transfusions. The narrators explain basic facts about AIDS, particularly in relation to necessary blood transfusions. They outline the ways to reduce the risks of contracting AIDS or other diseases from blood products. The video explains the use of autologous transfusions for elective procedures and ends with a plea for healthy donors. There is no discussion guide for this video.

Reviewers' Comments: The content, technical production, and instructional design of this videotape are excellent.

▲ For Ordering Information, see p. 214

❶ 1ST EDITION RECOMMENDED   ❷ 2ND EDITION RECOMMENDED   ○ NOT RECOMMENDED

CHILDREN AND ADOLESCENTS

BOOKS / MANUALS

❷ AIDS: Trading Facts For Fears

Consumer Reports Books
206 pages; paperback; photographs; 1989; $3.50; special rates / discounts; English.

This book is designed to answer questions about AIDS/HIV and encourage young adults to consider the issues. Topics include facts about AIDS, drugs, testing, after the test, treatment and support, and the future. Appendices with glossary and other resources are included.

Reviewers' Comments: This book contains factual material of excellent quality. The reading level is high, which makes this more appropriate for young adults than for children. The question and answer format is successful, and the positive approach to sexuality is refreshing. This is a good resource for high school libraries and college dormitories.

▲ For Ordering Information, see p. 218

❶ Andrea And Lisa

Health Education Resource Organization (HERO)
10 pages; stapled; illustrations; 1987; $.50, limited copies; English.

This comic book using a fairy-tale format, discusses AIDS/HIV and safer sex practices, specifically for sexually active teenager girls. It deals with transmission and lists local information resources.

Reviewers' Comments: This clever comic book provides direct, basic information about AIDS/HIV specifically to sexually active teenage women. It does not adequately warn the audience that condoms are not one-hundred-percent safe.

▲ For Ordering Information, see p. 220

◯ Learning About AIDS

Enslow Publishers

❶ Space Age Smarts

Florida Association of Pediatric Tumor Programs, Inc.
13 pages; illustrations; 1987; $1.95; English.

This comic book encourages common sense precautions for the prevention of the spread of AIDS/HIV. The teenagers, including one hemophiliac, discuss transmission, safer sex, the danger of IV drugs and the importance of hemophiliacs cleaning up their blood spills and disposing of needles. The comic book mentions condom use.

Reviewers' Comments: This engaging comic book is an original and effective way of treating hemophilia by discussing other teenager's concerns. It was great to see the hemophiliac shown leading a normal life with his friends.

▲ For Ordering Information, see p. 219

BROCHURES

❷ Advice From Teens On Buying Condoms

Center for Population Options
3 panels; special rates / discounts; 1988; English.

This brochure encourages sexually active teens and adults to buy condoms. Comic characters illustrate steps along a path to being smart and prepared. It suggests to readers that they are not alone, describes the kinds of stores where condoms can be bought, where to look for them in the store, and discusses the embarassment readers may feel when asking for condoms. On the back, specific advice on using a condom is provided.

▲ For Ordering Information, see p. 217

❶ AIDS: "Could I Get It?"

Dimension Communications Network (DCN)/RAMSCO Publishing Co.
3 panels; illustrations; $.20; special rates / discounts; 1986; English.

▲ For Ordering Information, see p. 218

❷ **AIDS: Facts For Teens**

Illinois Department of Public Health AIDS Facts for Life
2 panels; illustrations; free, limited copies; 1988; English.

The cover of this brochure displays a drawing of a student's locker on which "AIDS" is spray-painted in red. Interior copy describes what AIDS/HIV is, how it is transmitted, and those activites that do and don't present a risk. Condom use is advocated, and an Illinois AIDS hotline number is given.

▲ For Ordering Information, see p. 221

○ **AIDS: For Student Information**

Anne Arundel County Public Schools

○ **AIDS - Good News**

Good Samaritan Project

❷ **AIDS: It's No Joke**

Massachusetts Department of Public Health
3 panels; photographs; free, limited copies; 1988; English/Spanish.

This brochure uses simple language and photographs of black, white, Hispanic, and Asian teenagers to communicate its message. It explains how AIDS/HIV is and is not contracted and outlines prevention methods. Other important facts concerning symptoms and issues of pregnancy and AIDS/HIV are mentioned. A variety of Massachusetts phone numbers for more information is listed.

▲ For Ordering Information, see p. 222

❷ **AIDS Terminology Scramble**

D.C. Public Schools AIDS Education Office
1 page; free; 1988; English.

The top half of this leaflet contains a square composed of letters of the alphabet beneath which is a list of AIDS/HIV-related words. To solve the puzzle, directions are to find the words in the scramble. Sample words are "abstinence, rubber, AZT, and ELISA." The words in the scramble are not defined in this leaflet.

▲ For Ordering Information, see p. 218

○ **AIDS - What Every Student Should Know**

New Mexico AIDS Services, Inc.

❶ **The Best Way To "Score"! (Or How To Use A Rubber)**

Neon Street Center for Youth
4 panels; illustrations; Dec 1987; English.

▲ For Ordering Information, see p. 224

❶ **Break Away From AIDS**

Los Angeles County Dept. of Health Services AIDS Program Office
3 panels; illustrations; free; 1986; English.

▲ For Ordering Information, see p. 222

○ **Don't Let AIDS Catch You!**

American Institute for Teen AIDS Prevention, Inc.

❷ **Fact Sheet No.8 - Children And AIDS**

Gay Community AIDS Project
3 panels; $.10; 1988; English.

This brochure addresses parents' concerns regarding AIDS/HIV by explaining how the disease is and is not transmitted. It answers questions about the possibility of a child's exposure to HIV in settings such as school and playground. The reading level for this brochure is high.

▲ For Ordering Information, see p. 219

❶ **The Facts - AIDS And Adolescents**

Center for Population Options
1 page; $.17; Dec 1987; English.

▲ For Ordering Information, see p. 217

---

❶ 1ST EDITION RECOMMENDED   ❷ 2ND EDITION RECOMMENDED   ○ NOT RECOMMENDED

② **For Teens**

American Social Health Association
2 panels; 1988; cost not specified; English.

This brochure folds out into a small poster that addresses major topics on sexually transmitted diseases, with a special section on AIDS/HIV. It describes STD's generally, their symptoms, and how a person can reduce risk.

▲ For Ordering Information, see p. 215

② **HIV - Important News**

Special Immunology Service, Children's Hospital
2 panels; illustrations; free, limited copies; 1988; English.

This brief brochure for children conveys the message that, while people can die from AIDS/HIV, there is good news: the HIV virus is hard to catch--harder than a cold, flu, or chicken pox. It tells children that they can not catch the virus by playing with or hugging friends; using a drinking fountain or toilet seat; or from sharing pencil and paper, swimming pool, or sports equipment.

▲ For Ordering Information, see p. 228

① **Here's What Teenagers Are Saying About Condoms**

Planned Parenthood Alameda/San Francisco
4 panels; special rates / discounts; 1988; English.

▲ For Ordering Information, see p. 226

① **If You Know About AIDS You Don't Have To Panic - Get The Facts ... Not AIDS**

New York City Department of Health AIDS Education Training Unit
3 panels; illustrations; free, limited copies; Jan 1987; English.

▲ For Ordering Information, see p. 225

② **Teenagers And AIDS**

American Red Cross National Headquarters
7 panels; free; 1989; English.

This brochure contains information on safety at school, covering topics such as casual contact, bloody noses and blood on sports equipment, mosquitos, and kissing. It also gives information on sexual transmission of HIV and basic guidelines for protecting against transmission.

▲ For Ordering Information, see p. 215

② **Teens And AIDS**

NO/AIDS Task Force
3 panels; $.10; special rates / discounts; 1988; English.

This brochure answers basic questions about AIDS/HIV. It details transmission risks and the non-risks of casual contact. Readers are encouraged to avoid sex and drugs or to make those practices safer according to the guidelines provided. Readers are also encouraged to talk about AIDS/HIV with people they can trust. Local and statewide hotline numbers are provided.

▲ For Ordering Information, see p. 225

① **Teens And AIDS - Basic Information About Acquired Immunodeficiency Syndrome For Teens, Parents, And School Personnel**

Mississippi State Department of Health
4 panels; illustrations; Oct 1987; English.

▲ For Ordering Information, see p. 223

◯ **Teens And AIDS - For 15 To 19 Year Olds And Their Parents And Teachers**

Gay and Lesbian Community Center of Orange County AIDS Response Program

① **Teens And AIDS! - Why Risk It?**

ETR Associates/Network Publications
2 panels; illustrations; special rates / discounts; 1987; English.

▲ For Ordering Information, see p. 219

❷ **This Pamphlet Will Not Give You AIDS**

Illinois Alcoholism and Drug Dependence Association
2 panels; illustrations; special rates / discounts; 1988; English.

The cover of this brochure announces that "This pamphlet will not give you AIDS," while the content lists ways in which HIV is transmitted and statistics on infection in Illinois. Ways you can damage your immune system are also listed. Readers are encouraged to "say no" to drugs and unsafe sex and to help others by telling them that shooting drugs or having unsafe sex even once can transmit the virus. While the brochure contains information specific to Illinois; camera-ready art is available for agencies in other states who wish to reprint the materials.

▲ For Ordering Information, see p. 221

○ **What You Think You Know About AIDS...Could Be Dead Wrong!**

AIDS Prevention Project Dallas County Health Department

❷ **When A Young Friend Has The HIV Infection**

Special Immunology Service, Children's Hospital
3 panels; illustrations; free, limited copies; 1988; English.

This large-print brochure conveys to children the message that they will not catch AIDS/HIV by hugging or sitting next to a friend who has AIDS/HIV, and that the virus isn't spread by sneezing or drinking from the same water fountain. However, children are told that it's important not to touch their friend's blood and to wash their hands right away if they touch a cut. Children are encouraged to ask their parents if they have more questions.

▲ For Ordering Information, see p. 228

○ **You Can't Be Too Careful: Facts For Teens About AIDS**

Illinois State Medical Society

INSTRUCTIONAL PROGRAMS

○ **AIDS**

Carolina Biological Supply Company

❶ **AIDS: A Resource Guide - Upper Elementary/Middle School Junior High/Senior High AIDS Curriculum**

Nebraska Department of Education
3 volumes; illustrations; 1987; free, limited copies; English.

The package includes three curricula for AIDS/HIV education. The upper elementary curriculum discusses AIDS/HIV in the context of sexually transmitted diseases and covers transmission, symptoms, community resources, and common misconceptions. In addition to covering these subjects in more depth, the middle school-junior high curriculum discusses the HIV virus in relation to the human immune system and AIDS/HIV prevention. The material lists concepts, student objectives, activities, and resources. Appendices include information on communicable disease transmission, sexually transmitted diseases, AIDS/HIV transmission, symptoms, methods of prevention, a pronunciation glossary, and other resources. Much of the senior high curriculum is identical to "AIDS: What Young Adults Should Know - Instructor's Guide," published in 1987 by American Alliance for Health, Physical Education, Recreation and Dance. It includes educational objectives, lesson plans, descriptive outlines of learning opportunities, test questions, student worksheets, and handouts.

Reviewers' Comments: These curricula contain a wealth of information; however, they are somewhat out of sequence. They cover some unnecessary topics and fail to emphasize all of the important issues. The curricula are not appropriate to grade levels in every instance and require training for use.

▲ For Ordering Information, see p. 224

○ **AIDS & Young People**

Regnery Gateway, Inc.

❶ 1ST EDITION RECOMMENDED　❷ 2ND EDITION RECOMMENDED　○ NOT RECOMMENDED

❷ AIDS And Your World

Scholastic, Inc.
64 pages; paperback; charts, illustrations, photographs & graphs; 1988; $5.95; special rates / discounts; English.

This classroom text teaches students an understanding of AIDS/HIV as a pandemic, touching on social issues as well as basic information. The first of five chapters explains the syndrome and introduces students to some individuals who have it. The second chapter explains AIDS/HIV in a context of historical struggle against disease. Questions that AIDS/HIV raises about individual rights are explored in the next chapter. The fourth chapter encourages a sense of responsibility in students, to protect themselves from infection and to be understanding of those who have AIDS or HIV infection. The final chapter explains what the future holds regarding prevalence, treatments, and the possibility of a vaccine. The book contains skill activities in each chapter and a glossary of important concepts.

Reviewers' Comments: This is an excellent piece for the student population. It is nicely organized with review and discussion sections and adequate illustrations that break up the printed page and accent important points. Perhaps most important, this can be easily integrated by most teachers without a lot of training or rearrangement of curriculum time. The reading level is higher than average and should be evaluated for appropriateness by each teacher prior to use.

▲ For Ordering Information, see p. 228

❶ AIDS Curriculum - Grades 6-12

Eugene Public Schools School District 4J
45 pages; looseleaf; 1986; English.

This curriculum contains a middle school program (three 40-minute sessions) and a high school program (four 50-minute sessions) for use with units on sexually transmitted diseases. Upon completion, the students should be able to define AIDS, ARC, and HIV, explain the transmission of HIV, discuss methods to lower the risk of AIDS/HIV infection, identify false perceptions about the transmission of HIV, and discuss appropriate (for grade level) social and medical implications associated with AIDS/HIV. This curriculum provides lesson plans, listing objectives, content, time, activities, and resources for each day. It includes student handouts, homework assignments, lists of resources for further information on AIDS/HIV, and a glossary. One of the teacher resources provides information on preventive behaviors and discusses abstinence, monagamy, use of condoms, and the dangers of drug use, including sharing needles. The package also contains current guidelines regarding students with AIDS, HIV, and hepatitis B.

Reviewers' Comments: This curriculum is well organized and suitable for use in other school systems. It is easy for non-health educators to use, but should be part of a comprehensive school health program. A few minor inac-

curacies include the confusion of risk groups and behaviors, describing communicable diseases as being spread by the environment while listing AIDS as a communicable disease, and not specifying "latex" condoms.

▲ For Ordering Information, see p. 219

◯ AIDS Facts Curriculum - Magazine And Instructor's Guide

Classroom Connections, Inc.

◯ AIDS - Family Life, Grade 8 / SIDA - Vida Familiar, Grado 8

Sweetwater Union High School District

◯ AIDS - Family Life, Grade 10 / SIDA - Vida Familiar, Grado 10

Sweetwater Union High School District

❷ AIDS: The Preventable Epidemic

Oregon Health Division, HIV Program
216 pages; looseleaf; 1988; $25.00; English.

This manual is designed to help teachers, administrators and parents as they plan to organize and present appropriate AIDS/HIV-related materials in the classroom. It is divided into three grade level units: four through five, six thorough eight, and nine through twelve. The introduction states that a fourth unit for kindergarten through third grade will be available soon. Five or six lesson plans and copy-ready pages of activities and transparencies are included for each unit. A list of other resources is also provided. This curriculum has been reviewed in curriculum workshops and changes have been incorporated.

Reviewers' Comments: This is one of the best curriculum we've seen in content and design. The three-ring binder format is excellent and easily updated. The material is well-written and "user friendly." It includes good teacher education and preparation materials, along with an evaluation component that is well done. It is age-appropriate and has a good scope and sequence. This curriculum can be easily incorporated into a communicable disease unit of a comprehensive health program.

◯ AIDS - The Preventable Epidemic - A Teacher's Guide

State of New Mexico AIDS Prevention Program Health & Environment Department

❷ AIDS Prevention: Knowledge, Attitude, Behavior

Ohio Department of Health - AIDS Unit
92; stapled; Aug 1988; free, limited copies; English.

This curriculum is designed for teachers in middle, junior high, and senior high schools. It offers lessons and suggests student activities for topics such as characteristics of HIV, its transmission, high-risk behaviors, methods of prevention, and its social implications.

Reviewers' Comments: While this piece is disorganized and contains some outdated material, it has some activities that might be helpful in terms of attitudes and skills development. There is not enough information provided to teachers for discussions of sensitive topics, such as homosexuality and negotiating sexual activity, but a variety of exercises are offered that instructors could adapt to their classrooms.

▲ For Ordering Information, see p. 225

◯ AIDS: Suddenly Sex Has Become Very Dangerous

Goodday Video, Inc.

❶ AIDS Update

Globe Book Company, Inc.
43 pages; illustrations & photographs; 1988; $3.79; English.

This high school instructional program consists of five lessons about AIDS/HIV: The Facts; the Immune System and HIV; Interpersonal Relationships; Dealing with AIDS in the Community; and AIDS/HIV and the Future. It emphasizes written responses throughout each chapter's text, as well as in a chapter review. Not all of the activities relate directly to AIDS/HIV, but they give students opportunities for exploring personal values and testing their decision making skills. The book contains a pre-test and a glossary.

Reviewers' Comments: The overall structure of the student workbook is good and the chapter summaries are very useful. It does not, however, sufficiently cover AIDS prevention practices. It stresses abstinence and monogomy.

▲ For Ordering Information, see p. 220

❶ AIDS: What You And Your Friends Need To Know

Seattle-King County Department of Public Health
29 pages; looseleaf; illustrations; 1987; $15.00; English.

This package consists of a lesson plan for a high school unit on AIDS/HIV, slides, and a brochure. The lesson plan includes suggestions for one- and two- hour sessions for grades 9-10 and grades 11-12, and recommends videotapes that are appropriate for use in high school classrooms. The slides, with a companion script, illustrate the epidemiology of AIDS/HIV, transmission and reproduction of the virus, opportunistic diseases, "risk groups" and prevention. Other scripts in the plan include an attitude search, an acronym summary, answers to commonly asked questions about AIDS/HIV, and an evaluation survey. Five transparency masters illustrate statistics on the incidence of AIDS/HIV. The brochure gives a few of the basic facts on AIDS/HIV.

Reviewers' Comments: This multimodal program is a concise presentation of major AIDS/HIV epidemiological and scientific issues and it includes a good evaluation package. However, the coverage of risk reduction/safer sex practices is inadequate in detail.

▲ For Ordering Information, see p. 228

❶ AIDS: What Young Adults Should Know

American Alliance for Health, Physical Education, Recreation, Dance
20 pages; illustrations; 1988; student guide $2.50, instructor's guide $8.95; special rates / discounts; English.

This Curriculum includes guides for students and teachers and is designed for three class sessions in grades 7-12. The guides present information on the cause of AIDS/HIV, sexual transmission of the virus, the HIV antibody test, and symptoms of ARC and AIDS. The curriculum dispels behaviors misconceptions about the disease and identifies high risk behaviors. Strategies for prevention focus on those related to sexual behavior, such as condom use and avoidance of IV drug abuse. The Student Guide includes a summary of the information, a glossary, self-tests, and a list of information sources. It also discusses what individuals can do to promote AIDS/HIV prevention efforts and to support people with AIDS/HIV. In addition to information on these subjects the Instructor's Guide includes educational objectives, lesson plans, descriptive outlines, learning opportunities, test questions, student worksheets, handouts, and answers to common AIDS questions asked by young adults.

Reviewers' Comments: These guides present vital information in an accessible, concise format. They provide opportunities for values clarification and, if the exercises in the Instructor's Guide are repeated over time, a useful means of monitoring attitude and behavior trends. Used alone, the Student Guide is probably not very effective

---

❶ 1ST EDITION RECOMMENDED   ❷ 2ND EDITION RECOMMENDED   ◯ NOT RECOMMENDED

beyond giving factual information. Major weaknesses include no discussion of sexual decision-making or communication issues and the use of the term "risk groups."

▲ For Ordering Information, see p. 214

❷ Aunt Rita's Patient: A Story About AIDS

American Red Cross St. Paul Area Chapter
93 pages; stapled; illustrations; 1988; special rates / discounts; English.

This program provides children in grades four through six with the information they need to respond to the AIDS/HIV epidemic safely. The program consists of a student workbook and a teacher's guide. The workbook follows a storyline about two children learning about AIDS/HIV and includes exercises and activities which help students understand AIDS/HIV vocabulary, the immune system, how the virus is and is not transmitted, and other basic concepts. The teacher's guide explains how to use the program in a group process and includes additional activities, assignments, and background information useful in answering student questions.

Reviewers' Comments: This should be used as a supplement to a comprehensive school health curriculum. The objectives are attainable but not measurable. It offers no information on the time needed for implementation.

▲ For Ordering Information, see p.

❶ Curriculum Recommendations On Acquired Immune Deficiency Syndrome For Michigan Students - Grades 7-8, 9-10, 11-12

Michigan Department of Education
200 pages; looseleaf; graphs; 1988; free, limited copies; English.

This three-volume, comprehensive curriculum on AIDS, for students in grades 7-8, 9-10, 11-12, respectively, was developed jointly by the Michigan departments of Education and Public Health. Each volume includes a set of lesson objectives, detailed lesson plans, teacher and student resources, bibliographies for students and teachers, a glossary, student worksheets, and transparencies.

Reviewers' Comments: This curriculum includes good student activities and exercises which are grade-level appropriate, combined with accurate, well-organized content, presented simply and clearly. The approach to both information and behavioral issues is excellent and not heavily value-laden, taking students through logical thought processes and application. The emphasis on compassion and care for persons with AIDS/HIV is particularly noteworthy. Communication of AIDS/HIV information by and among peers also is stressed. This curriculum is readily transferrable to other school systems.

▲ For Ordering Information, see p. 223

❶ Educator's Guide To AIDS And Other STD's

Health Education Consultants
looseleaf; illustrations; 1989; $25.00; English.

This educator's guide presents AIDS in the context of other sexually transmitted and communicable diseases in general. It offers a suggested organization plan, fact sheets on several diseases including AIDS, activities for students, evaluation questionnaires, and a separate section containing only AIDS/HIV materials. In its discussion of the virus, the guide covers myths and facts about AIDS/HIV and risk behavior. It proposes abstinence from sex and drugs as the most effective prevention method but also emphasizes responsible sexual behavior. The student activities include an action plan for persons with sexually transmitted diseases, an exercise for practicing "saying no" skills, and a section on prevention strategies.

Reviewers' Comments: This is a thorough approach with numerous resources, but it does need teacher amplification.

▲ For Ordering Information, see p. 220

❶ Health - AIDS Instructional Guide - Grades K-12

The State Education Department Bureau of Curriculum Development
looseleaf; charts; Dec 1987; $3.50; English.

This curriculum provides a framework for AIDS/HIV instruction within a comprehensive program stressing positive health behavior. Chapter topics include integrated lesson development plans for different grade levels: K-3, 4-6, 7-8, and 9-12. Appendices cover condom information, adolescent pregnancy prevention projects, current AIDS/HIV information, and include a glossary.

Reviewers' Comments: This fine curriculum is flawed by unrealistically recommending abstinence as the only prevention option. Therefore it should be used with supplementary material on safer sex for sexually active teenagers.

▲ For Ordering Information, see p. 229

◯ Health Education Curriculum Supplement Acquired Immune Deficiency Syndrome

D.C. Public Schools AIDS Education Office

❷ Into Adolescence: Learning About AIDS

ETR Associates/Network Publications
232 pages; paperback; charts & illustrations; 1988; $19.95; special rates / discounts; English.

A 14 lesson module for grades five through eight focuses on giving students a solid understanding of disease transmission and prevention. Emphasizing that AIDS/HIV education remains part of a comprehensive health education program, this curriculum provides teachers with concrete behavioral objectives and specific stagies for an effective, age-appropriate AIDS/HIV education unit.

Reviewers' Comments: This program contains some scientific inaccuracies which need to be addressed. For example, gonorrhea is referred to as the number one sexually transmitted disease; epidemics are said to always be fatal; the factsheet on polio needs updating. Good public health information and debates are included. The teaching methods are excellent, and the objectives are very good. The reading level is high and should be adapted to continue targeting grades 5 through 8. The worksheets included are good. The program does not address sexual identity/orientation.

▲ For Ordering Information, see p. 219

❷ K-6 AIDS Education Supplement To Michigan Model For Comprehensive School Health Education

Michigan Department of Education
1989; English.

This instructional program contains guidance for teachers on addressing AIDS/HIV issues and questions raised by young students. While this program does not intend to address AIDS/HIV formally in kindergarten and first grade, it does suggest ways to handle questions when they arise. The lessons contained in the program are for grades 2 through 6, and they follow a logical progression of vocabulary building, activities, and story lines that are metaphors for immunology and HIV infection and thus convey physiological concepts of AIDS/HIV.

Reviewers' Comments: This instructional program is an excellent incorporation of AIDS/HIV education into comprehensive health education. Support materials are well integrated, and there is a good message of caring and compassion for persons with AIDS/HIV. Its format is complex and somewhat difficult to use. The program also assumes that teachers will have access to adequate and appropriate inservice preparation.

▲ For Ordering Information, see p. 223

❶ Learn & Live - A Teaching Guide On AIDS Prevention

Massachusetts Department of Public Health
17 pages; looseleaf; Aug 1987; English.

This AIDS prevention teaching guide, with eight lesson plans, written for adolescents in grades 9-12, may be adjusted for junior high school students. Specially designed to be integrated into existing curricula, it suggests presenting units on communicable diseases and human sexuality before teaching about the AIDS virus. The guide lists answers to the most commonly asked question about AIDS, its epidemiology, transmission, symptoms, ARC, incubation period, prevention, and HIV antibody testing. The guide includes handouts for students and four appendices: a resource listing, fact sheet, the Massachusetts school attendance policy, and the "U.S. Surgeon General's Report on AIDS." It provides information on specific modes of transmission and prevention including risky sexual practices and use of condoms.

Reviewers' Comments: This is an excellent teaching tool for use with students and is easily incorporated into existing curricula. The format is complex and may discourage some teachers from using it. This guide borrows heavily from another source, "Teaching AIDS," as noted in the acknowledgements.

▲ For Ordering Information, see p. 222

◯ Lesson Plan On AIDS

Boston Public Schools
The School Committee of the City of Boston

◯ New Pathways To Health Lessons For Teaching About AIDS And Other STD's - High School

Los Angeles Unified School District

❶ Special Topic Curriculum Resource Packet AIDS, Secondary Level

Connecticut Department of Education
47 pages; stapled; 1987; free; English.

This secondary level instructional guide provides lesson plans, quizzes, and masters for overhead transparencies. AIDS/HIV background information is provided along with video and print resources to be used in conjunction with the lessons. Among the subjects covered are: what AIDS/HIV is, how it is transmitted, information on HIV antibody tests, and transmission prevention. Open discussion with students is encouraged. A glossary of terms is included.

---

❶ 1ST EDITION RECOMMENDED   ❷ 2ND EDITION RECOMMENDED   ◯ NOT RECOMMENDED

Reviewers' Comments: This is a good guide overall, although it needs to be updated. Reformating it for use in a three ring binder would facilitate revision, updating, and use. It contains very good pre- and post tests. There is an inaccuracy in one of the transparencies. It states that the "AIDS virus is not spread through... objects." Needles are objects, and the message of the transparency should be clarified.

▲ For Ordering Information, see p. 217

❷ Special Topic Curriculum Resource Packet Primary And Elementary Levels

Connecticut Department of Education
29 pages; saddle stitched; 1988; free; English.

The primary and elementary school instructional guide is divided by age groups: pre-school through Kindergarten, grades 1-3, and grades 4-6. It provides teachers with discussion guides, developmental characteristics for each age group, and a section on parent/child communication. Subjects are modified for each group and include a description of AIDS/HIV, how the disease is transmitted, and preventive measures. Also included are an introductory section of background facts on the AIDS virus and appendicies with difficult questions that students may ask, sample parent information sheets, and a glossary of terms. Video and print resources are listed.

Reviewers' Comments: This is useful as a format from which to develop a curriculum, but the responsibility for doing so rests with the teacher. It lacks sample lesson plans and updated resource lists. It provides good information on test results and their meaning; however, the information on safer sex should be more specific. It includes helpful information on safe IV drug use. The concepts for each developmental level were appropriate.

▲ For Ordering Information, see p. 217

❶ STD - Sexually Transmitted Diseases - Teacher's Guide

Abbott Laboratories
16 pages; looseleaf; illustrations; 1987; $5.00; English.

This high school instructional program includes six lesson plans on sexually transmitted diseases including AIDS. It includes a special AIDS supplement which provides accurate information and corrects myths and misinformation. Topics include causes, symptoms, effects and treatment of specific diseases, understanding risks, seeking help, informing partners, and making decisions.

Reviewers' Comments: This instructional program contains a large amount of information for only six lessons. The graphics are excellent but the statistics need updating.

▲ For Ordering Information, see p. 213

◯ STD Teacher's Guide And AIDS Supplement

American Social Health Association

◯ Suggested Lesson Plan On AIDS-Supplement to Resource Unit For "Family Life Education, Grade 7"

Chicago Public Schools Bureau of Science

◯ Teaching About AIDS - A Teacher's Guide

R & E Research, Inc.

❶ Understanding AIDS

Lerner Publications Co.
64 pages; hardcover; illustrations; 1987; $9.95; special rates / discounts; English/Spanish.

This book, primarily intended for adolescents, explains facts about AIDS, its origin and transmission, homosexuality, blood transfusions, hemophilia, ARC, drug abuse, condom use, and current treatment options. Each of these topics is explored through a storyline to illustrate the feelings that revolve around this disease. A glossary is included.

Reviewers' Comments: This is a library book appropriate for young adolescents. There are a few statements presented as fact that are not well-founded, e.g., that sexual preference is inborn, that half of all IV drug users are HIV infected, and that one person in ten is gay. The doctors portrayed appear condescending to their patients. The Spanish version is excellent and enjoyable to read. It presents good factual and medical information. This version is somewhat explicit and is therefore more appropriate for young adolescents than for children.

▲ For Ordering Information, see p. 222

◯ Understanding AIDS (Computer Assisted)

Substance Abuse Education, Inc.

◯ What You Need To Know About AIDS

PSI Associates, Inc.

MULTICOMPONENT PROGRAM

❶ AIDS Prevention Program For Youth

- **Answers About AIDS**
  16 min.; VHS 3/4; Sep 1987; $19.95; English.

- **Don't Forget Sherrie**
  30 min.; VHS 3/4; 1988; $19.95; English.

- **A Letter From Brian**
  29:21 min.; VHS 3/4; Sep 1987; $19.95; English.

- **Information For Students (Student Workbook)**
  32 pages; paperback; 1988; special rates / discounts; English.

- **Information For Teachers / Leaders**
  64 pages; paperback; 1988; special rates / discounts; English.

- **What Every Parent Should Know About AIDS**
  64 pages; free; 1988; English.

American Red Cross National Headquarters

The American Red Cross AIDS Prevention Program for Youth is a multi-component family and school-based education program for junior and senior high school students. The program package includes a series of videos, a student workbook, a teacher's curriculum guide, and a pamphlet for parents.

"Answers about AIDS" features U.S. Surgeon General Koop in a classroom setting giving an overview of the AIDS epidemic and answering questions from students. He explains his views against quarantines and mandatory testing. He also discusses children with AIDS in schools, reliability of the antibody test, and transmission of the virus. Dr. Koop recommends abstinence as the only fully safe sexual behavior for teenagers and condom use for those that are sexually active. He emphasizes that the epidemic can be controlled only through education. An accompanying 12-page video discussion guide lists suggested questions and answers for group discussion before and after viewing the video, and a short glossary of terms.

The video "A Letter from Brian" provides information on reducing the risk of contracting AIDS/HIV. In a dramatic story, a teenager learns that an ex-boyfriend contracted the virus while using IV drugs. She and her friends discuss AIDS/HIV, peer pressure to use drugs and have sex, and whether to use condoms. An IV drug user also describes getting AIDS/HIV from sharing needles. The story ends with the teenager and her boyfriend deciding to postpone sex. The video is interspersed with factual narration by actor Michael Warren and Surgeon General Koop, a brochure by the same name accompanies the video. It describes the video, outlines the American Red Cross position on adolescent sexuality education, and provides basic information in question-and-answer format.

"Don't Forget Sherrie," provides urban youth with information on reducing the risk of AIDS/HIV. In a dramatic story, a teenage man learns that his ex-girlfriend contracted AIDS/HIV while using IV drugs. Several scenes deal with the dilemmas that he and his new girlfrined must resolve. The story ends with the young man deciding to be tested. The video is interspersed with factual narrative by actor Michael Warren and Surgeon General Koop.

The workbook "Information for Students" and the companion curriculum guide, "Information for Teachers/Leaders," refer specifically to the videotape, "A Letter from Brian," but also may be used more generally with other program materials. The workbook and curriculum guide are organized in a question and answer format, covering AIDS symptoms, risk factors and behaviors, transmission, testing, and prevention. The emphasis is on avoidance, saying no to sex and drugs, but condom use and high-risk sexual practices are also covered. The workbook and guide include self-tests and crossword puzzles. The teachers' guide also includes tips on relating the video to the workbook exercises and facilitating class discussions. A four-page glossary and sources of additional instruction materials are also included. The pamphlet, "What Every Parent Should Know about AIDS," provides basic information about AIDS.

Reviewers' Comments: Overall, this ambitious program is an important contribution to AIDS/HIV education for young people. In conjunction with the accompanying curriculum and workbooks, the videotapes are helpful vehicles for stimulating class discussions on sexual values and behaviors. "Answers about AIDS" provides clear, accurate, and frank answers to a variety of specific questions about transmission. It assumes, however, that the audience has a basic knowledge of AIDS/HIV. The lecture/discussion format may not hold the attention of high school students. "A Letter from Brian" effectively portrays, on the students' level, what they need to hear about AIDS and the possibility of infection. Primarily reflecting the white, middle class community, it is, nonetheless, culturally sensitive. "Don't Forget Sherrie" is particularly well suited for black and urban youth and is excellent in modelling and promoting communication in relationships. The importance of testing as a solution/resolution for AIDS/HIV, however, is somewhat overdrawn.

▲ For Ordering Information, see p. 215

---

❶ 1ST EDITION RECOMMENDED   ❷ 2ND EDITION RECOMMENDED   ○ NOT RECOMMENDS

❶ AIDS - What We Need to Know

- **AIDS - Answers For Parents**
  20 pages; 1988; special rates / discounts; English.

- **AIDS Level I - Instructional Program**
  327 pages; spiral; illustrations & graphs; 1988; $43.00; English.

- **AIDS Level II - Instuctional Program**
  425 pages; spiralbound; illustrations & graphs; 1988; $52.00; English.

- **AIDS Level I - Workbook For Students**
  69 pages; paperback; illustrations & graphs; Dec 1987; $8.00; English.

- **AIDS Level II - Workbook For Students**
  94 pages; paperback; illustrations & graphs; 1988; $9.00; English.

Pro - Ed Publishing

This two-level curriculum for junior and senior high school students consists of student workbooks, instructors' manuals, and a parents' booklet. The Level I Workbook for grades 7-9 includes four chapters: What is AIDS? How is AIDS spread? How do we protect ourselves and others from AIDS? What issues does AIDS raise? The chapters are concise and allow for class discussions, role plays, and written homework assignments. The workbook's last section includes review tests, worksheets, additional case studies, and a glossary.

The Level II Workbook for grades 10-12 is similar in format to Level I but is expanded for a more mature audience. A chapter on responsible behavior discusses safe and unsafe sex, IV drug use, AIDS/HIV and pregnancy, and long-term relationships. Instructors' manuals for Level I and II include comprehensive teaching plans, a more detailed analysis of AIDS/HIV, plus sections on the immune system, transmission of the virus, public policy and AIDS/HIV, financing the crisis, public and private precautions, and research. More than 50 black-line-master drawings, applicable as teaching transparencies or posters, are included along with a resource list and glossary.

The parents booklet provides basic information about AIDS/HIV, explains the curriculum's particular approach to AIDS/HIV education, and assists parents in guiding their child in learning about AIDS/HIV and in developing behavior. All components use some explicit anatomical terminology when discussing sexual behaviors and practices.

Reviewers' Comments: This excellent package is comprehensive and well-organized, with good graphics and resource materials. It covers basic information about AIDS and prevention, as well as other important issues such as confidentiality, social and economic costs of the disease, research, homophobia, drugs, and the role of religion and other support systems. The exercises are well planned to raise awareness and clarify individual feeling and values. The instructors' manuals provide more detail regarding the disease. The parents' booklet provides a balanced presenta-

tion of facts and feelings associated with AIDS/HIV, including tips on how to talk to teenagers about AIDS/HIV.

▲ For Ordering Information, see p. 227

❶ Facts, Choices, Prevention: An Educational Package on AIDS

- **Administrators Guide To AIDS Education**
  1988; $3.75; English.

- **Choices: Learning About AIDS**
  20 min.; VHS 3/4; 1988; $125.00; English.

- **Guide To Teaching About AIDS**
  1988; $5.00; English.

- **What You Should Know About AIDS**
  12 pages; paperback; 1988; $.69; English.

- **What You Teenager Will Be Learning About AIDS**
  12 pages; paperback; 1988; $1.25; English.

National Safety Council

This is a multicomponent educational package on AIDS/HIV for junior and senior high school students. Collectively, these materials can be used to establish, implement, and evaluate education programs tailored to the individual community.

The "Administrator's Guide to AIDS Education" describes the process of developing and assessing AIDS/HIV education programs in schools, emphasizing community involvement in the process.

The teacher's guide, "Guide to Teaching about AIDS," provides suggestions for teaching, lecture "scripts," discussion guides, and student work sessions.

The student's booklet, "What You Should Know about AIDS,: and the related 20-minute video, "Choices: Learning about AIDS" use a straightforward approach, incorporating teenage expressions and some slang to describe sexual behaviors and practices. The video and booklet present the facts and dispel myths about AIDS/HIV and the way it is spread; discuss protective behaviors; and strongly encourage voluntary testing, open discussions with peers and sexual partners, and individual responsibility in prevention of the disease.

The parents' booklet, "What Your Teenager Will Be Learning about AIDS," repeats the coloful design and straightforward approach of the student booklet in describing curriculum content. It also covers questions about AIDS-infected children in schools, emphasizes the necessity and urgency for good teenage education programs, and highlights the role of parents in this process. The package components may be purchased as a set or individually.

Reviewers' Comments: The excellently produced video in this package is very effective as a vehicle for discussion and as a peer teaching tool. It demonstrates tolerance, compassion, and communication in a believable way, and provides good multicultural images. It is excellent for behavior modeling for both males and females. The student booklet is a good basic information source. It reinforces the video message and is most effectively used in conjunction with it. The parents' booklet also provides useful basic information on AIDS/HIV and on the scope of this particular educational program. It is most suitable for parents with at least a high school education.

▲ For Ordering Information, see p. 224

❷ Kids Poster and Guide

- **AIDS Is Not Spread By Things We Touch**

- **You Know What? You Can't Get AIDS From:**
  17 x 22; illustrations; color; 1987; $3.00; English.

Minnesota AIDS Project

The poster shows a cartoon strip that reads at the top, "Hey! You know what? You CAN'T get AIDS from:" followed by cartoons of things from which you can not contract AIDS/HIV such as eating in restaurants, using toilets in public places, mosquito bites, or giving hugs and kisses. The last cartoon reads "AIDS is not spread by things we touch."

The 12 page teaching guide explains that the poster is meant as a springboard for discussion of AIDS/HIV and is designed to reassure children that they are not at risk for AIDS/HIV. The guide also reassures adults who may be reluctant to discuss AIDS/HIV with children and explains what it is, how it's transmitted, treatment options, and questions children may ask, along with answers.

Reviewers' Comments: The poster is colorful and eye catching; the guide is useful. Together they make an effective instructional tool.

▲ For Ordering Information, see p. 223

❷ Understanding And Preventing AIDS

- **Understanding And Preventing AIDS**
  125 pages; 1988; $5.95; English.

- **Understanding And Preventing AIDS -
  A Teacher's Guide**
  32 pages; stapled; 1988; English.

- **Understanding And Preventing AIDS**

Childrens Press

The book, geared to upper elementary through middle school students, starts with stories about people with AIDS/HIV, then presents the speculated causes and history. How the virus attacks the immune system is specifically discussed and illustrated. Historical and social perspectives of a "new plague," are presented along with stories that convey a real sense of tragedy about contracting the disease.

Medical research for cures and controls is also discussed. The book includes a quick reference to AIDS/HIV, a guide to prevention methods, suggested reading, and a list of information resources.

The video is a narrated series of photographs and illustrations. Part one discusses scientists' relatively recent awareness of AIDS and that no cure is expected for a long time. It explains how the virus works and that death is usually the result of another disease the body cannot fight off. This part of the video also tells why AIDS/HIV is called "a sexually-transmitted" disease, describes how the virus is and is not passed on, and suggests ways to avoid contracting the disease.

A screening of part two by teachers prior to classroom use is recommended by the producer because of content. This section describes protection measures, including a look at condoms for those who will not abstain from sex. A one page guide is provided with the video that includes a program summary, student objectives, suggested readiness activities, suggested follow-up activities, and additional information sources.

The Teacher's Guide provides lesson plans and ancillary material. The four daily lesson plans include suggestions for teacher preparation, readiness activities for the students, and specifics for class discussion. For the students, there is a unit pretest, reading guides with questions, and a pop quiz.

Reviewers' Comments: Overall the book is a good presentation of AIDS/HIV information and is well written with accurate information and illustrations that add to the text. The text does refer to risk groups instead of risk behavior and uses the term "victim" throughout. The local resource list is an effective tool.

The teacher's guide provides useful methods for reinforcing the materials from the textbook; however, teaching objectives are not clear. It refers incorrectly to "AIDS infection" rather than "HIV infection," and several of the suggested questions emphasize high-risk groups rather than high-risk behaviors.

The video did not meet minimum screening criteria.

▲ For Ordering Information, see p. 217

---

❶ 1ST EDITION RECOMMENDED ❷ 2ND EDITION RECOMMENDED ○ NOT RECOMMENDED

PAMPHLETS

❷ A Close Encounter

New York State Department of Health
14 pages; illustrations; 1988; special rates / discounts; English.

The heroines of this comic book are teenagers Jackie and her friend Tanya. After Tony gets Jackie stoned, Tanya tries to convince her not to go out with him again. Their teacher gives a talk about AIDS/HIV and how you contract it, and Tanya asks her for help with Jackie. In a flashback, we see that Tony used IV drugs a year ago. Jackie goes out with him again, but when he gives her a laced joint, she runs away. Tanya tells her she could have become infected with the AIDS virus if she'd had sex with Tony, and Jackie says she never wants to be that out of control again.

Reviewers' Comments: This comic book engages and holds the reader's interest, and seemingly is geared to adolescents who live in urban areas.

▲ For Ordering Information, see p. 225

◯ AIDS Coloring Cartoon Book

Coronado Neighborhood Council

❷ AIDS News

People of Color Against AIDS Network
16 pages; illustrations; 1988; $.25, limited copies; English.

This comic book contains cartoon strips about many different issues related to AIDS/HIV. In a humorous way the reader is shown how the virus is and is not transmitted, how lovers have to talk about HIV and condom use, symptoms of infection, and how to stay healthy. Social acceptance for someone who has AIDS/HIV virus is also depicted.

Reviewers' Comments: This is targeted largely to an in-school population. The story line seems geared to youth, while the language is slightly more sophisticated.

▲ For Ordering Information, see p. 226

◯ Be AIDS Aware Coloring Book

American Red Cross Columbus Area Chapter

❷ Corey's Story

Minnesota AIDS Project
8 pages; illustrations; 1987; $.50; English.

This comic book is the story of how Corey insists that her boyfriend wear a condom before she has sex with him for the first time. He leaves, insulted, but after seeing a cartoon about condom use and infection prevention on TV and talking to a friend, he returns convinced that Corey was right. The comic book ends with the line "And they lived happily ever...well, anyway, they lived!"

Reviewers' Comments: Corey's Story is engaging and generalizeable to a broad teenage audience. It uses vernacular, direct language and visual presentation to illustrate condom use and the importance of safer sex. There is occasional use of profanity.

▲ For Ordering Information, see p. 223

❷ Daily Care Of Infants And Children With AIDS And HIV Infection

Wisconsin Division of Health, AIDS/HIV Program
13 pages; 1988; free; English.

This pamphlet provides guidelines for the care of children with AIDS and HIV infection to protect against other infections and to protect the caretaker from the unlikely possibility of HIV transmission. The guidelines encourage routine hand washing to prevent infections and provides good health practices for feeding, diapering, and the use of potty chairs and toilets. Treatment and prevention of common illnesses, accidents, and ways to prevent skin rashes in the HIV infected child are presented. Routine cleaning, laundering, housekeeping and play activities are discussed.

Reviewers' Comments: This offers good recommendations, but the options (e.g. use of gloves) are not realistic for many people such as low-income child caregivers. The technical language may be too difficult for home health-care workers or non-professionals in health care facilities.

▲ For Ordering Information, see p. 231

❶ Get The Facts

State of Florida Department of Health and Rehabilitative Services - Broward County Public Health Unit
16 pages; illustrations; 1986; free, limited copies; English.

This comic book, written primarily for students in grades 7-12, their parents, and teachers, includes definitions of AIDS/HIV and ARC, "risk groups," modes of transmission, symptoms, and prevention. It attempts to dispel the myths surrounding the disease, such as transmission through casual contact. The comic book advocates safer sex practices and healthy lifestyles, and stresses the importance of research and counseling. It discourages drug abuse and unsafe sex.

Reviewers' Comments: This publication refers to high-risk groups rather than to high-risk behaviors. Its reading level may be high for average seventh grade students. It uses the outdated HTLV-III term, but its comic book format may attract student' attention.

▲ For Ordering Information, see p. 228

❷ Let's Talk About AIDS: An Information And Activities Book

Channing L. Bete Co., Inc.
   7 pages; illustrations; 1988; special rates / discounts; English.

Three cartoon characters, two boys and a girl, discuss AIDS/HIV and then appear throughout this short workbook to explain AIDS/HIV to children and young adolescents. Included are games and exercises such as decoding a short list of words to find the names of several viruses; a review that uses clues to answer a crossword puzzle on how HIV is transmitted; decoding a message about various kinds of casual contact that don't spread the virus; and completing a maze while avoiding "running into" ways of getting HIV. A final crossword puzzle encourages young readers to be friendly to people with AIDS/HIV.

Reviewers' Comments: This book is good for use as a teaching component in a health course for elementary school children. There is an emphasis on compassion and the book provides teachers with a number of good discussion points. The terms HIV and AIDS are used interchangeably in the text; this needs to be corrected with a definition of the HIV virus that leads to AIDS.

▲ For Ordering Information, see p. 217

❶ Let's Talk About Sex

National Hemophilia Foundation
   8 pages; illustrations; 1988; free, limited copies; English.

This pamphlet candidly discusses sex for teenagers and college students, including the dangers of AIDS to people with hemophilia. The pamphlet addresses the first sexual experience, different types and methods of sexual activity, safe sex, and the importance of using condoms properly.

Reviewers' Comments: The language of the pamphlet is informal. The content is excellent and appropriate for teenagers. While thorough, it requires high reading level skills and the copy format is dense.

▲ For Ordering Information, see p. 224

❶ Making Responsible Choices About Sex

Channing L. Bete Co., Inc.
   16 pages; illustrations; 1987; special rates / discounts; English.

This pamphlet offers adolescents guidance on whether to enter into a sexual relationship and the consequences of that decision. It encourages adolescents to think about their sexuality, values, and expectations before deciding. It advocates abstinence until the adolescent can determine that all consequences of having sex will be positive. The negative consequences mentioned are sexually transmitted diseases including AIDS/HIV, pregnancy, feelings of guilt, and unexpected emotional reactions.

Reviewers' Comments: This pamphlet is most appropriate for white, heterosexual pre-adolescents who are not yet experimenting with sex. It treats psychological issues underlying love and sex clearly, although it doesn't address safer sex. The graphics are simplistic.

▲ For Ordering Information, see p. 217

❶ Rappin' - Teens, Sex And AIDS

Multicultural Prevention Resource Center (MPRC)
   4 pages; illustrations; Dec 1987; $1.00; English.

This comic book, designed for young women, particularly urban teenage blacks and Latinos, covers the topics of safe sex, pregnancy prevention, the AIDS virus, and personal responsibility in dealing with these issues. Carmen and Tanya discuss the dilemmas of their newly-pregnant friend Consuela and problems of their own with their boyfriends' attitudes on the use of birth control pills and condoms. They seek advice from the school counselor, who is friendly and forthright in her discussion of these issues.

Reviewers' Comments: The content is excellent and the slang is very appropriate for the audience. It is sensitive to females and does not sterotype them.

▲ For Ordering Information, see p. 223

❷ Risky Business

San Francisco AIDS Foundation
   19 pages; illustrations; 1988; English.

This comic book contains two stories. The first, "AIDS VIRUS," illustrates the release of a deadly monster virus that goes forth to destroy the earth and to combat Mr. T-cell. The story then shifts to a group of high school students discussing HIV infection; how to clean needles in bleach; and condoms, including where to buy and how to apply them.

The second comic, "RISKY BUSINESS," portrays teens as they think and talk about sex. It conveys information about

---

❶ 1ST EDITION RECOMMENDED   ❷ 2ND EDITION RECOMMENDED   ○ NOT RECOMMENDED

the transmission and symptoms of AIDS/HIV. The back cover has questions and answers, and a glossary of words used in the book.

Reviewers' Comments: The language in this comic book is direct and appropriately humorous. However, the depiction of a student's reaction to testing HIV positive is not credible, and ignores the possibility of a false positive result.

▲ For Ordering Information, see p. 227

❶ Teens And AIDS - Playing It Safe

American Council of Life Insurance
12 pages; illustrations; 1987; special rates / discounts; English.

This brochure offers adolescents basic information about AIDS/HIV, models for discussing AIDS/HIV, and guidance for making choices. With each turn of the page a different conversation is "overheard," in which topics are discussed such as fear and judgment of people with AIDS/HIV, use of rubbers, and making one's own choices about sex and drugs. It offers boldly printed facts about protection. National hotline numbers are provided as well as information about getting tested.

Reviewers' Comments: This pamphlet provides information that is useful to young people and is well presented. The elementary information about "Who has AIDS right now?" discusses risk groups instead of risk behaviors, and future revision of this is recommended.

▲ For Ordering Information, see p. 214

◯ What Young People Should Know About AIDS

Channing L. Bete Co., Inc.

◯ You Should Know About AIDS

Portnoy Enterprises

◯ A Bad Reputation Isn't All You Can Get...

AIDS Prevention Project Dallas County Health Department

◯ AIDS: The Ultimate Going Away Present

AIDS Prevention Project Dallas County Health Department

◯ Don't Let Love Sweep You Off Your Feet

AIDS Prevention Project Dallas County Health Department

❷ Getting Any

Indiana State Board of Health
35 x 18; photographs; color; Sep 1988; special rates / discounts; English.

This poster is an enlarged photograph of several high school students of various cultural backgrounds. It explains six reasons to say no when your friends ask, "getting any?" among them pregnancy, reputation, STDs and AIDS/HIV. Each reason appears beneath one of the teens in the photo as a seeming caption for that person's situation, thus emphasizing to young viewers that they are vulnerable to those problems; the surest way to avoid them is to not have sex. The Indiana State AIDS/HIV hotline number is included.

Reviewers' Comments: While this poster is visually appealing, it is somewhat busy and, as a consequence, the message may be diluted.

▲ For Ordering Information, see p. 221

◯ Its OK To Say No

New York City Department of Health AIDS Education Training Unit

◯ The More You Score The Greater Your Chances Of Losing The Game

AIDS Prevention Project Dallas County Health Department

❷ **My Boyfriend Gave Me AIDS And I Was Only Worried About Getting Pregnant**

Oregon Health Division, HIV Program
16 x 20; photographs; black & white; 1988; $5.00; English.

This black and white poster features a photograph of a teenage girl whose expression is serious. The starkness of the image emphasizes the messages of the text. The poster warns, "AIDS is a killer" and urges sexually active adolescents to protect themselves against infection.

Reviewers' Comments: This poster clearly conveys its message, which is a very needed one for the sexually active teenage population.

▲ For Ordering Information, see p. 226

❷ **Series: You Won't Get AIDS (In A Restaurant, From A Bug Bite, From Hide 'N' Seek, From A Public Pool)**

CDC National AIDS Information and Education Program
16 x 22; illustrations; color; Oct 1988; free; English.

This series presents drawings that illustrate the captions, "You Won't Get AIDS in A Restaurant"; "You won't Get AIDS From A Bug Bite"; "You Won't Get AIDS From Hide 'N' Seek"; and "You Won't Get AIDS From A Public Pool." The copy beneath the drawings adds that HIV is not spread through casual contact. The National AIDS Hotline number is listed for further information.

Reviewers' Comments: This series seems to be geared to children rather than adults and the images vary in their effectiveness. The copy at the bottom of the posters is awkward because of the sentence structure.

▲ For Ordering Information, see p. 216

PUBLIC SERVICE ADS (TV, RADIO, PRINT)

○ **AIDS Is Scary, But A Zit Is Real. Right?**

CDC National AIDS Information and Education Program

❷ **AIDS Radio Public Service Campaign - "Teens"**

Connecticut State Department of Health
60 sec.; 1988; special rates / discounts; English.

In this radio PSA, we hear party noises in the background and a conversation between a girl and her brother. When he gives her a condom she protests that she isn't going to get pregnant or sleep with anyone with AIDS/HIV. She asks her brother if he thinks it's ok to fool around since he's given her a condom. He replies, "Only fools fool around." The slogan for the PSA is, "Say no to sex, or yes to a condom."

Reviewers' Comments: These messages are appropriately targeted to teens with an effective slogan. The presentations are catchy and upbeat. Purchasers should note that the tape credits the State of Connecticut Health Deparment.

▲ For Ordering Information, see p. 218

○ **AIDS Rap Song**

Indiana State Board of Health

❶ **Minnesota Aidlines Public Service Announcements On AIDS**

Hennepin County Administration
30 sec.; TV; color; Aug 1987; $75.00; English.

This videotape contains three 30-second messages directed at teenagers. The first shows teens dancing together and warns against sharing needles and having sex without a condom. The second message, picturing people from diverse ages, races, and both sexes, stresses that anyone can get AIDS/HIV. In the third PSA, a young man with AIDS reflects on how he has been hurt by people avoiding him. The messages give a number to call for more information. Printed texts of the three announcements accompany the video.

Reviewers' Comments: All three excellent public service announcements present strong, clear messages.

▲ For Ordering Information, see p. 220

❶ 1ST EDITION RECOMMENDED   ❷ 2ND EDITION RECOMMENDED   ○ NOT RECOMMENDED

VIDEOS / FILMS

❷ A Is For AIDS

Perennial Education, Inc.
   15 min.; VHS; 1988; $275.00; special rates / discounts;
English.

This video is designed to give children an overview of the
AIDS/HIV and to calm their fears of contracting the disease. Two girls and a boy take a fantasy journey to see
Andy Answer, the animated scientist-dog, in his lab. On
his video screen, Andy introduces the three children to a
girl and a boy who have AIDS/HIV--one got the virus from
her mother and the other from a blood transfusion. The
children with AIDS talk about what it's like and their
friends talk about being their friends. Andy also shows
how the virus works in the body and explains that it is not
transmitted through casual contact.

*Reviewers' Comments: The video introduces sex as a
means of transmission, so teachers need to be prepared to
respond appropriately to children regarding the topic. The
video inaccurately implies that not all blood is tested for the
HIV antibody. The animation is excellent, particularly the
portion depicting how HIV affects the immune system.
This video, if accompanied by appropriate and adequate
teacher facilitation, is recommended for grades 2 through 4.*

▲ For Ordering Information, see p. 226

❶ A.I.D.S.

**Walt Disney Educational Media Company
   c/o Coronet/MTI Film & Video**
   18 min.; VHS; 1987; $345.00; English.

In this videotape, hosted by Ally Sheedy, doctors and
health educators answer high school students' common
questions about AIDS/HIV. Computer graphics illustrate
the impact of the AIDS virus on the human immune system. The script suggests that abstinence from drug use and
sex is the best method of prevention, but it also discusses in
forthright language safer sex practices. A discussion guide
is available.

*Reviewers' Comments: This video provides good basic
medical and clinical information for junior and senior high
school students. It requires updating since it provides no
informataion on current treatment options and uses the
phrase "risk categories" rather that "risk behaviors."*

▲ For Ordering Information, see p. 231

❶ AIDS Alert

Creative Media Group Health Alert Division
   22 min.; VHS 3/4; 1987; $125.00; English.

Dr. Richard Keeling introduces and closes this cartoon
video with warnings that AIDS/HIV is a serious health
problem. He separates the facts about this disease from the
fear of contracting it. He advises both men and women to
carry condoms. Dr. Goodhealth, one of the cartoon characters, answers questions on the origin of AIDS/HIV, how
the virus is and is not transmitted, the HIV antibody test,
signs and symptoms of HIV and AIDS, and prevention. He
advises not to shoot drugs or at least not to share needles,
and to practice safer sex. A discussion leader's guide accompanies the video.

*Reviewers' Comments: The content does not match the
approach. The content of this video targets high school students, but the visual approach and style suits elementary
students or possibly 7th to 9th graders.*

▲ For Ordering Information, see p. 218

❷ AIDS And The Immune System

Churchill Films
   12 min.; VHS 16mm; 1988; $225.00; rental fee:
$60.00/3 days; special rates / discounts; English.

This video was designed to be used in teaching about the
immune system for the intermediate grades. Examples
show a girl with a splinter in her finger, another with the
flu, and a boy who carries the AIDS virus. In this context,
children learn through animation and live action how white
cells kill bacteria and viruses, how antibodies assist, and
how HIV destroys killer white cells, weakening the immune system so the body can't protect itself from disease.
Vaccination and antibiotics are discussed.

*Reviewers' Comments: This is appropriate for grades 4
and up. It addresses the immune system in an age-appropriate, innovative way. This is an excellent example of
how HIV/AIDS can be incorporated into health curricula
for this age group. There is good multi-ethnic representation.*

▲ For Ordering Information, see p. 217

❶ AIDS: Answers For Young People

Churchill Films
 18 min.; VHS; 1987; $275.00; rental fee: $60.00/3
 days; English.

In this video, teenage peer counselors, a health educator, a physician, a 12-year-old hemophiliac boy with AIDS, and several other persons with AIDS answer the questions from seventh grade students. It uses animation to explain how the virus attacks the immune system. The film allays worries about being exposed to the virus through casual contact. It details how the virus is transmitted, particularly through contaminated IV drug needles and unprotected sex. It urges young people not to experiment with sex as the only sure way to avoid sexual transmission.

Reviewers' Comments: The video makes good use of peer educators, persons with AIDS, discussions, and interviewers. It deals with the questions concerning HIV transmission in a forthright manner and is a good program for teens and their parents.

▲ For Ordering Information, see p. 217

◯ AIDS In Your School

Perennial Education, Inc.

❶ AIDS In Your School

Pergrine Productions
 23 min.; VHS; Jan 1987; $320.00; English/Spanish.

With music and fast-moving graphics, this videotape, designed for teenagers, features two teenage hosts and Dr. Mervyn Silverman. He explains the human immune system and how HIV attacks and destroys that system. He also discusses transmission and symptoms of AIDS/HIV. Three people with AIDS/HIV relate how it has changed their lives and that they want to be treated normally. The video discusses frankly, the importance of practicing safer sex and sharing information about AIDS/HIV. This video also is available in Spanish.

Reviewers' Comments: This comprehensive video may attempt to cover too much in 23 minutes. It uses an expert, rather than student peers, for transmitting factual information. The graphics quality is mixed, and the video is slow in places.

▲ For Ordering Information, see p. 226

❶ The AIDS Movie

Durrin Films / New Day Films
 26:03 min.; VHS; Oct 1986; $390.00; English.

This video addresses how the AIDS/HIV issue affects high school aged people. David Brumbach, an AIDS educator, speaks before a high school class with interview segments from three persons with AIDS interspersed: a 30-year-old married woman and former drug user, a young gay black man, and a woman who had several bisexual lovers. Brumbach reviews the main facts about AIDS/HIV: what it is and does, symptoms, modes of transmission (risk behaviors) and non-transmission (casual contact), and prevention (including safe sex and condoms). The three persons interviewed offer their personal experiences and insights, and warn against needlessly engaging in risk behaviors. It strongly discourages drug use, but for users, recommends never sharing needles. It emphasizes that AIDS/HIV does not discriminate among its hosts, but that exposure to the virus can be avoided. There is a discussion guide available.

Reviewers' Comments: This video presents a strong and realistic prevention message. The interviews with the three persons with AIDS are the highlight of the program. Viewers will empathize with the real people portrayed.

▲ For Ordering Information, see p. 218

◯ AIDS: The Disease And What We Know

Sunburst Communications, Inc.

❷ AIDS: Learn For Your Life

New Dimension Media, Inc.
 24 min.; VHS; 1987; $350.00; rental fee: $40.00/day;
 English.

This video is for use in high school AIDS/HIV education classes. They cover a range of AIDS/HIV topics, including how HIV is and is not transmitted, condom use, and relevant statistics. The video presents dramatization and information from professionals. A 50 page teacher's guide is included.

Reviewers' Comments: The experts tend to be a bit judgemental, but the peer narrative is excellent in this video that deals with sensitive topics. The physician shows some subtle biases and prejudices, e.g. "normal intercourse," and some of the material is heavily fatalistic. Latex condoms are not specified in the discussion of condoms and spermicides with nonoxynol-9 are not identified.

▲ For Ordering Information, see p. 224

❶ 1ST EDITION RECOMMENDED   ❷ 2ND EDITION RECOMMENDED   ◯ NOT RECOMMENDED

❷ AIDS: Let's Talk

New Dimension Media, Inc.
1989; $295.00; rental fee: $40.00/day; English.

Developed under the guidance of the Centers for Disease Control, the Michigan Department of Health, and the Michigan Department of Education, this video is designed to help dispel irrational fear of AIDS/HIV for students in grades three through six. It conveys that the virus is difficult to contract and does not spread easily. The serious nature of the AIDS epidemic and why some children have become infected are explained by other young people and life-size puppets. Children are assured that doctors are searching for a cure and that they do not need to avoid other children who have the disease.

Reviewers' Comments: This video by and for kids is racially inclusive, with older children modeling for younger children. The puppet show for intermediate students is a good teaching technique and is age-appropriate. The instructor should note some negative health messages, i.e., unhealthful foods, fighting, and arguing. The hesitation about "kids with AIDS didn't do anything wrong," might imply that adults did. Overall the video is accurate, well-produced, uses humor effectively, and contains age-appropriate information.

▲ For Ordering Information, see p. 224

❶ AIDS: Protect Yourself

Harris County Medical Society Houston Academy of Medicine
15:49 min.; VHS; 1987; $30.00; rental fee: $8.00/14 days; English.

This videotape makes use of young people to dramatize AIDS/HIV prevention methods. Rock-and-roll background music will attract adolescents. It is a companion piece to the "AIDS Survival Guides" from the same producer. No discussion guide is available.

Reviewers' Comments: The videotape is excellent in content and above avarage in instructional design and technical production. The booklet, "AIDS Survival Guides" (available from same distributor) is a useful resource with this video.

▲ For Ordering Information, see p. 220

❷ AIDS: Taking Action

New Dimension Media, Inc.
22 min; VHS; 1987; $275.00; rental fee: $40.00/day; English.

Designed for children in grades seven through nine, this video presents information about the transmission and prevention of AIDS/HIV and explains the difference between HIV, ARC, and AIDS. It opens with several teenagers who make false assertions about how AIDS/HIV is transmitted. An older, more authoritative teenager counters these statements by presenting information on how it is and is not transmitted, addressing irrational fears, and emphasizing the difficulty of contracting the virus. Other young adolescents offer advice on how junior high students can become more active in disseminating correct information about AIDS/HIV. A 16 page teacher's guide is included.

Reviewers' Comments: This well-done video uses a good sense of humor, nice technique and culturally sensitive material to empower students with specifics on how to take action. The messages are age-appropriate and compassionate, demonstrating good support from the students. The peer education is very effective, although peer pressure could be better utilized. The video has the potential to apply across generations. The price is a bit high.

▲ For Ordering Information, see p. 224

❷ AIDS: Teens Taking Control

Family Planning Council of Western Massachusetts, Inc.
20 min.; VHS; 1988; $50.00; rental fee: $35.00/1 week; English.

The video is aimed at upper-level middle class high school students, encouraging assertiveness among adolescents in situations involving drugs and sex. Adolescents wrote and acted in vignettes showing difficult situations such as saying no to drugs, negotiating abstinence with a partner, convincing a boyfriend to use condoms, buying condoms in a drug store, and visiting a famiy planning clinic. A health educator intermittently gives information about HIV infection.

Reviewers' Comments: This video receives high ratings for content accuracy. It deals with medical information as well as the psychosocial aspects of HIV risk, STDs, and other adolescent sexuality concerns. It contains positive sexuality messages. The vignettes regarding teenage drug use and sexual situations are frank and explicit. The video would need careful discussion and debriefing after viewing as there is much information given in a relatively short time. It would be very appropriate for college level students.

▲ For Ordering Information, see p. 219

❷ AIDS: What Everyone Needs To Know

Churchill Films
19 min.; VHS 16mm; 1987; $275.00; rental fee: $60.00/3 days; special rates / discounts; English/Spanish.

This newly updated edition of an earlier AIDS/HIV teaching film explains the facts about AIDS/HIV: how HIV is and is not transmitted, what high risk behaviors are, and why it is neccessary to avoid them. Animation explains the immune system, showing how HIV disables it. The film stresses prevention, noting that abstinence and avoiding used IV drug needles are the sure ways to prevent infection by the AIDS virus.

Reviewers' Comments: This is appropriate for junior high and high school students. The animation of the immune system may be too simple for some and the death scene may be upsetting for students who have not been exposed to these issues before.

▲ For Ordering Information, see p. 217

❷ The Body Fights Disease

Churchill Films
13 min.; VHS; 1988; $230.00; rental fee: $60.00/3 days; special rates / discounts; English.

This film describes how the body protects itself against germs, first by the barriers of skin and mucous membrane, then by the immune system. An explanation of HIV and how it disables the immune systems is given. Extensive animation illustrates the action of white blood cells, particularly the role of lymphocytes in producing antibodies and as killer cells. The film discusses immunization, antibiotics, and particularly, the importance of basic good health.

Reviewers' Comments: This is recommneded for junior high; younger students may be confused and or bored by the material. A good explanation of the immune system is included, but the technical production does not enhance the instructional effectiveness of the content.

▲ For Ordering Information, see p. 217

❷ Don't Get It

University of Massachusetts Medical Center
4:30 min.; VHS; 1989; $55.00; English/Spanish.

This video is written and performed by adolescents to educate their peers on the AIDS/HIV. It is set in an alley in which musicians rap to an audience of city youth. The words focus on modes of transmission and raising awareness of the disease. A segment in which adolescents deliver ten statements that give additional information on transmission and methods of risk reduction is included. In the Spanish version of the video these statements are subtitled. The band and the audience include black, Latino, and white adolescents.

Reviewers' Comments: While this video is good for use as an attention-getter and is captivating, it should be used only as a motivational piece. An extensive follow-up discussion is necessary to provide accurate information and to deal with issues raised.

▲ For Ordering Information, see p. 231

❷ Don't Get It: Teenagers And AIDS

Human Relations Media
30 min.; VHS; 1988; $159.00; special rates / discounts; English.

This documentary opens with excerpts from a music video about AIDS/HIV and safer sex and continues with statements by health professionals, interviews with teenagers, and images from the Names Project Quilt. It presents a montage of teens talking to teens and experts talking to teens on how HIV is transmitted and how transmission can be prevented.

Reviewers' Comments: This video is engaging and enhanced by popular music. While it addresses a multicultural audience, it does not show children of color in "teaching" roles. Its content and visuals are disjointed in several places, and there are minor inaccuracies (one is "infected with AIDS," there is a test "to tell you if you have AIDS"). In general, it is an adequately produced film, but not highly recommended.

▲ For Ordering Information, see p. 221

◯ Don't Let AIDS Catch You!

American Institute for Teen AIDS Prevention, Inc.

◯ An Educational Approach To AIDS

Carolina Biological Supply Company

---

❶ 1ST EDITION RECOMMENDED ❷ 2ND EDITION RECOMMENDED ◯ NOT RECOMMENDED

❷ Everyone Can Avoid AIDS

Milestone Productions
20 min.; VHS; 1988; $395.00, special rates / discounts; English

This video features clay and animated figures. The multi-ethnic audience of all ages listens to a talk on AIDS by "Dr. Prevention," who emphasizes that while AIDS is dangerous, it is preventable and can't be transmitted by casual contact. She outlines the ways in which AIDS is transmitted and illustrates its effect on the immune system. She encourages a caring attitude towards those with AIDS, and the initially hostile audience is eventually won over by the clear message. No discussion guide is included.

▲ For Ordering Information, see p. 223

❷ Face To Face With AIDS

Novela Health Foundation
31 min.; VHS; 1988; $250.00; English.

This video, starring Latino youth, shows the complex patterns of behavior that can lead to transmission of the HIV virus. When a man finds out he has AIDS from earlier intravenous drug use, the aunt who has been helping out since his wife died leaves out of fear and his daughter has to take care of him. As her father deteriorates and her friend's boyfriend finds out he's HIV positive from sharing needles, misconceptions about AIDS/HIV are confronted, up-dated information is given, and a compassionate response to a person with AIDS/HIV is shown. It is also available as a fotonovela.

Reviewers' Comments: This video incorporates elements of the Latino culture: family, homosexuality, virginity. It is emotionally powerful and uses appropriate humor. The acting is excellent as is the illustration of peer counseling. It provides concise information on transmission and prevention methods. The video is a little long and can be overwhelming.

▲ For Ordering Information, see p. 225

❷ Facing AIDS: Teens Ask A Young Man What It's Like

New York State Department of Health
20 min.; VHS; 1988; $20.00, limited copies; special rates / discounts; English.

The setting of this video is a small auditorium where adolescents, ages 13-15, listen to a speaker who has AIDS. He explains the behavior that may have led to his HIV infection: his one-time experiment with IV drug use and a homosexual experience. He also speakes of the social consequences of being a person with AIDS. The teens question him about the AIDS virus, its symptoms, treatments that are available, and prevention. The questions and answers are wide-ranging and are supplemented in a teachers' guide that contains the entire transcript.

Reviewers' Comments: The multicultural audience contrasts sharply with the single white educator and many of the questions seem staged. Though all the right questions are asked, the long interview format makes the film boring. Several educators are needed to create a racial and sexual balance.

▲ For Ordering Information, see p. 225

❷ A Million Teenagers

Churchill Films
22:30 min.; VHS 16mm; 1985; $360.00; rental fee: $60.00/3 days; special rates / discounts; English/Spanish.

This video presents information about chlamydia, PID, NGU, herpes, and AIDS/HIV. Through live action and detailed animation, the film illustrates how sexually transmitted diseases are transmitted, how they are treated, and how using good sense can help control them.

Reviewers' Comments: This is a good mult-ethnic presentation for grades 8 and up. The video makes good use of peer educators. Illustrations and a few actual photographs of sexual anatomy are used for instructional purposes. The STD content is good with the exception of the AIDS/HIV section, which needs improvement.

▲ For Ordering Information, see p. 217

❶ Sex, Drugs And AIDS

O.D.N. Productions, Inc.
18 min.; VHS; 1986; $325.00; English.

Actress Rae Dawn Chong, host and narrator, explains vital information about the transmission of HIV through drug injections and sexual intercourse. The film clarifies the difference between casual and sexual contact. Documentary-style segments illustrate and amplify the central message that young people can reduce their risk of getting AIDS/HIV. The film's objectives are to overcome fear and anxiety about casual contact, identify unsafe behavior, encourage abstinence or condom use, and foster a humane approach to persons with AIDS/HIV. There is a discussion guide available.

Reviewers' Comments: Overall, this is an excellent and pertinent film, appropriate for high school students. However, people of color are not adequately represented and the term "high-risk groups" is used rather than "high-risk behaviors," and no instruction is provided on cleaning IV drug "works." It is a more comprehensive version than "The Subject Is AIDS" described below.

▲ For Ordering Information, see p. 225

❶ The Subject Is AIDS

O.D.N. Productions, Inc.
18 min.; VHS; 1987; $325.00; English.

For the most part, this videotape and "Sex, Drugs, and AIDS," described above, share the same content. This videotape however, was edited to advocate the practice of sexual abstinence among teenagers as the primary means of AIDS prevention. An introduction by Surgeon General C. Everett Koop was also added. There is a discussion guide available.

Reviewers' Comments: This film succeeds as an effective peer education tool. The explanations provided are concise and appropriate for the teenage viewer. The video is suited more to teens who are not sexually active.

▲ For Ordering Information, see p. 225

❶ What Is AIDS?

The J. Gary Mitchell Film Company c/o Coronet/MTI Film & Video
15 min.; VHS; 1988; $335.00; English.

This video explores many of the AIDS/HIV issues and questions relevant to elementary school students. It provides children with a basic understanding of the body's immune system and how it works. It describes the AIDS virus as "a tricky son-of-a-gun" that does not "play fair," and fools the body's immune system into thinking the virus is not an enemy. The program also focuses on what can be done to prevent AIDS/HIV and dispels many of the myths surrounding the disease. The video features a father talking to two pre-adolescent little leaguers (a boy and girl) over pizza. Through live-action dramatizations, many of which include the use of baseball-related analogies and cartoon-like viruses, this program prepares young people to understand the facts about AIDS/HIV and what they can do to help prevent the spread of the disease. A discussion guide accompanies the video.

Reviewers' Comments: This video is an excellent educational tool for younger children to learn about AIDS/HIV. Creative and entertaining, it uses excellent analogies and wonderful characters to explain the immune system and transmission of the disease. Its approach is nonjudgemental and compassionate.

▲ For Ordering Information, see p. 229

◯ Young People And AIDS

Channing L. Bete Co., Inc.

❶ 1ST EDITION RECOMMENDED   ❷ 2ND EDITION RECOMMENDED   ◯ NOT RECOMMENDED

COLLEGE AND UNIVERSITY STUDENTS

BROCHURES

❶ AIDS: What Everyone Should Know

American College Health Association
5 panels; illustrations; $.45, limited copies;
special rates / discounts; 1987; English.

▲ For Ordering Information, see p. 214

❶ Deciding About Sex...The Choice To Abstain

ETR Associates/Network Publications
3 panels; illustrations; 1986; English.

▲ For Ordering Information, see p. 219

❷ On With Condoms

Madison AIDS Support Network
4 panels; photographs; $.17; 1988; English.

This brochure is targeted to college and university students asking questions such as "Did you think you were safe from AIDS/HIV because you're a student at a wholesome midwestern university?" It mixes humor with facts on safe sex and offers guidelines on how to stay satisfied and healthy, tips on condom use, a buyer's guide to condoms, and what to say when a partner refuses to use a condom. A table is also provided listing "safe," "possibly safe," and "not safe" sex behaviors.

▲ For Ordering Information, see p. 222

❷ What Are Sexually Transmitted Diseases?

American College Health Association
6 panels; $.50; special rates / discounts; 1988; English.

This brochure features a chart of the most common sexually transmitted diseases, their symptoms, available treatments, and related complications. Special boxes discuss the use of antibiotics, interrelated STDs, incurable STDs, and safer sex.

▲ For Ordering Information, see p. 214

INSTRUCTIONAL PROGRAMS

❶ Medical, Psychological, And Social Implications Of AIDS: A Curriculum For Young Adults

State University of New York at Stony Brook - Dept of Allied Health Professions, SUNY AIDS Education Project
150 pages; paperback; graphs; Feb 1987; $25.00; English.

This curriculum attempts to reduce fears and anxieties about AIDS/HIV in young adults. For each of nine sessions it contains specific objectives, an outline of information , instructional activities, lecture guides, and student activities. Specific topics include symptoms of AIDS/HIV, epidemiology, risk reduction, psycho-social problems of people with AIDS/HIV, specifics of safer sex, specific recommendations for IV drug users, employment of HIV-infected persons, HIV screening, and ethical responsibilities of people at risk for AIDS. The price of the curriculum includes periodic updates, information references and resources, and unlimited consultant services in project offices.

Reviewers' Comments: This is a good curriculum for older persons as well as young adults. It is not a packaged or self-instructional unit and it requires training of instructors prior to use. The teaching strategies, such as the student activities, can be adapted to different community settings.

▲ For Ordering Information, see p. 228

❷ Teaching AIDS: A Resource Guide On Acquired Immune Deficiency Syndrome

ETR Associates/Network Publications
159 pages; paperback; 1988; English.

This comprehensive curriculum helps teachers approach the topic of AIDS/HIV from several viewpoints. It provides basic AIDS/HIV information and teaching strategies with a guide for using the curriculum, and it details several plans for teaching whose use depends on the goals of the class. Examples are "AIDS - The Basic Unit," "Public Response to AIDS," and "STDs and AIDS." The curriculum includes materials such as related worksheets for optional use in the various lesson plans plus helpful hints and information useful in responding to difficult or controversial questions. A glossary and a list of AIDS/HIV information resources such as hotlines are included.

Reviewers' Comments: This overemphasizes lecture and discussion and does not provide enough experiential activities. It also addresses the origin of AIDS/HIV, which is too loaded a topic to discuss properly in a curriculum. It is, however, well organized and easy to use, and it contains a wealth of useful information.

▲ For Ordering Information, see p. 219

MICROFILMS / SLIDES

❷ AIDS: What College Students Need To Know

AIDS Research and Education Project, Psychology Department California State University at Long Beach
44 slides; graphs; 1987; $15.00; English.

There are thirty slides in this set, whose topics range from the history of AIDS/HIV and a definition of the acronym to immunology, statistics, transmission, testing, and legal issues. The slides are accompanied by an outline and a comprehensive speaker's supplement that guides the presentation facilitator in answering questions students might have.

Reviewers' Comments: This is best for a fairly educated audience and requires a strong facilitator who can update statistics. The presentation consists of simple word slides. State laws are specific to California.

▲ For Ordering Information, see p. 213

MULTICOMPONENT PROGRAMS

❷ Safer Sex Kit
Brochures, Condoms, Latex Sheet

Dartmouth College Department of Health Education
1987; special rates / discounts; English.

The purpose of these kits is to increase students' awareness that they can contract AIDS/HIV. The kits contain two brochures - "AIDS: Questions and Answers" and "Safer Sex," as well as items necessary for practicing safer sex, including a rubber dam, a condom, and a container of sper-

micidal lubricant. The "AIDS: Questions and Answers" brochure was developed by Dartmouth's College Health Service to answer questions most often asked by Dartmouth students. The "Safer Sex" brochure was developed by the Charlottesville AIDS Resource Network and includes a discussion of safe versus risky or dangerous sexual practices and provides information on condoms, lubricants, drugs, and alcohol.

Reviewers' Comments: This is an innovative awareness tool. The kit needs to include more instruction on how to use its components (condom, dental dam); there are no illustrations. There is also no mention of spermicide use in the literature of the kit.

▲ For Ordering Information, see p. 218

PAMPHLETS

○ AIDS - A Primer For Students

Truckee Meadows Community College - AIDS Education Project

❶ Sex On Campus: Sexually Transmitted Disease, Surviving The Epidemic Of The 1980's

College Satellite Network
16 pages; illustrations & photographs; Sep 1987; $1.50, limited copies; English.

This pamphlet examines AIDS/HIV and other sexually transmitted diseases as they impact college and university students. It discusses, among other issues, AIDS/HIV testing, public policy issues, and the concerns of persons with AIDS/HIV. It includes national and local hotlines and other resources, including organizations, publications, films, and videotapes. It carries endorsements from several health and educational organizations.

Reviewers' Comments: This readable magazine presents diverse and interesting content. It provides the personal as well as the public policy perspectives on AIDS. It articulates AIDS and other STD prevention guidelines in a straight forward manner.

▲ For Ordering Information, see p. 217

❶ 1ST EDITION RECOMMENDED   ❷ 2ND EDITION RECOMMENDED   ○ NOT RECOMMENDED

POSTERS

◯ **AIDS (HIV) Virus Electron Micrographs Chart**

Carolina Biological Supply Company

❷ **Alka Seltzer/Condom**

AIDS Research and Education Project,
Psychology Department California State
University at Long Beach
17 x 11; illustrations; color; 1988; $.75;
special rates / discounts; English.

This poster seeks to raise awareness among college students about the seriousness of AIDS/HIV. One side of the poster shows a glass with a seltzer tablet; on the other side is a condom packet. The message reads, "This (seltzer) works the morning after. . . this (condom) doesn't." Condom use or abstinence is recommended as a means of protection from HIV transmission.

Reviewers' Comments: The message offers facts and choices in an interesting manner and is medically accurate. It does not, however, specify latex condoms.

▲ For Ordering Information, see p. 213

❷ **College Success**

AIDS Research and Education Project,
Psychology Department California State
University at Long Beach
11 x 17; illustrations; color; 1988; $.75;
special rates / discounts; English.

This poster depicts the "essentials for college success": some basic school supplies and, disproportionately larger than the other items, a condom. It encourages the use of condoms coupled with spermicide during sex and urges the viewer to learn the facts about AIDS/HIV and safer sex.

Reviewers' Comments: The accurate message promotes safer sex but does not offer choices. It does not specify latex condoms.

▲ For Ordering Information, see p. 213

❷ **Could He Be The One?**

AIDS Research and Education Project,
Psychology Department California State
University at Long Beach
11 x 17; illustrations; color; 1988; $.75;
special rates / discounts; English.

This poster uses an illustration depicting many standing men arranged as a question mark. They are all colored red except for the single black figure which is the "dot" of the question mark. The text explains that HIV can be spread unwittingly, that someone who has it might not know it, and that you can't tell by looking at someone whether or not he is infected. It stresses the need to talk with sexual partners about safer sex and sexual histories and urges the viewer to "Limit (his/her) risk by getting to know (his/her) partner's past." The poster includes the phone number of the AIDS Research & Education Project.

Reviewers' Comments: The poster effectively attracts one's attention, but the text is somewhat wordy. To be medically accurate, the condom should be specified as latex.

▲ For Ordering Information, see p. 213

❷ **Don't Miss Out On Your Future**

AIDS Research and Education Project,
Psychology Department California State
University at Long Beach
11 x 17; illustrations; color; 1988; $.75;
special rates / discounts; English.

This poster uses the ghostly image of a bodiless cap and gown to convey its poignancy to the college-aged. It's message, "Don't throw away four years of hard work for one night of passion," intends to raise awareness of AIDS/HIV and related issues on college campuses. The copy encourages safer sex as a means of protecting that four year investment.

Reviewers' Comments: The graphics are appealing, but the approach is one which uses "scare tactics." Condoms are not specified as being latex, and the safer sex guidelines refer to having sex with one partner rather than one uninfected partner.

▲ For Ordering Information, see p. 213

❷ **How To Keep From Getting Lovesick**

AIDS Administration for the State of Maryland
Maryland C.A.R.E.S.
11 x 14; photographs; color; 1988; free; English.

Focusing primarily on teenagers and young adults, this poster is geared toward young heterosexuals who are either considering becoming or already are sexually active. Beneath a photograph of a young man and woman holding hands, a caption advises that those who choose to have sexual intercourse should use condoms.

Reviewers' Comments: The photograph transmits a sense of romanticism, but would be more effective if it were clearer. To be medically accurate, the condom should be specified as "latex."

▲ For Ordering Information, see p. 213

VIDEOS / FILMS

○ AIDS: What Are the Risks?

Human Relations Media

❷ AIDS-Wise, No Lies

Current-Rutledge
　22 min.; VHS; 1988; $250.00; rental fee: $50.00/1 use; special rates / discounts; English.

This video was designed to be presented on the third day of a five day lesson plan as outlined in the accompanying study guide. Each lesson includes objectives and suggestions for meeting those objectives, including quiz questions, quotes from individuals in the video, and exercise material. In the video, adolescents and adults express their views and concerns about AIDS/HIV. The participants include young musicians who describe their fears of contracting the virus, an IV drug user who relates her anxieties on taking the HIV antibody test, a housewife and a former teacher who relate how having the disease has affected their lives, and a gay man seriously ill with AIDS.

Reviewers' Comments: Through a series of vignettes, this video sets the stage for good classroom discussion with the emphasis on "what you do, not who you are." The technical quailty is very good and helps to make this video appealing. A few minor misleading statements will need to be pointed out by the facilitator, but otherwise this is an excellent tool for AIDS/HIV education.

▲ For Ordering Information, see p. 218

❶ Discussing AIDS Prevention On A College Campus

The Exodus Trust
　19 min.; VHS; 1986; $150.00; English.

In this video, a university health educator explains how to avoid AIDS to six college students. The educator describes safer sex techniques and demonstrates, with an anatomical model, how to use a condom effectively. She stresses the importance of good communication with sexual partners and responsible decision-making regarding sexual activity. An accompanying viewer's guide provides questions for group discussion. The video uses explicit language and demonstrations when discussing sexual behaviors and protective measures.

Reviewers' Comments: This video, suitable for senior high school students as well as college students, is excellent in content, but suffers in its use of a lecture format. The presentations on sexuality, safer sex, and need for communication between partners are extremely well done. Its discussion of safe sex products is informative, and it is one of the few videos that explain and demonstrate condom usage.

▲ For Ordering Information, see p. 229

○ Responsible AIDS Information At Dartmouth (RAID) Road Show

Dartmouth College Department of Health Education

❶ The Search For The AIDS Virus: An Interview With Dr. Robert Gallo

Carolina Biological Supply Company
　28 min.; VHS; 1986; $149.95; English.

This videotape features an interview with Dr. Robert Gallo of the National Cancer Institute. Dr. Gallo describes his involvement in AIDS research and the events that led to the isolation of the AIDS virus. He also presents his opinion regarding blood tests for the AIDS virus antibody. He speculates on the prospects for an AIDS vaccine, how such a vaccine would work, and the possibility of a cure for AIDS. No discussion guide is available.

Reviewers' Comments: This highly technical but good documentary is best suited for a high school or college science program.

▲ For Ordering Information, see p. 216

❶　1ST EDITION RECOMMENDED　　❷　2ND EDITION RECOMMENDED　　○　NOT RECOMMENDED

GAY AND BISEXUAL MEN

BROCHURES

○ **AIDS And HIV Infection**

Memphis / Shelby County Health Department

❷ **AIDS: Reducing The Risk For Gay And Bisexual Men**

Howard Brown Memorial Clinic
   4 panels; special rates / discounts; 1988; English.

Along with basic descriptions of the AIDS virus, its affect on the immune system, and means of transmission, this brochure concentrates on safer sex practices for gay and bisexual men. Protective measures for specific types of behavior are listed. Some information on the risks associated with IV drug and alcohol abuse is also included. The Illinois AIDS Hotline number is listed.

▲ For Ordering Information, see p. 221

○ **AIDS - Reducing Your Risks**

Columbus AIDS Task Force

❶ **Are You Man Enough? / ¿Que Tan Hombre Es Usted?**

Community Outreach Risk Reduction Education Program (CORE)
   8 pages; illustrations; $.35; May 1988; English/Spanish.

▲ For Ordering Information, see p. 217

❷ **Brothers Loving Brothers Safely**

D.C. Commission of Public Health
   1 panel; photographs; special rates / discounts; 1987; English.

This brochure encourages gay and bisexual men to practice safer sex. One side contains a photograph of two black men, who are nude from the waist up, embracing. The reverse explains safer sex practices and provides local phone numbers for more information on AIDS.

▲ For Ordering Information, see p. 218

○ **Fact Sheet No. 6 - Poppers and AIDS**

Gay Community AIDS Project

○ **Fight The Fear With The Facts**

Whitman-Walker Clinic

❶ **Great Northwest Sex**

Cascade AIDS Project
   4 panels; illustrations; 1987; English.

▲ For Ordering Information, see p. 216

○ **Guidelines & Recommendations For Healthful Gay/Lesbian & Bisexual Activity**

The National Coalition of Gay Sexually Transmitted Disease Services

❶ **Guidelines For Safer And Healthier Sex**

AIDS Task Force of Central New York
   4 panels; Jan 1986; English.

▲ For Ordering Information, see p. 213

○ **Healthy Sex Is Fun**

Wellness Networks, Inc. - Flint

○ **How To Be A Life Saver / Cómo Ser Un Salvavidas**

Gay and Lesbian Community Services Center

❷ How to Use a Rubber

Community Outreach Risk Reduction Education Program (CORE)
5 panels; illustrations; $.10; 1988; English.

This mini-brochure is designed for gay and bisexual men with poor or no reading skills. It uses a series of 9 drawings to illustrate key points of condom use for anal intercourse.

▲ For Ordering Information, see p. 217

❷ An Important Message For Gay And Bisexual Men

San Francisco AIDS Foundation
2 panels; illustrations; $.50; special rates / discounts; 1988; English.

The brochure folds out into a poster. It strongly encourages the elimination of unsafe sex practices and includes a blunt description of what unsafe sex is. It contains a message of hope and inspiration to do all that can be done to stop the spread of AIDS/HIV and counters common excuses for practicing unsafe sex.

▲ For Ordering Information, see p. 227

○ Latest Facts About AIDS - Gay And Bisexual Men And AIDS

American Red Cross National Headquarters

❶ Nothing But The Facts: AIDS Risk-Reduction Guidelines For Gay Men

St. Louis Efforts for AIDS
3 panels; free, limited copies; 1986; English.

▲ For Ordering Information, see p. 228

❶ An Ounce Of Prevention Is Worth A Pound Of Cure / SIDA/AIDS Se Puede Prevenir

Gay Men's Health Crisis, Inc.
5 panels; illustrations; special rates / discounts; 1986; English/Spanish.

▲ For Ordering Information, see p. 219

○ Play Safe! Warning! Sexually Explicit Material Contained Inside

Wellness Networks, Inc. - Flint

○ Rod's Bar Card

Madison AIDS Support Network

❶ SEX

Philadelphia AIDS Task Force
3 panels; $.15; 1985; English.

▲ For Ordering Information, see p. 226

❷ Safer Sex

Health Issues Taskforce of Cleveland
Card; $.05; 1988; English.

This wallet-sized card discusses the risks in specific sexual practices and offers guidelines for practicing safer sex.

▲ For Ordering Information, see p. 220

○ Safer Sex - You Don't Have To Do It Alone - We're All In This Together

Whitman-Walker Clinic

❶ Safer Sex Can Be Sensuous

Tidewater AIDS Crisis Taskforce
4 panels; illustrations; $.15; Apr 1987; English.

▲ For Ordering Information, see p. 229

❷ Safer Sex Is Bringing Men Together

Health Issues Taskforce of Cleveland
4 panels; illustrations; $.10; 1988; English.

This brochure offers detailed guidelines for safer sex as a creative and healthy experience. It uses explicit sexual language to discuss the risks of specific sexual practices and ways to reduce risk. It also notes the hazards of alcohol and drug use in the context of AIDS/HIV prevention, and provides instructions on proper use of condoms. The emphasis is on safer sex practices for general healthful living and community responsibility. The brochure also describes the Task Force's Safer Sex House Party program.

▲ For Ordering Information, see p. 220

❶ 1ST EDITION RECOMMENDED   ❷ 2ND EDITION RECOMMENDED   ○ NOT RECOMMENDED

❶ Staying Healthy: AIDS Information For Gay Men - We're All In This Together

Whitman-Walker Clinic
3 panels; illustrations; 1987; English.

▲ For Ordering Information, see p. 231

❶ Warning!!!!! Explicit Unsafe Sex Information

Tampa AIDS Network
Card; free, limited copies; Apr 1987; English.

▲ For Ordering Information, see p. 229

❶ What Are The Symptoms Of AIDS?

Whitman-Walker Clinic
1 panel; 1987; English.

▲ For Ordering Information, see p. 231

❶ You Don't Have To Say No

Long Island Association For AIDS Care, Inc.
Special rates / discounts; Feb 1987; English.

▲ For Ordering Information, see p. 222

INSTRUCTIONAL PROGRAMS

◯ AIDS Education For The Health Care Worker (Computer Assisted)

Substance Abuse Education, Inc.

PAMPHLETS

❷ AIDS Safe S & M

Community Outreach Risk Reduction Education Program (CORE)
5 pages; Nov 1988; $.50; English.

This pamphlet discusses in detail most common S&M sexual activities, explaining methods to reduce risks associated with each activity.

Reviewers' Comments: This pamphlet is well done and appropriate for both men and women. It's discussion of the topic is frank and candid. There is space available for listing local resources. The print size is too small, but otherwise it is well designed.

▲ For Ordering Information, see p. 217

❶ Face AIDS With Facts

Gay and Lesbian Community Services Center
16 pages; photographs; 1987; free; English.

This pamphlet provides basic information about the origin and spread of the AIDS virus and the means of lessening the risk of infection. It describes risky sexual behaviors in general terms and provides names and addresses of AIDS/HIV service providers and referral services in southern California.

Reviewers' Comments: Suited for well-educated adults, this pamphlet holds the readers interest and has a positive tone. It is lengthy enough to treat a range of issues, but brief enough to be read in five to ten minutes. The comprehensive resource section lacks resources for the Latino community.

▲ For Ordering Information, see p. 219

◯ The Hot 'n Healthy Times

Eroticus Publications

❷ What Gay And Bisexual Men Should Know About AIDS

Channing L. Bete Co., Inc.

16 pages; illustrations; 1987; special rates / discounts; English/Spanish.

Addressed to gay and bisexual men, this pamphlet describes what AIDS/HIV is and the importance of learning about it. Simple diagrams show how HIV affects the immune system, and describe typical diseases, including Pneumocystis carinii and Kaposi's sarcoma, as well as ways that HIV can affect the nervous system. A chart showing percentages of various groups who have contracted AIDS/HIV is included. How AIDS/HIV is transmitted, typical symptoms and treatments are described. AIDS/HIV prevention methods are listed and hotlines for more information are given.

Reviewers' Comments: The information is presented in a simple, direct and unbiased manner. Page four is almost too simple and therefore misleading.

▲ For Ordering Information, see p. 217

POSTERS

❷ Don't Love Your Partner To Death

D.C. Commission of Public Health

11 X 17; photographs; black & white; 1987; special rates / discounts; English.

This poster urges gay and bisexual men to have safer sex. It shows a photograph of the unclothed upper bodies of two black males embracing with a caption advising the use of condoms. It lists local Washington, D.C. phone numbers for more information.

Reviewers' Comments: This poster goes straight to the point, but is not clear on why one needs to use a condom in relationship to HIV transmission.

▲ For Ordering Information, see p. 218

❷ Good Boys

Willamette AIDS Council

14 x 20; photographs; color; 1987; $500.00; special rates / discounts; English.

In this poster, a man poses enticingly, wearing only his rain slicker and galoshes, over the message "Good Boys Always Wear Their Rubbers." Produced for a state-wide media campaign in Oregon but rejected for being "too risque."

Reviewers' Comments: This poster makes great use of humor to present a sexy, fun, pointed message. The only problem is that the message is to "protect yourself" when it should more appropriately be "protect yourself and your partner."

▲ For Ordering Information, see p. 231

❷ Last Night These Men Slept With Each Other And A Hundred More Without Knowing It

AIDS Administration for the State of Maryland Maryland C.A.R.E.S.

11 x 14; photographs; color; 1988; free; English.

Geared to homosexual males, this poster warns that ignorance about a partner's former sexual encounters may be risky. Beneath a photograph of two casually dressed men gazing into the distance, the caption encourages personal responsibility for one's actions and advocates the use of condoms as a safety measure.

Reviewers' Comments: The message can be read to imply that "sleeping with" others is unsafe. It might be seen as a message against "promiscuity" rather than one in favor of condom use.

▲ For Ordering Information, see p. 213

❶ Meet The Safety Pin

Northwest AIDS Foundation

16 x 24; photographs; color; free, limited copies; English.

The central image in this photo-poster is a pin-on-button of the black-on-yellow international traffic warning for an S-curve. A bright red textured fabric forms the background for the pin. The text says, "Your chance to tell the world that you follow the new rules of the road. Free and available here, insist on safer sex. You'll find yourself in great company. Please be safe. The Northwest AIDS Foundation."

Reviewers' Comments: Ths poster was produced as part of the Seattle "Rules of the Road" campaign and is appropriate and meaningful only in that context.

▲ For Ordering Information, see p. 225

---

❶ 1ST EDITION RECOMMENDED　❷ 2ND EDITION RECOMMENDED　○ NOT RECOMMENDED

❶ A Rubber Is A Friend In Your Pocket / Un Amigo Es Un Condón En El Bolsillo

Gay Men's Health Crisis, Inc.
 17 x 22; illustrations; color; 1987; $3.50; special rates / discounts; English/Spanish.

In Spanish and English, this poster promotes a condom as "A Friend In Your Pocket." It pictures a man's back blue jeans-pocket with the raised "O" shape of a condom showing through. Both English and Spanish versions meet the selection criteria.

Reviewers' Comments: For the gay audience, this poster provides good reinforcement for condom usage. It does not give specific information about how to use a condom.

▲ For Ordering Information, see p. 219

❶ Rubbers Are Bringing Men Together Again

Gay Men's Health Crisis, Inc.
 17 x 23; photographs; color; 1986; $3.50; special rates / discounts; English.

The bold, red captions, "Rubbers Are Bringing Men Together Again" (top) and "Condoms. Use Them" (bottom), are superimposed on a black-and-white photo of two male torsos, nipples touching.

Reviewers' Comments: The image and text of this poster effectively convey the message that the use of condoms need not detract from sexual pleasure.

▲ For Ordering Information, see p. 219

❶ Rules Of The Road

Northwest AIDS Foundation
 8 x 14; color; free, limited copies; English.

This series of posters addressed to gay and bisexual men employs the black-on-yellow traffic sign with varying symbols (e.g. "Dead End," "Detour") and text to convey information about AIDS/HIV. The information they convey include the importance of knowing about and following safer sex practices and avoiding drug and alcohol excesses. Each poster also displays the Sexual Safety Card which lists safest, possibly safe, and unsafe sexual practices. The card may be cut out of the poster.

Reviewers' Comments: Although the posters contain a large amount of information, they are eye-catching. They address a variety of safe sex issues with a frank, positive, and reassuring tone.

▲ For Ordering Information, see p. 225

❶ Safe Sex Is Coming...

Pittsburgh AIDS Task Force, Inc.
 17 x 23; photographs; color; Jun 1987; free, limited copies; English.

This poster advertises safer-sex workshops for gay and bisexual men in the Pittsburgh area. It features the obliquely lit and deeply shadowed black and white photo of the torso of a man who is reaching under his t-shirt to place his hand on his chest. The phrase "Safe Sex is Coming..." will be viewed as a double-entendre by the sexually active.

Reviewers' Comments: Although this poster is primarily an advertisement, it may alert viewers to the need for concern for safer sex.

▲ For Ordering Information, see p. 226

❷ We Can Live Together

Cascade AIDS Project
 22 x 21; photographs; black & white; 1988; $2.00, limited copies; special rates / discounts; English.

This poster is a low resolution photo of two men expressing joyful, casual affection. Across the top are the words, "We can live. Together." It urges gay men to continue to respond positively and responsibly to the threat of AIDS/HIV. Local and statewide hotline numbers for more information are provided.

Reviewers' Comments: This is a very positive message for gay men; the production is also good.

▲ For Ordering Information, see p. 216

❷ You Will See

Columbus AIDS Task Force
 19 x 25; black & white; 1988; free; English.

The black and white poster says, "You will see... (a long list of mostly male names) at the bar tonight because they Play Safe." The Columbus AIDS Task Force and local hotline numbers are included.

Reviewers' Comments: This has a simple message, but the graphics on the bottom line make the copy unclear.

▲ For Ordering Information, see p. 217

VIDEOS / FILMS

○ **Condom Commercials**
San Francisco AIDS Foundation

○ **For Our Lives**
Focus International

○ **Safe Sex - Here We Come**
San Francisco AIDS Foundation

○ **What's Next**
Gay Men's Health Crisis, Inc.

GENERAL COMMUNITY

AUDIO TAPES

❷ One Woman

Development Through Self-Reliance, Inc.
8:25 min.; 45 RPM Record; 1988; $5.00; special rates / discounts; English.

This song, performed by Oliver Motukdzi, a Zimbabwean musician, encourages listeners to "stay with one woman" to prevent AIDS/HIV. It was performed on the World AIDS Day telecast Dec. 1, 1988.

Reviewers' Comments: This record may appeal only to a narrow audience attracted to reggae music and is most appropriate for sexually active, heterosexual adults. It uses a simple medium to present a simple message of monogamy. It lacks a sense of living with AIDS/HIV and is fatalistic. It is recommended that other instructional materials be used in conjunction with the song to increase its educational value.

▲ For Ordering Information, see p. 218

BROCHURES

◯ The Acquired Immune Deficiency Syndrome

AID Atlanta, Inc.

◯ The Acquired Immune Deficiency Syndrome - Straight Or Gay, What You Know About It May Save Your Life.

AID Atlanta, Inc.

◯ Acquired Immune Deficiency Syndrome - What You Know About It May Save Your Life

Tidewater AIDS Crisis Taskforce

❷ AIDS

Anne Arundel County Public Schools
3 panels; free; 1988; English.

This brochure provides basic information about the transmission, symptoms, and prevention of AIDS/HIV. It identifies high-risk "groups" and describes two of the most common opportunistic infections. The prevention measures suggested include communication with sex partners, condom use, and abstinence from IV drug use.

▲ For Ordering Information, see p. 215

◯ AIDS

Washington State Office on HIV\AIDS

❶ AIDS: Acquired Immune Deficiency - What Everyone Needs To Know

AIDS Foundation Houston, Inc.
4 panels; graphs; free, limited copies; 1986; English.

▲ For Ordering Information, see p. 213

❶ AIDS - An Essay In Prophecy

Cristo AIDS Ministry
3 panels; free, limited copies; Oct 1985; English.

▲ For Ordering Information, see p. 218

❶ AIDS And Straight People

New York City Department of Health AIDS Education Training Unit
1 panel; free, limited copies; Feb 1987; English.

▲ For Ordering Information, see p. 225

◯ AIDS And The Antibody Test

New York City Department of Health AIDS Education Training Unit

❶ AIDS And The Safety Of The Nation's Blood Supply

American Red Cross National Headquarters
6 panels; free; Jan 1987; English/Spanish.

▲ For Ordering Information, see p. 215

❷ AIDS And TB

Hawaii State Department of Health STD/AIDS Prevention Program
3 panels; illustrations; free; 1988; English/English.

This brochure advises that Filipinos, Koreans, and other immigrants to Hawaii coming from countries where tuberculosis is still prevalent should take a TB test and an AIDS/HIV test, since a person with both AIDS and TB can die very quickly without proper care. Testing sites and AIDS hotline numbers in Hawaii are listed. The English version of this brochure meets minimum screening criteria, as do the Chinese, Ilocano, Visayan, and Tagalog translations. Translations in Japanese, Thai, Korean, and Cambodian did not meet acceptance criteria. Language reviewers were unable to assess Vietnamese, Laotion, Samoan, Tongan, and Hawaiian translations.

▲ For Ordering Information, see p. 220

◯ AIDS - Be In The Know

Cristo AIDS Ministry

❷ AIDS Discrimination Is Illegal In New York City

New York City Commission on Human Rights/AIDS Discrimination
3 panels; free; 1988; English/Spanish.

This pamphlet describes several situations in which discrimination occured against people with AIDS or people thought to have AIDS, explaining that such discrimination is forbidden by law. The work of the AIDS Discrimination Division is described and phone numbers are provided for those who seek assistance in remedying an incident of AIDS-related discrimination. Some information about transmission is also provided. The English, Spanish, and Creole versions of this meet the minimum acceptance criteria.

▲ For Ordering Information, see p. 225

◯ AIDS - Do You Know The Facts? Are You Sure?

Arizona Department of Health Services Office of Health Promotion and Education

◯ AIDS: Facts / AIDS - Hechos

Chicago Department of Health AIDS Program

❷ AIDS Facts Card

Massachusetts Department of Public Health
Card; free, limited copies; 1987; English/Spanish.

This wallet card presents basic AIDS/HIV facts primarily regarding transmission and prevention. It advocates education as an infection preventing tool and provides several Massachusetts phone numbers for more information to English speaking and Spanish speaking readers.

▲ For Ordering Information, see p. 222

❶ AIDS - Facts Of Life / AIDS Hechos Vitales

Sacramento AIDS Foundation
4 panels; free, limited copies; Feb 1988; English/Spanish.

▲ For Ordering Information, see p. 227

◯ AIDS Facts: The Antibody Test / SIDA Realidad: Examen Anticuerpos

Chicago Department of Health AIDS Program

◯ AIDS: Fear And Facts

Public Affairs Committee, Inc.

◯ AIDS - How To Avoid It / AIDS Cómo Evitar Contraerlo

Connecticut Department of Health Services AIDS Program

❷ AIDS - How You Can Prevent Its Spread

Krames Communications
4 panels; illustrations; 1987; $1.10; special rates / discounts; English/Spanish.

This pamphlet uses color illustrations and text to describe AIDS, ARC, high and low risk behavior, and how AIDS/HIV is and is not transmitted. It encourages the reader to educate others about AIDS/HIV and to support AIDS/HIV research and education efforts.

▲ For Ordering Information, see p. 222

❶ 1ST EDITION RECOMMENDED   ❷ 2ND EDITION RECOMMENDED   ◯ NOT RECOMMENDED

❶ AIDS In Your Neighborhood

New York City Department of Health AIDS Education Training Unit
3 panels; illustrations; free, limited copies; Feb 1987; English/Spanish.

▲ For Ordering Information, see p. 225

❷ AIDS Information

Hawaii State Department of Health STD/AIDS Prevention Program
4 panels; free; 1988; English.

General information about AIDS/HIV is provided in this brochure, including what the virus is, symptoms, modes of transmission, risk groups, AIDS/HIV prevention methods, testing, and treatment. Hotline numbers are listed for Hawaii.

▲ For Ordering Information, see p. 220

◯ AIDS Information

Merced County Health Department

❶ AIDS Information That Everyone Ought To Know

Virginia Department of Health - AIDS Program
3 panels; Jun 1987; English.

▲ For Ordering Information, see p. 231

**❶ AIDS - Learn And Live /
Aprenda Y Viva - SIDA**

Massachusetts Department of Public Health
6 panels; free, limited copies; Sep 1987; English/Spanish.

▲ For Ordering Information, see p. 222

**❶ AIDS Lifeline - The Best Defense Against AIDS Is Information /
AIDS / Cable De Salvamento - La Mejor Defensa En Contra El AIDS Es Información**

San Francisco AIDS Foundation
3 panels; free, limited copies; 1987; English/Spanish.

▲ For Ordering Information, see p. 227

❶ AIDS: Prevention Is Your Business

Dimension Communications Network (DCN)/RAMSCO Publishing Co.
2 panels; illustrations; $.20; special rates / discounts; 1986; English.

▲ For Ordering Information, see p. 218

◯ AIDS: Protect Yourself And Those You Care About

New York State Department of Health

❶ AIDS Questions And Answers

Denver Disease Control Service
3 panels; illustrations; free, limited copies; Sep 1986; English.

▲ For Ordering Information, see p. 218

❶ AIDS - Questions, Answers

American Social Health Association
4 panels; free, limited copies; special rates / discounts; 1987; English.

▲ For Ordering Information, see p. 215

◯ AIDS: Reducing The Risk

AIDS Foundation Houston, Inc.

**◯ AIDS-Related Complex - Putting It In Perspective /
Complejo Relacionado Con El SIDA (AIDS) Y Sus Manifestaciones**

Gay and Lesbian Community Services Center

❶ AIDS Risk - A Reference Guide

Health Education Resource Organization (HERO)
1 panel; $.15, limited copies; 1987; English.

▲ For Ordering Information, see p. 220

❷ AIDS / SIDA

AIDS Project Los Angeles
4 panels; $.25; special rates / discounts; 1988; English/Spanish.

This brochure defines AIDS/HIV and opportunistic infections. It includes a list of symptoms but stresses that symptoms do not necessarily indicate a diagnosis of AIDS. It discusses high-risk behaviors, how to take precautions against transmission of HIV, and how to offer help through community organizations. Southern California AIDS Hotline numbers are listed.

▲ For Ordering Information, see p. 213

○ AIDS - The Best Defense Against AIDS Is Information.

San Mateo County AIDS Project

❶ AIDS - The Equal Opportunity Syndrome

Dallas County Health Department
3 panels; illustrations & photographs; free, limited copies; 1987; English/Spanish.

▲ For Ordering Information, see p. 218

○ AIDS - The Facts

Idaho Department of Health and Welfare AIDS Program

○ AIDS: The Facts

American Red Cross National Headquarters

❷ AIDS: The Facts

Dimension Communications Network (DCN)/RAMSCO Publishing Co.
2 panels; $.20; special rates / discounts; 1986; English.

In bulleted paragraphs, this brochure describes the AIDS virus and modes of transmission, and clears up various myths about transmission, including the idea that HIV is spread by non-sexual, casual contact (e.g., touching dishes, linens, etc., that have been used by an infected person). The U.S. Public Health Service AIDS hotline is listed for further information.

▲ For Ordering Information, see p. 218

❷ AIDS: The Facts

NO/AIDS Task Force
2 panels; $.10; special rates / discounts; 1988; English.

This brochure provides very basic AIDS/HIV information. It defines AIDS and describes HIV transmission, including information about blood transfusions, blood donation, and casual contact. Questions such as "Can you tell if someone has the virus?" and "What are some of the symptoms of AIDS?" are answered. Local and statewide hotline phone numbers are included.

▲ For Ordering Information, see p. 225

○ AIDS: The Facts And The Fallacies

University Hospitals of Cleveland

❷ AIDS: The More We Know, The Less We Have To Fear

D.C. Commission of Public Health
3 panels; special rates / discounts; 1988; English/Spanish.

This brochure is designed to provide basic information about AIDS/HIV to the general community. It explains what AIDS/HIV is, what behaviors spread the virus, that there is no risk in casual contact, how to protect yourself and others, what the signs and symptoms are, counseling and testing, and that AIDS/HIV-related descrimination is illegal. Several D.C. phone numbers are listed for information and testing.

▲ For Ordering Information, see p. 218

❶ AIDS: The New Epidemic

Abbott Laboratories
4 panels; illustrations; free, limited copies; Apr 1987; English.

▲ For Ordering Information, see p. 213

❶ AIDS: What Everyone Needs To Know

North Central Florida AIDS Network
3 panels; illustrations; free, limited copies; Sep 1987; English.

▲ For Ordering Information, see p. 225

○ AIDS - What Everyone Should Know

New Mexico AIDS Services, Inc.

❶ 1ST EDITION RECOMMENDED   ❷ 2ND EDITION RECOMMENDED   ○ NOT RECOMMENDED

❶ AIDS: What Everyone Should Know

New York City Department of Health AIDS Education Training Unit
3 panels; illustrations; English/Spanish.

▲ For Ordering Information, see p. 225

❶ AIDS: What You Should Know

Tennessee Department of Health and Environment
3 panels; free; English.

▲ For Ordering Information, see p. 229

❷ AIDS: Why Take Chances?

Wisconsin Division of Health, AIDS/HIV Program
3 panels; free; 1988; English.

This brochure informs the general population on basic facts about AIDS/HIV. Activities that can and cannot transmit HIV are included. Ways to protect oneself from infection by not sharing needles, abstaining from sexual contact, limiting the number of sexual partners, and using condoms are also included. Persons who are described as at higher risk for the virus are urged to discuss the need for an HIV antibody test with a physician.

▲ For Ordering Information, see p. 231

◯ America Responds To AIDS Point Of Purchase Materials

CDC National AIDS Information and Education Program

◯ Answers About AIDS

St. Louis Efforts for AIDS

◯ Answers To Commonly Asked Questions About AIDS

Greater Cincinnati AIDS Task Force University of Cincinnati Medical Center

◯ Cook County Hospital: Questions & Answers

Cook County Hospital AIDS Service

❶ Could I Get AIDS?

Maryland Department of Health and Mental Hygiene AIDS Administration
3 panels; illustrations; free, limited copies; May 1987; English.

▲ For Ordering Information, see p. 222

❶ Could I Get AIDS?

St. Paul Division of Public Health
3 panels; charts; Oct 1987; English.

▲ For Ordering Information, see p. 228

◯ Current Information About Sexual Behavior Relating To Potential HIV Infection

County of Riverside Department of Health

◯ Do You Know The Facts? Questions And Answers About Acquired Immune Deficiency Syndrome

AIDS Task Force of Winston-Salem

◯ Exploring Another "Religious" Myth...AIDS And Africa

Cristo AIDS Ministry

❷ Fact Sheet No. 12 - I Know Someone With AIDS: Can I Shake Hands With Them? Can They Serve Me Food?

Gay Community AIDS Project
3 panels; $.10; 1988; English.

This brochure presents quotes from research journals suggesting that there is no evidence that HIV is spread through casual contact. A list of resources is included.

▲ For Ordering Information, see p. 219

◯ Fact Sheet No. 2 - How Is HIV ("The AIDS Virus") Transmitted?

Gay Community AIDS Project

❷ **Fact Sheet No. 5 - Saliva And AIDS**

Gay Community AIDS Project
3 panels; $.10; 1988; English.

This brochure is designed to help answer the question of whether HIV can be transmitted by saliva. Quotes from studies published in the New England Journal of Medicine, the New York Times, and others are used to support the view that saliva is not a vehicle for the transmission of HIV. A list of other GCAP fact sheets and publications and how to obtain them is provided.

▲ For Ordering Information, see p. 219

❶ **Fact Versus Fiction: Ten Things You Should Know About AIDS**

San Francisco AIDS Foundation
2 panels; free, limited copies; English.

▲ For Ordering Information, see p. 227

◯ **The Facts About...AIDS**

South Carolina Dept. of Health and Environmental Control Bureau of Preventive Health Services

❶ **Facts You Should Know About AIDS**

Texas Medical Association Committee on Sexually Transmitted Diseases
4 panels; free, limited copies; Dec 1987; English.

▲ For Ordering Information, see p. 229

◯ **Facts About AIDS / Datos Sobre SIDA**

U.S. Government, Centers for Disease Control - National AIDS Hotline, National AIDS Information / Education Program

◯ **Facts The Public Should Know About AIDS**

Columbus AIDS Task Force

◯ **The Facts...AIDS**

Georgia Department of Human Resources

❶ **HIV (AIDS Virus) Infection**

Mississippi State Department of Health
3 panels; illustrations; free, limited copies; Oct 1987; English.

▲ For Ordering Information, see p. 223

◯ **Idaho Women And AIDS**

Idaho Department of Health and Welfare AIDS Program

❶ **Imagine...What If Sex Could Be Better...And Safer**

Maryland Department of Health and Mental Hygiene AIDS Administration
4 panels; illustrations; free, limited copies; 1987; English.

▲ For Ordering Information, see p. 222

◯ **Is AIDS God's Wrath On Homosexuals?**

Cristo AIDS Ministry

❶ **Kids And AIDS**

New York City Department of Health AIDS Education Training Unit
1 page; free, limited copies; Feb 1987; English.

▲ For Ordering Information, see p. 225

◯ **Latest Facts About AIDS - AIDS, Sex, And You**

American Red Cross National Headquarters

◯ **Latest Facts About AIDS - Facts About AIDS And Drug Abuse**

American Red Cross National Headquarters

◯ **Living With Safer Sex - AIDS - A Matter Of Choices And Chances**

Oak Lawn Counseling Center AIDS Program

❶ 1ST EDITION RECOMMENDED ❷ 2ND EDITION RECOMMENDED ◯ NOT RECOMMENDED

② Love In The 1980's

Planned Parenthood of New York City
4 panels; $.50; special rates / discounts; 1988; English.

This flyer provides information on the proper use of condoms and contraceptive foam. In simple language it emphasizes the importance of practicing safer sex and gives information about birth control options.

▲ For Ordering Information, see p. 226

❶ Myths And Facts About AIDS

Cascade AIDS Project
2 panels; free; 1988; English.

▲ For Ordering Information, see p. 216

◯ New Lepers

Cristo AIDS Ministry

❶ No-Nonsense AIDS Answers

Blue Cross and Blue Shield Association
2 panels; photographs; $.35; 1987; English.

▲ For Ordering Information, see p. 216

◯ Person To Person

AIDS Administration for the State of Maryland Maryland C.A.R.E.S.

❶ Q And A About AIDS

Seattle-King County Department of Public Health
7 panels; illustrations; $.15; Apr 1986; English.

▲ For Ordering Information, see p. 228

◯ Questions & Answers - AIDS / Preguntas Y Respuestas: El SIDA

Philadelphia AIDS Task Force

② Safe Acts: Facts About AIDS

Howard Brown Memorial Clinic
3 panels; special rates / discounts; 1988; English.

This brochure answers commonly asked questions about AIDS/HIV including what the virus is, how it is transmitted, high risk behavior, and how transmission can be prevented. Basic information on testing for the HIV antibody is included. The Illinois AIDS Hotline and numbers of the Howard Brown Memorial Clinic are listed.

▲ For Ordering Information, see p. 221

❶ Save Lives. Give Blood. It's Safe. It's Necessary.

American Association of Blood Banks National Office
2 panels; illustrations; special rates / discounts; 1988; English.

▲ For Ordering Information, see p. 214

② Social Security Card

Illinois Alcoholism and Drug Dependence Association
card; illustrations; special rates / discounts; 1987; English.

This wallet card provides general information about AIDS/HIV and its relationship of AIDS to sex and drugs. It encourages readers to seek the "social security" gained through transmission prevention behaviors. It contains information specific to Illinois; however, camera-ready art is available for agencies in other states who wish to reprint the materials.

▲ For Ordering Information, see p. 221

② Some Facts About AIDS

Ohio Department of Health - AIDS Unit
4 panels; free, limited copies; Mar 1987; English.

This brochure offers the general community an overview of AIDS/HIV--its definition, causes, transmission, and prevention. Testing, symptoms, treatment, and pregnancy are also covered. Ohio and national hotline numbers are included.

▲ For Ordering Information, see p. 225

❷ **Symptoms Of AIDS And ARC**

Illinois Alcoholism and Drug Dependence Association
Card; illustrations; special rates / discounts; 1987; English/Spanish.

This folding wallet-sized card displays nine symptoms related to HIV infection including general symptoms and symptoms of related infections. The symptom descriptions are simple, concise, and accompanied by illustrations. It contains resource information specific to Illinois; however, camera-ready art is available for agencies in other states who wish to reprint the materials. The Spanish translation meets the minimum acceptance criteria.

▲ For Ordering Information, see p. 221

❷ **Those Who Think. . .**

Damien Ministries
1 page; illustrations; free, limited copies; 1987; English.

This leaflet shows a picture of a man who looks like a priest or minister compassionately embracing a person who is suffering. In black calligraphy letters, the message reads: "Those who think AIDS is a plague sent by God have never met our God."

▲ For Ordering Information, see p. 218

○ **Understanding AIDS**

CDC National AIDS Information and Education Program

❷ **Understanding And Preventing AIDS**

Krames Communications
3 panels; illustrations; $.50; special rates / discounts; 1987; English/Spanish.

This brochure uses illustrations and text to describe what AIDS/HIV is, how it affects the body, low risks behaviors, and behavior with no risk of viral transmission. Also included is a true-false test that measures the reader's knowledge of AIDS/HIV.

▲ For Ordering Information, see p. 222

○ **Update: Information On AIDS**

Wellness Networks, Inc. - Flint

○ **What Do We Know About AIDS?**

ETR Associates/Network Publications

❶ **What Everyone Should Know About AIDS**

North Carolina AIDS Control Program
4 panels; free; Oct 1987; English.

▲ For Ordering Information, see p. 225

❶ **What Everyone Should Know About AIDS And HIV / Lo Que Todos Deben Saber Acerca Del AIDS Y El HIV**

Texas Department of Health Bureau of AIDS and STD Control
3 panels; illustrations; free; Nov 1987; English/Spanish.

▲ For Ordering Information, see p. 229

○ **What Everyone Should Know About AIDS - Information For The General Public**

Montana Department of Health & Environmental Sciences Montana AIDS Program

○ **What Is AIDS?**

Washington State Office on HIV\AIDS

❷ **What You Should Know About AIDS**

U.S. Government, Centers for Disease Control AIDS Information/Education Program
4 panels; 1987; English.

This brochure provides facts about AIDS/HIV, how to protect yourself and your family, and what to tell others. It is a component of the America Responds to AIDS public awareness campaign.

▲ For Ordering Information, see p. 230

❶ 1ST EDITION RECOMMENDED ❷ 2ND EDITION RECOMMENDED ○ NOT RECOMMENDED

◯ **What You Should Know About HIV Antibody Testing**

Connecticut State Department of Health

❶ **What You Should Know About The AIDS Virus But Were Afraid To Ask**

Tidewater AIDS Crisis Taskforce
3 panels; illustrations; $.10; Dec 1987; English.

▲ For Ordering Information, see p. 229

◯ **What You Should Know About The Antibody Test**

ETR Associates/Network Publications

◯ **What's Safe And What's Not**

Northwest AIDS Foundation

◯ **Why Be In The Dark About AIDS**

Health Issues Taskforce of Cleveland

◯ **You Can Prevent AIDS - Fight The Fear With The Facts**

Connecticut Department of Health Services AIDS Program

❶ **Your Health Is Our Concern**

American Dental Association Division of Communications
2 panels; photographs; free, limited copies; 1986; English.

▲ For Ordering Information, see p. 214

❶ **Your Test Is Positive**

Mississippi State Department of Health
2 panels; free, limited copies; Oct 1987; English.

▲ For Ordering Information, see p. 223

INSTRUCTIONAL PROGRAMS

◯ **AIDS - Acquired Immune Deficiency Syndrome**

Maryland Department of Health and Mental Hygiene AIDS Administration

◯ **Maryland C.A.R.E.S Training Curriculum**

AIDS Administration for the State of Maryland Maryland C.A.R.E.S.

MULTICOMPONENT PROGRAMS

❶ AIDS Facts For Life

- **Brochures**
  1987; free, limited copies; English.
- **General Purpose Fact Sheet**
  8 1/2 x 11; 1987; free, limited copies; English.
- **Media Fact Sheet**
  8 1/2 x 11; 1987; free, limited copies; English.
- **Poster**
  17 x 22; 1987; free, limited copies; English/Spanish.
- **Wallet Card**
  1987; free, limited copies; English.

**Illinois Department of Public Health
AIDS Facts for Life**

This public service campaign kit contains a series of information and educational materials issued under the unifying theme "AIDS - Facts for Life." It includes: 1) a two-sided media fact sheet with basic and medical facts on AIDS/HIV; 2) a two-sided general purpose fact sheet in the form of a 10-question quiz; 3) a wallet-size card with seven basic AIDS/HIV facts and an Illinois State AIDS Hotline number; 4) English and Spanish language versions of a 17" x 22" poster, presenting 10 facts on AIDS/HIV; and 5-7) three multi-paneled brochures, in question and answer format, providing basic facts on HIV-antibody testing; answers to the 10 most frequently asked questions about AIDS/HIV; and details on procedures for premarital blood tests for AIDS required in Illinois since January 1988.

Reviewers' Comments: This visually attractive set of print materials provides information relevant to the general public rather than to any specific population. The media fact sheet is quite technical and would need adaptation for use in mass media. The brochure on antibody testing is particularly well done. The kit is specific to citizens of Illinois, although certain components could serve as models for other public service campaigns.

▲ For Ordering Information, see p. 221

❶ AIDS Media Campaign

Michigan Department of Public Health Special Offices on AIDS Prevention
Jan 1988; English.

8 TV spots and 12 radio spots of varying lengths;
(4) 8 1/2" x 11" posters, 1-color photographs;
(4) 6 1/4" x 10" print ads.

This AIDS/HIV prevention multi-media campaign focuses on IV drug users and their significant others, high school and college students, and the general public of Michigan. Of the eight TV commercials, three address public fears about AIDS/HIV and people with AIDS/HIV. Three commercials urge teenagers not to share dirty needles or have sex with someone who shares needles and to use condoms. Two other TV commercials warn sex partners of drug users who share needles. The radio commercials present similar messages. The print ads urge parents to educate their children about AIDS/HIV and advocates condom use, safe sex behaviors, and sanitary drug use habits. The campaign stresses education, drug abstinence, and monogamy as preventive measures. It opposes mandatory testing for the AIDS virus.

Reviewers' Comments: These ads and posters present the dangers of AIDS/HIV in a powerful manner. Particularly effective are the messages aimed at IV drug users.

▲ For Ordering Information, see p. 223

◯ AIDS 101 Slideshow

San Francisco AIDS Foundation

◯ AIDS Visual Education Packet Transparancies And Outline For Presentation

AIDS-Related Community Services

❶ 1ST EDITION RECOMMENDED ❷ 2ND EDITION RECOMMENDED ◯ NOT RECOMMENDED

PAMPHLETS

◯ **AIDS**

T.H.E. Clinic Asian Health Project

◯ **AIDS: Acquired Immune Deficiency Syndrome**

Nevada AIDS Foundation

◯ **AIDS Alcohol And Drugs**

Washington State Office on HIV\AIDS

◯ **AIDS: Education For A Safe Future**

The Knowledge Well

◯ **AIDS Information Booklet - Family Edition**

Center One Anyone In Distress

◯ **AIDS: 100 Questions And Answers**

National Sheriffs' Association

❷ **AIDS: Questions And Answers**

Planned Parenthood Federation of America
13 pages; stapled; Jan 1987; $.75; English.

This pamphlet provides technical information about AIDS and addresses questions regarding its causes and transmission, high-risk populations, symptoms, diagnosis, antibody testing, methods of prevention (e.g. "safer sex" guidelines), what pregnant women should do if they are exposed to HIV, and blood transfusion/donation. A final section discusses the ingredients for a supportive environment and addresses myths that surround the disease. It also lists additional resources and hotline numbers.

Reviewers' Comments: The information on AIDS and birth control, syringe cleaning techniques, and care and community support for people with AIDS is particularly valuable. It does, however, require high reading comprehension.

▲ For Ordering Information, see p. 226

❶ **Answers About AIDS**

American Council on Science and Health
60 pages; charts; Feb 1988; $2.00; English.

This pamphlet answers some of the most frequently asked questions about AIDS/HIV. It covers symptoms, risk factors, high-risk groups, fatality rates, causes and methods of virus transmission, clinical manifestations, development of the disease, racial aspects of AIDS/HIV epidemiology, and the economic impact of AIDS/HIV. It also discusses the origin of AIDS/HIV, the safety of the blood supply, HIV antibody testing, treatment possibilities, and the status of vaccine development. It lists precautions for heterosexuals, homosexuals, and IV drug users. References are updated through January 1988.

Reviewers' Comments: This publication may be too detailed for the general public, but it is an excellent resource for health care professionals, educators and physicians.

▲ For Ordering Information, see p. 214

❷ **A Closer Look At AIDS**

Health Councils of Pasco-Pinellas and West-Central Florida, Inc.
32 pages; Sep 1988; free, limited copies; English.

This pamphlet contains basic information on AIDS/HIV, how it is spread, and its prevention and treatment. AIDS/HIV in the workplace, schools, and day care centers are briefly addressed. A resources section lists Florida support groups, patient care, counseling and testing sites, educational materials, and both local and national AIDS organizations.

Reviewers' Comments: This pamphlet is recommended only for residents of West-Central Florida to whom the listed resources apply. There is good information on proper precautions and Florida resources. However, the reading level (10th grade) is high, and the terminology is problematic. As examples, the words "illicit" and "illegal" are used in relation to drug use, which is value-laden beyond the concerns of AIDS/HIV prevention; and the terms "AIDS virus" and "HIV" are used interchangeably without full explanation.

▲ For Ordering Information, see p. 220

◯ **Handbook On Acquired Immune Deficiency Syndrome**

Medical Surveillance, Inc. MED-ED Productions

○ Knowledge Protects

Maryland Department of Health and Mental Hygiene AIDS Administration

❷ Living With AIDS: A United Church Of Christ Perspective

United Church Board for Homeland Ministries AIDS Program
20 pages; photographs; 1988; $.60; English.

This booklet contains a series of articles reporting the involvement of church members in the fight against AIDS/HIV, the care of persons with AIDS/HIV, the dissemination of AIDS/HIV information, and the building of support relating to AIDS/HIV issues within the religious community. Each article is accompanied by a personal statement by, and a photograph of, the involved person or family.

Reviewers' Comments: This provides the church community with information which encourages involvement in providing care and support of people with AIDS/HIV. The content was accurate, except for the use of the term "HTLV III" rather than "HIV."

▲ For Ordering Information, see p. 230

❶ Medical Answers About AIDS

Gay Men's Health Crisis, Inc.
70 pages; May 1987; $2.00; special rates / discounts; English.

This pamphlet serves as a general, rather than detailed, guide to the known facts about AIDS/HIV for the general public, for persons with AIDS/HIV and those at risk for HIV, their families and friends, and health care providers. It covers definitions, modes of transmission, symptoms, diagnosis and treatment, prevention, and risk reduction. It also discusses the future of the AIDS epidemic. Appendices supply more detailed background information of The Centers for Disease Control's classification system for HIV/AIDS infections and case definition for adults and children. This section also includes information relating to homosexuality, civil liberties, and the preventive medicine of AIDS/HIV.

Reviewers' Comments: This booklet is thorough and offers very accurate information on every aspect of AIDS/HIV. It takes complex medical information and translates it adequately for educated non-medical readers.

▲ For Ordering Information, see p. 219

○ Microscopic Monster

National AIDS Prevention Institute

❶ 100 Questions And Answers About AIDS/ 100 Preguntas y Respuestas - SIDA/ AIDS

New York State Department of Health
22 pages; Apr 1988; special rates / discounts; English/Spanish.

This pamphlet uses a question and answer format to cover AIDS/HIV-related topics such as high-risk "groups", transmission, incidence, diagnosis and treatment, AIDS/HIV in children, prevention, care for AIDS/HIV patients, testing, human rights issues, and risk reduction. Hotline numbers for New York state counseling and testing programs are listed.

Reviewers' Comments: The content is accurate and although it contains statistics and resources which are specific to New York, most of the information is appropriate for distribution in any state.

▲ For Ordering Information, see p. 225

❶ Protecting Yourself From AIDS

Channing L. Bete Co., Inc.
16 pages; 1988; special rates / discounts; English/Spanish.

This pamphlet provides a general overview of AIDS/HIV, with emphasis on protection. It explains the acronyms "AIDS" and "HIV" and outlines ways the virus is and is not transmitted. It emphasizes that anyone who has sex with an infected partner is at risk and suggests sex should be restricted to one faithful partner who doesn't use IV drugs. Abstinence, safer sex activities only, or condom use if there is a possibility a sexual partner may be infected are recommended. Details of safe condom use are given. AIDS/HIV symptoms, the HIV antibody test, and what to do if the test is positive are described.

Reviewers' Comments: This pamphlet provides accurate, up-to-date information and presents useful alternatives for those who feel they might be HIV infected. It is a clear overview which serves as a good introduction to HIV antibody testing. Its weaknesses are that it does not urge the reader to find out more about the pros and cons of HIV antibody testing, and it appears biased toward opting to take the test. The written information is inconsistent with the graphic presentation, which is very simple and seems suited for a younger audience.

▲ For Ordering Information, see p. 217

---

❶ 1ST EDITION RECOMMENDED   ❷ 2ND EDITION RECOMMENDED   ○ NOT RECOMMENDED

❶ Questions And Answers About Acquired Immune Deficiency Syndrome (AIDS)

Maine Department of Human Services Office on AIDS

21 pages; Mar 1987; English.

This pamphlet presents 91 questions and answers about AIDS/HIV, covering all aspects of the disease. It discusses public policy, the quarantine and isolation of people with AIDS/HIV, mandatory versus voluntary testing, and prejudicial treatment of children and teachers with AIDS/HIV in the public schools. It uses frank language to describe sexual practices. The pamphlet provides AIDS/HIV statistics and resources for the state of Maine.

Reviewers' Comments: The pamphlet contains good policy information and thorough coverage of AIDS/HIV issues.

▲ For Ordering Information, see p. 222

❶ What Do You Know About AIDS? - The National AIDS Awareness Test

Metropolitan Life Insurance Company

12 pages; 1987; free; English.

In true/false and multiple-choice formats, this brochure offers the 55 questions and answers about AIDS/HIV used in the videotape, "What Do You Know About AIDS? The National Awareness Test." The self-administered test briefly conveys how AIDS/HIV is spread, how to avoid infection, and the results of infection. It also gives facts on the numbers of people affected, the cost of AIDS care, and HIV antibody tests. It discusses sexual behaviors in general terms.

Reviewers' Comments: This awareness test is easily usable by anyone with a moderate reading level, although it does contain references to points that might be familiar only to persons already knowledgeable about AIDS/HIV (e.g., a reference to AZT, an AIDS medication). The statistics may need updating.

▲ For Ordering Information, see p. 223

❶ What Everyone Should Know About AIDS

Channing L. Bete Co., Inc.

8 pages; illustrations; 1985; special rates / discounts; English/Spanish.

An overview of AIDS/HIV issues, this pamphlet is directed to the general public, using a mixture of cartoons and sentences scattered around the page in various typefaces. AIDS is defined and the importance of knowing about AIDS to prevent disease and separate fact from myth is emphasized. Described are: HIV and its modes of transmission, its effects on the body, methods of protection, and treatments.

Reviewers' Comments: The high level of written information in this pamphlet is inconsistent with the graphic presentation, which is very simple and seems suited for a much younger audience.

▲ For Ordering Information, see p. 217

POSTERS

❶ AIDS Does Not Discriminate / El SIDA No Discrimina

New York State Department of Health
11 x 13 1/2; photographs; color; English/Spanish.

This full-color photo-poster pictures nine individuals of different sexes, cultural groups, ages, and occupations. The text states, "Anyone can get AIDS from sexual contact or sharing needles with an infected person. But we know how to prevent AIDS. Learn how to protect yourself." Both Spanish and English versions of this poster meet the selection criteria.

Reviewers' Comments: This colorful poster elicits the viewer's attention and effectively expresses the mutli-ethnic importance of AIDS/HIV.

▲ For Ordering Information, see p. 225

◯ AIDS Doesn't Care

Massachusetts Department of Public Health

❷ AIDS Posters

Health Issues Taskforce of Cleveland
8 1/2 x 11; black & white; 1987; free, limited copies; English.

These six black and white posters convey basic facts about HIV infection, its transmission, and prevention. The posters are titled: We've Got AIDS Too, AIDS Does Not Discriminate, It's Not Easy To Get AIDS, How AIDS Multiplies, Controlling AIDS Is Up To You, AIDS Is No One's Fault/Everyone's Concern. They were designed for display in offices, clinics, schools and other public areas. Some are specific to the Cleveland community; others can be used nationwide. The posters are available in various sizes.

Reviewers' Comments: The posters convey a great deal of information in a small space, using small type. While specific to the Cleveland area, these can serve as models for other areas.

▲ For Ordering Information, see p. 220

❶ AIDS: The Equal Opportunity Syndrome

Oak Lawn Counseling Center AIDS Program
18 x 24; photographs; English.

This poster shows a photograph of a black woman's hand clasping a white man's hand. Above this, the message reads: "AIDS - The Equal Opportunity Syndrome." The remaining text reads "Get the Facts" and lists a local hotline number.

Reviewers' Comments: The bi-racial handshake speaks to the multi-ethnicity of AIDS/HIV, but might also appear to be addressing bi-racial brotherhood.

▲ For Ordering Information, see p. 225

◯ Anyone Can Get AIDS

Brooklyn AIDS Task Force

◯ Choose Your Life

Brooklyn AIDS Task Force

❶ Does Someone You Know Have To Get AIDS Before You'll Help?

Long Island Association For AIDS Care, Inc.
11 x 14; photographs; color; 1987; special rates / discounts; English.

This poster shows a middle-aged woman comforting a young man as they clasp hands over a table. The poster appeals for AIDS volunteers who can staff hotline phones, work in education programs, be a "buddy," or contribute money to the sponsoring agency.

Reviewers' Comments: The quality of the poster is good, although it appeals to one's sense of guilt for motivation.

▲ For Ordering Information, see p. 222

❷ Fight The Fear With Facts

AIDS Project Los Angeles
17 x 13 1/2; photographs; black & white; 1986; $2.00; special rates / discounts; English.

This poster displays a black and white photograph of a candellight AIDS vigil. The headline reads "Fight The Fear With Facts," and provides a toll-free number for AIDS/HIV information.

Reviewers' Comments: This serves primarily to convey a California state hotline telephone number.

▲ For Ordering Information, see p. 213

❶ 1ST EDITION RECOMMENDED   ❷ 2ND EDITION RECOMMENDED   ◯ NOT RECOMMENDED

❶ Graphic Message Display

Health Education Learning Programs, Inc.
5 x 6; photographs; color; Feb 1987; $12.00.

This display kit includes 12 message-cards (one for each month) which fit into the plexiglas, stick-on frame. Intended for office or restaurant restroom walls, the slogans and graphics convey warnings about alcohol and drug use and about AIDS/HIV, its causes, transmission, and methods of prevention. A toll-free hotline number appears on each card.

▲ For Ordering Information, see p. 220

❶ His Father Disowned Him

Long Island Association For AIDS Care, Inc.
11 x 14; photographs; color; 1987; special rates / discounts; English.

This poster shows a troubled, upper-middle class, young, white man with a Kaposi's sarcoma lesion on his forehead. The poster mentions his isolation and ostracism in bold white letters superimposed on the black and white photograph. This poster is primarily the organization's appeal for volunteers for its people with AIDS support programs.

Reviewers' Comments: This poster presents an effective message to address the need for volunteeers, but may imply that the person with AIDS is a "victim."

▲ For Ordering Information, see p. 222

❶ I'm Not Gay, I Don't Shoot Drugs - I Got AIDS

Long Island Association For AIDS Care, Inc.
11 x 14; photographs; color; 1987; special rates / discounts; English.

This poster depicts, in a black-and-white photograph, a young woman with her arms folded. The young woman has tears in her eyes and has a pained and indignant expression as she states, "I'm not gay. I don't shoot drugs. I got AIDS." This poster reinforces the idea that HIV is indiscriminate in whom it infects. The poster invites the viewer to contact the Long Island Association for AIDS Care for more information about AIDS/HIV.

Reviewers' Comments: In addition to encouraging the viewer to obtain more information, the poster underscores the need for all sexually active adults to be concerned about AIDS/HIV.

▲ For Ordering Information, see p. 222

❶ Ignore AIDS And It Will Bury The Rest Of You

Oregon Health Division, HIV Program
22 1/2 x 30; illustrations; color; 1988; $5.00; English.

Stark modern art depicts rigid block figures with their heads beneath the ground. The message, "Ignore AIDS and it will bury the rest of you," urges readers not to stick their heads in the sand regarding the risk of AIDS/HIV.

Reviewers' Comments: This poster will probably have the greatest impact upon those persons with a relatively sophisticated artistic sense. It will be useful in raising consciousness about the gravity of the AIDS epidemic; no referral numbers or other information are included.

▲ For Ordering Information, see p. 226

◯ It's Very Difficult To Learn About AIDS. You Have To Make A Phone Call.

Long Island Association For AIDS Care, Inc.

❷ Keep Columbus Beautiful

Columbus AIDS Task Force
19 x 25; photographs; black & white; 1988; free; English.

The center of this poster is a photograph of condoms and condom packages. large letters above the picture say, "KEEP COLUMBUS BEAUTIFUL," and below, "USE THESE." Columbus Task Force and hotline numbers are included.

Reviewers' Comments: This is a very comprehensive guide with an excellent discussion about sex for people who are diagnosed as HIV positive. The reading level is high and there is not enough material on discrimination. Overall it is a good handbook, but may be overwhelming for people who have tested positive recently.

▲ For Ordering Information, see p. 217

❶ My Daughter Died Of AIDS. And Now I Have To Live With The Fact That I Never Helped Her.

Long Island Association For AIDS Care, Inc.
11 x 14; photographs; color; 1987; special rates / discounts; English.

In the dark black-and-white photgraphic poster, a grieving middle-aged father in a working man's plaid flannel shirt knits his brow and laces his fingers before him, confessing that he failed to help his daughter before she died of AIDS. By sharing this father's anguish and self-recrimintion, the poster urges the viewer to volunteer for the Long Island Association for AIDS Care's support programs for persons with AIDS/HIV.

Reviewers' Comments: Although this poster relies upon guilt to convey its message, it nevertheless succeeds in evoking compassion for people with AIDS/HIV and their families.

▲ For Ordering Information, see p. 222

❶ No One Can Afford To Ignore AIDS - You Owe It To Yourself To Get The Facts

Idaho Department of Health and Welfare AIDS Program
17 x 11; photographs; color; free; English.

This small poster features a black and white photograph of a large group of people who represent a broad spectrum of Idaho's citizens. With everybody smiling and standing very close, the image reinforces the idea that AIDS/HIV does not discriminate among those whom it infects, and that it is a community concern that people face together.

Reviewers' Comments: The poster does make its point that AIDS/HIV is a community concern. A single hotline number would be helpful and less confusing to viewers.

▲ For Ordering Information, see p. 221

◯ Protegete Contra SIDA / Protect Yourself Against AIDS

Los Angeles Centers for Alcohol & Drug Abuse

◯ Some Diseases Are Getting Away With Murder

Columbus AIDS Task Force

❶ Some People Think You Can Catch AIDS From A Glass

San Francisco AIDS Foundation
8 1/2 x 17; photographs; color; 1986; free, limited copies; special rates / discounts; English.

This poster, suitable for general display, shows a drinking glass. The brief text explains how AIDS/HIV is and is not transmitted. The poster can be personalized with any local hotline number for out-of-state orders.

Reviewers' Comments: Forceful and unequivocal, this poster is excellent for dispelling myths about HIV tranmission through casual contact.

▲ For Ordering Information, see p. 227

❷ Stop Worrying About How You Won't Get AIDS, And Worry About How You Can

CDC National AIDS Information and Education Program
16 x 22; black & white; Oct 1988; free; English.

With the caption, "Stop Worrying About How You Won't Get AIDS. And Worry About How You Can," this all-print poster lists 36 ways in which you can not contract HIV (e.g., from a toilet seat, from a hug, from a kiss, etc.) and three major ways the virus can be transmitted (i.e., from sharing drug needles with an infected person, by being born to an infected mother, from sexual intercourse with an infected partner).

Reviewers' Comments: This is a very good approach to "casual contagion" fears, and the design helps to delineate the differences between myth and reality. The statement that you can "get AIDS from sexual intercourse with an infected person" is a bit misleading and there is no referral for more information.

▲ For Ordering Information, see p. 216

◯ This Four-Letter Word

Columbus AIDS Task Force

❶ We Need A Cure For People Who Turn Their Backs On AIDS

Birmingham AIDS Outreach, Inc.
9 x 13; photographs; color; English.

This poster shows a photograph of five people with their backs turned to the camera. The message states that ignoring AIDS will not make the disease go away. Knowledge and compassion will "cure" ignorance and fear. The poster includes a Birmingham telephone number for more information or assistance.

Reviewers' Comments: Though visually appealing, the poster does not indicate that education is one way to overcome ignorance and inattention. This is an effective tool for soliciting volunteers.

▲ For Ordering Information, see p. 215

❶ 1ST EDITION RECOMMENDED   ❷ 2ND EDITION RECOMMENDED   ◯ NOT RECOMMENDED

❷ Yes Or No

Hawaii State Department of Health STD/AIDS Prevention Program
16 x 20; color; 1988; free; English.

This poster is a checklist of ways you can and can not contract HIV. Items listed are: handshakes, drinking cups, mosquito bites, toilet seats; having sex; and sharing drug needles. The appropriate box indicating "yes" or "no" is marked for each. AIDS hotline numbers are listed for Hawaii.

Reviewers' Comments: This is an adequate treatment for an all print poster, but is misleading since it implies that all sex is risky, rather than qualifying unprotected sex. The English version meets minimum acceptance criteria, as do the Chinese, Ilocano, Visayan, Tagalog, and Cambodian translations. Reviewers were unable to assess other translations: Japanese, Thai, Korean, Vietnamese, Laotion, Samoan, Tongan, and Hawaiian.

▲ For Ordering Information, see p. 220

❶ You Can't Get AIDS

Texas Department of Health Bureau of AIDS and STD Control
8 1/2 x 11; illustrations; color; Mar 1987; free, limited copies; English.

Developed by the American Red Cross, this poster uses four simple drawings to illustrate that HIV is not spread through casual contact, hugging, eating in restaurants, or using public restrooms. It adds, "Don't let fear get in the way of facts. Take the time to learn about AIDS."

Reviewers' Comments: This poster effectively presents its simple, clear message.

▲ For Ordering Information, see p. 229

❷ You Can't Get AIDS From A Glass

AIDS Project Los Angeles
11 x 17; photographs; color; 1987; $2.00; special rates / discounts; English.

Beneath the headline stating that some people think AIDS/HIV can be contracted from a glass, this poster displays a photograph of a glass with the caption "You can't." Additional text informs readers on the basics of how AIDS/HIV is and is not spread, to dispel fear about the risk of exposure to HIV through casual contact. It displays Northern and Southern California hotline numbers.

Reviewers' Comments: The print is small and may be difficult to read. Although not very attractive, the poster conveys its message simply and directly.

▲ For Ordering Information, see p. 213

PUBLIC SERVICE ADS (TV, RADIO, PRINT)

○ AIDS: Fight The Fear With Facts

AIDS Project Los Angeles

❶ AIDS Public Service Announcements - 1987

New York City Department of Health AIDS Education Training Unit
30 sec.; TV; color; Dec 1987; free, limited copies; English/Spanish.

This videotape contains nine 30-second messages. Five contain the message, "If you think you can't get it, you're dead wrong." 1) A young woman dressing to go out, puts a condom in her purse; 2) A mother (Black) thinks her child is too young for sex but tells him/her to use a condom if he/she is having sex; 3) A woman walks out on a man who refuses to use a condom; 4) In Spanish, same as 2. but mother is Latino; 5) In Spanish, same as 3. One PSA containing the message, "Don't get stuck with AIDS, " shows a funeral procession for a baby who dies of AIDS transmitted from an IV drug user father to the mother to the baby.

Three use the message, "Don't ask for AIDS - don't get it": 1) A rock video shows male prostitutes and a male and female embracing on a bench; 2) An AIDS patient lies in bed and describes symptoms; 3) A young mother with a baby wants to turn the clock back because both are HIV infected.

Reviewers' Comments: All are adequate for target audiences. The producer's product description lists three PSA's in Spanish, but only two were on the preview copy.

▲ For Ordering Information, see p. 225

❶ AIDS Radio Public Service Announcements

New York City Department of Health AIDS Education Training Unit
60 sec.; Dec 1987; free, limited copies; English.

This audiotape contains seven one-minute HIV prevention scenarios. Four carry the message, "If you think you can't get it, you're dead wrong." They emphasize the need to practice safe sex by using condoms. Two of the scenarios caution, "Don't ask for AIDS, don't get it." Of these, one describes the symtoms of AIDS and the ways it is spread; the other warns young women of the risks of transmitting AIDS in pregnancy. One final segment urges drug users with AIDS to stop using drugs or sharing "works." Its message warns, "Don't get stuck with AIDS."

Reviewers' Comments: Aimed at illuminating different high-risk behaviors, these PSAs are excellent in content, design, and technical production.

▲ For Ordering Information, see p. 225

❶ AIDS: We Need To Know. We Need To Care.

National Association of Social Workers
Multimedia; color; 1987; free, limited copies; English.

This multi-media information kit on AIDS/HIV is part of the 1988 National Association of Social Workers public service campaign. The goal of the campaign is to raise public awareness about the psychological and social problems arising from the AIDS/HIV epidemic. This public service package includes a brochure presenting the basic facts about AIDS; a large poster; five public service announcements suitable for print, radio, and television; and a price list of resources. The specific topics of these materials range from AIDS/HIV education in the schools, parent/child discussions, and the emotional needs of people with AIDS/HIV, to safer sex practices.

Reviewers' Comments: The artwork is particularly attractive. The kit is aimed primarily toward social workers.

▲ For Ordering Information, see p. 223

❷ Call For Help Newspaper Print Ads

CDC National AIDS Information and Education Program
Print; black & white; Oct 1988; free; English.

These two print ads have texts which read: "If He Won't Wear A Condom, Call For Help." and "If You're Having Trouble Understanding AIDS, Call For Help." There is space provided for government agencies and AIDS organizations to include appropriate hotline numbers. Similar spots have been developed for radio and TV in both English and Spanish. The print ads are for newspaper use and are only available in 2 col. x 3" size.

Reviewers' Comments: These ads are clear, simple, and direct, and they are effective means of providing numbers for assistance and information.

▲ For Ordering Information, see p. 216

❷ Heard Much About AIDS Lately?

CDC National AIDS Information and Education Program
Multimedia; black & white; Oct 1988; free; English.

This America Responds To AIDS print ad presents a photograph of "Barbara" who is sitting under a hair dryer reading a magazine. The title question opens a dialogue with her in which she explains her resistance to talking about AIDS/HIV. The ad encourages uninhibited public discussion of AIDS/HIV. It provides the number for the National AIDS Hotline and is available in a variety of sizes; a radio PSA is also available. Government agencies and AIDS organizations are free to localize it to meet their needs.

Reviewers' Comments: This ad conveys a good message, but uses a sterotypical image which trivializes the woman and her concerns.

▲ For Ordering Information, see p. 216

◯ How Would You Deal With It If One Of You Got AIDS?

CDC National AIDS Information and Education Program

❷ Mosquitos

Indiana State Board of Health
30 sec.; TV; black & white; Sep 1988; special rates / discounts; English.

In this PSA the "Dragnet" theme is heard while a detective enters an older couple's home where the wife has taken extreme precautions to protect against mosquitos she fears could carry HIV. The detective tells her to "get the facts ma'am." Indiana's AIDS Hotline telephone number is provided.

Reviewers' Comments: This PSA is light-hearted and engaging. The message is particularly clear. Problems are that the female is portrayed as hysterical, and the audio is muddy.

▲ For Ordering Information, see p. 221

◯ No Matter What Shape You're In, Anyone Can Get The AIDS Virus.

CDC National AIDS Information and Education Program

❶ 1ST EDITION RECOMMENDED   ❷ 2ND EDITION RECOMMENDED   ◯ NOT RECOMMENDED

② Protect Yourself / Stop The Epidemic

AIDS Project Los Angeles
TV; 1986; special rates / discounts; English.

ID: 00:30 min. each except "comedian", 00:60 min.

These five television public service announcements stress the importance of taking informed precautions against HIV transmission. A stand-up comic tells a story of a drowning man refusing available help, likening it to the refusal to face facts and take sensible precautions against HIV; a Black family discusses the importance of teenagers adopting safer sex practices; a teenage girl talks about her dreams of marriage; a young boxer refers to AIDS as a "dream killer;" and a young man working on a car comments on the risk of contracting the disease through sex with many partners. All spots focus on the neccessity of personal responsibility in the prevention of AIDS/HIV.

Reviewers' Comments: These spots do not instruct on prevention, but they do "stop and grab" you. The boxer sequence borders on stereotyping. The use of humor is welcome.

▲ For Ordering Information, see p. 213

VIDEOS / FILMS

○ **AIDS...A 20th Century Crisis**

Performance Matters, Inc. c/o Printed Matter, Inc.

❶ AIDS - Can I Get It?

Light Video Television, Inc.
18 min.; Nov 1987; $9.95; English.

This videotape uses interviews with experts, people with AIDS (called friends with AIDS), and people on the street to dispel myths and present facts about AIDS/HIV. Topics include how AIDS is and is not transmitted, the effect of the virus on the immune and neurological systems, the safety of the blood supply, and autologous transfusions. The experts discuss sexual transmission of HIV and safe and unsafe sexual practices. They also explain HIV antibody testing and azidothymidine (AZT) treatment and discuss hopes for a vaccine.

Reviewers' Comments: The techical production of this videotape is excellent and the content and instructional design are good. It appears to overemphasize the need to be tested and to express an inappropriate level of optimism about AZT.

▲ For Ordering Information, see p. 222

○ **AIDS - Medical Education For The Community**

Medical Surveillance, Inc. MED-ED Productions

○ **AIDS Risk Self-Assessment**

Planned Parenthood of Maryland

○ **AIDS You Can't Catch It Holding Hands**

Health Matters, Inc.

○ **AIDS And The American Family**

Medical Action Group, Inc. c/o Freeman Marketing

❶ AIDS And The Arts

Films for the Humanities & Sciences, Inc.
20 min.; VHS; 1987; $149.00; English.

This video examines the devastating effects of AIDS on the arts community. A prominent dancer who has since died of AIDS talks about how the disease has altered his work and his relationship with his male dancing partner and lover. It also features Elizabeth Taylor and playwright Harvey Fierstein.

Reviewers' Comments: This film uses the documentary approach. It is a good kickoff for a discussion of AIDS/HIV in the Arts. It also sensitively demonstrates the need for emotional and financial support for people with AIDS. The film engages the viewer. Good technical quality characterizes the film.

▲ For Ordering Information, see p. 219

❶ AIDS...What You Need To Know

Future Vision
43:30 min.; VHS; Oct 1987; $19.95; English/Spanish.

This is a video production of Surgeon General C. Everett Koop's Report on AIDS. Dr. Koop is the primary narrator of this comprehensive overview of facts about AIDS/HIV: how it is transmitted, the relative risks of infection, and how to prevent it. He stresses the need for education about AIDS/HIV and for every citizen to excercise appropriate prevention measures. No discussion guide is available.

Reviewers' Comments: The technical production of this rather lengthy video is occasionally distracting, e.g. blurry video effects. In addition, several spokespersons appear on-camera without identification.

▲ For Ordering Information, see p. 219

◯ AIDS: ABC News Special Assignment

ABC Video Enterprises, Inc. c/o Coronet/MTI Film & Video

❶ AIDS: Fight Fear With Fact

Connecticut Department of Health Services AIDS Program
18.40 min.; VHS; 1987; English.

Two Connecticut State health educators explain how HIV affects the immune system and the statistical relationship among AIDS, ARC, and HIV-positive diagnoses. It explains how the virus can be transmitted through sexual activity and drug use. It discusses risky sexual behavior in general terms and recommends preventive measures. It

urges drug users to get off drugs. There is no discussion guide available.

Reviewers' Comments: The videotape presents some information specific to Connecticut. The video is above average in content and instructional design.

▲ For Ordering Information, see p. 218

❶ AIDS: In Search Of A Miracle

Columbia University Graduate School of Journalism Seminars on Media and Society
60 min.; VHS; Sep 1986; $85.00; English.

Moderated by Professor Arthur R. Miller of Harvard Law School, this video features a panel of 16 nationally known leaders and decision makers who debate ethical, legal, and social AIDS/HIV-related questions. Casting the guests as officials in a hypothetical metropolis, the program answers questions about how the virus is contracted, testing practices, testing requirements, AIDS patients' acceptance in the community, sexually explicit education at the grade school level, and distribution of self-destructing needles for drug use. The program is one of a five-part series on public television entitled, "Managing Our Miracles--Health Care in America." There is no discussion guide available.

Reviewers' Comments: This discussion of ethical, legal, and social issues presents hypothetical situations which a local leader may encounter. It does not address medical topics but is engaging, believable, and of good technical quality. It uses outdated HTLV-II terminology.

▲ For Ordering Information, see p. 217

◯ AIDS: Our Worst Fears

Films for the Humanities & Sciences, Inc.

❶ AIDS: Profile Of An Epidemic - Update

Indiana University Audio-Visual Center
60 min.; VHS; 1986; $180.00; English.

This television program, produced by WNET/New York and hosted by Ed Asner, strives to educate, alleviate fear and superstition, and help foster humane regard for persons with AIDS. Staff from the Centers for Disease Control and the New York Hospital-Cornell Medical Center provide basic facts of the disease, describe the functions of the immune system, and dispel myths about HIV transmission. Personal profiles of five persons with AIDS dramatically illustrate the impact of the disease on individuals and family members. The video emphasizes the importance of caregiving, therapy, and support for persons with AIDS. There is no discussion guide available.

❶ 1ST EDITION RECOMMENDED   ❷ 2ND EDITION RECOMMENDED   ◯ NOT RECOMMENDED

Reviewers' Comments: Intended for a television audience, this video is suitable as a general introduction to the subject, but may be too long for other, more informed audiences.

▲ For Ordering Information, see p. 221

❶ AIDS: An Enemy Among Us

Churchill Films
45 min.; VHS; 1987; $295.99; rental fee: $60.00/3 days; English.

Sixteen-year-old Scott must come to terms with the fact that he has contracted HIV through a blood transfusion. This video-drama presents important facts about AIDS/HIV and portrays the anger, fear and uncertainty that surround it. Gladys Knight plays an immunologist who helps dispel the myths and explain the facts to Scott's family, classmates, and community. The film encourages safe sex and responsible behavior and affirms abstention from sex and drugs.

Reviewers' Comments: This somewhat melodramatic video may be effectively used as a means of sensitizing teens to the issues surrounding AIDS/HIV. It is, however oriented primarily to a white, middle-class audience.

▲ For Ordering Information, see p. 217

❷ AIDS: You Don't Have To Get It!

Louisville and Jefferson County Board of Health
16 min.; VHS; Jul 1988; $99.00; rental fee: $29.00/5 days; English.

This video outlines three stages of the disease, its symptoms, how it is and is not contracted, and ways to protect yourself. The film is a mix of a narrator's description of the facts, personal interviews with people who have lost family members to AIDS, "man-on-the-street" interviews that illustrate what average people know about AIDS/HIV, and brief public service spots - each with a different message. It provides Louisville Board of Health phone numbers.

Reviewers' Comments: The video is suitably formated, and it covers a range of important issues. There are some informational overstatements such as, "When you have AIDS, you WILL die."

▲ For Ordering Information, see p. 222

❷ About AIDS

Channing L. Bete Co., Inc.
15 min.; VHS; 1987; $195.00; special rates / discounts; English.

This video is designed to answer some common questions about AIDS/HIV and motivate people to protect themselves. Comments from four authorities on the subject are interspersed with animated cartoon illustrations of various points. "Man in the street" comments from a wide variety of people illustrate the public's attitudes, knowledge, and lack of correct knowledge. Issues covered include: what AIDS is, who gets it, misconceptions about transmission, routes of transmission, testing, and protection. A leaders guide answers common questions that may arise and provides a quiz. Also included is a poster that reads: "Know how to protect yourself from AIDS. Use a latex condom. Never shoot drugs."

Reviewers' Comments: This is geared toward a high education level: grade 12+, and the cartoon format is inconsistent with the language and interview segments.

▲ For Ordering Information, see p. 217

❶ About AIDS

Pyramid Film and Video
15 min.; VHS; 1986; $125.00; rental fee: $55.00/3 days; special rates / discounts; English.

This 15-minute videotape on the AIDS/HIV virus and its transmission uses computer graphics, microphotographs, anatomical drawings and live-action sequences to illustrate the narration. It covers the following topics: origin of AIDS/HIV, a description of the virus, the effect of the virus on the immune system, signs and symptoms of AIDS, how HIV is and is not transmitted, and precautions that reduce the chance of infection. It describes the fragility of the virus and it's susceptibility to heat and detergents. Responsible sexual behavior, use of condoms, and using reputable professionals for acupuncture and tattooing are advised. It warns against IV drug use and particularly the sharing of needles. The producers indicate no discussion guide is available.

Reviewers' Comments: This video is suitable for those seeking medical information on AIDS/HIV. It gives precise explanation of medical issues, but focuses on high risk groups rather than behaviors. The discussion of "risk groups" and of one of the theories of the purported origin of AIDS/HIV can be interpreted as prejudicial.

▲ For Ordering Information, see p. 227

❶ Beyond Fear

American Red Cross National Headquarters
60 min.; VHS; 1986; $45.00; English/Spanish.

This videotape, available in 60-minute or 30-minute versions, has three segments dealing with AIDS/HIV: the Virus, the Individual, and the Community. Each segment addresses issues related to the title topic, from the nature of the virus, the safety of the blood supply, status of research, family issues, and community outreach. A Spanish-voice dubbed version is available. The video has a companion multi-component discussion guide.

Reviewers' Comments: Although somewhat outdated (HTLV III), this video is a comprehensive, instructional tool, whose basic messages are reinforced in varied ways. It recognizes multi-ethnic concerns but lacks much youth involvement. The 60 minute version is probably too long for most audiences.

▲ For Ordering Information, see p. 215

◯ Did You Know? -- Quick Facts About AIDS

AIDS Research and Education Project, Psychology Department California State University at Long Beach

❶ Heroism: A Community Responds

John Canalli
30 min.; VHS; 1987; English.

This video celebrates the efforts of community volunteer and support groups for persons with AIDS and HIV infection in the San Francisco area. Representatives from these groups and organizations describe their activities and successes. A number of people with AIDS describe how they have been positively affected by the San Francisco effort.

Reviewers' Comments: This videotape is important as a volunteer recruitment film. It will help expand public awareness about the work being done in at least one community to help those with AIDS. It extensively discusses controversial healing methods.

▲ For Ordering Information, see p. 221

◯ Introduction To AIDS

Indiana State Board of Health

◯ Legal Issues And AIDS

Indiana State Board of Health

❷ Living With AIDS

New Jersey Network
30 min.; VHS 3/4; 1988; $95.00; rental fee: $50.00/2 weeks; English.

This documentary provides interviews with IV drug users, people with AIDS, physicians who treat children with the disease, a foster parent who has adopted several of those children, New Jersey's Health Commissioner, and a director of a research laboratory. It covers issues such as AIDS/HIV education in the schools, the compensation for medical costs of AIDS patients, the need for more facilities for AIDS patients, and discrimination against people who have contracted the disease. It also reports statistics on the prevelance of the disease and describes the stages of infection, identifying symptoms.

Reviewers' Comments: The documentary format includes stark images and discussions. The medical information is accurate throughout and is explicit. The positive approach to those in treatment and the compassionate responses are effective and compelling. This film will be good for both drug users and professionals new to the field.

▲ For Ordering Information, see p. 225

❶ Living With AIDS

Carle Medical Communications
23 min.; VHS; 1987; $385.00; rental fee: $65.00/3 days; special rates / discounts; English.

This video shows the final six weeks in the life of 22-year old Todd Coleman who died of AIDS in San Francisco. In the film, Coleman reveals his feelings in open, emotional conversation. Coleman's male lover, his doctor, and several volunteers who were with Coleman during the last months of his life also describe their feelings. As described, this video "demystifies the disease by personalizing it and its human impact."

Reviewers' Comments: This well-done, moving story conveys the impact of AIDS/HIV and addresses the issue of homophobia. It does not, however, provide any information on preventing this disease. No discussion guide is provided.

▲ For Ordering Information, see p. 216

❶ 1ST EDITION RECOMMENDED   ❷ 2ND EDITION RECOMMENDED   ◯ NOT RECOMMENDED

❷ On The Brink: An AIDS Chronicle

Centre Productions c/o Barr Films
60 min.; VHS; 1988; $485.00; rental fee: $60.00/3 days; English/French.

This video, which is feature-length, covers a broad range of AIDS-related issues, is international in scope, and includes a wide range of perspectives from policy-makers, to physicians, and AIDS patients. A sample of those who offer opinions includes: the World Health Organization AIDS Task Force Director, educators from the Gay Mens Health Crisis (GMHC) in New York; prostitutes in Amsterdam, Holland; a missionary from Central Africa; and physicians and researchers from the Pasteur Institute, Paris, France; the Center for Tropical Diseases, Antwerp, Belgium; and Abbott Laboratories, USA. Topics include: prevention; prejudice towards AIDS patients; origins of the disease, depicting the situation in Central Africa; diagnosis, related diseases, and treatment; AIDS research; living with AIDS from the perspective of AIDS patients; drug addiction as related to AIDS; ethics; and the reactions of those who work with AIDS patients.

Reviewers' Comments: This is appropriate for people already fairly knowledgeable about AIDS/HIV. Although some of the information is dated and the editing is poor, the treatment of research/clinical issues is thoughtful and effective. This video could be used for training staff and volunteers who are new to the field.

▲ For Ordering Information, see p. 217

◯ On The Trail Of A Killer

New Jersey Network

❶ Safe Sex For Men And Women - How To Avoid Catching AIDS

Cinema Group Home Video For Apex Productions
60 min.; VHS; Sep 1987; $29.98; English.

This video describes AIDS/HIV transmission and prevention. The videotape deals with real-life situations experienced by sexually active people. It dispels common misconceptions and assesses the AIDS/HIV-related risks of various sexual practices, particularly in relationships established since 1977. The tape features interviews with Dr. Laura Schlessinger, a marriage and family therapist, and Dr. Michael Gottlieb, a prominent clinical researcher and one of the first physicians to diagnose AIDS. Hosted by actress Morgan Fairchild, the tape provides useful information for families, young adults, students, and the general public. There is no discussion guide available.

Reviewers' Comments: Well-acted, well-scripted vignettes dramatize effective communication about AIDS/HIV between potential heterosexual sexual partners. Fairchild handles the moderator's role in a comfortable, conversational manner. The videotape emphasizes risky behaviors, not risk groups.

▲ For Ordering Information, see p. 217

❷ Seize The FDA

Gay Men's Health Crisis, Inc.
28 min.; VHS; 1988; $79.95; special rates / discounts; English.

This video documents events on October 11, 1988, when hundreds of AIDS activists from around the U.S. seized control of the Food and Drug Administration in Rockville, Maryland. It addresses the issues that motivated this non-violent direct action and presents a clear summary of the gay community's objections to current FDA practices for approving new and investigational drugs related to AIDS/HIV.

Reviewers' Comments: This presentation is split between being an educational film about FDA policy and being a documentary of empowerment. It explains problems and inequities in drug trials, encourages activism, and provides a sense of empowerment by showing collective actions taken to address the AIDS epidemic. The information about the FDA is presented at too scientific a level and is difficult to comprehend. More background on this issue is needed, and the material on the FDA could easily be dated. Background on the demonstration is also lacking. Demonstrators are overwhelmingly young, white, gay, and middle class; the video is best geared toward this population as there is some potential for negative stereotyping among general audiences.

▲ For Ordering Information, see p. 219

❷ Testing The Limits: Part One

Testing The Limits Collective
29:45 min.; VHS; Mar 1988; special rates / discounts; English.

This video is the first of a chronological series of documentaries about AIDS activism in New York City. From scenes of recovering IV drug users distributing condoms in the South Bronx to civil disobedience at Federal Plaza, the tape chronicles communities' efforts to take control of the epidemic. Spanning March to August 1987, Part 1 examines government accountability with respect to civil liberties, education, and health care.

Reviewers' Comments: This video presents a realistic and balanced portrayal of the diversity of the impact of AIDS/HIV in New York City. However, it tries to cover too many topics and ends up appearing somewhat superficial and disorganized. Issues of needle distribution and testing, especially, need more background. It contains some candid language about safe sex practices that might be offensive to some. While some of the issues have the potential for going out of date, and the tape is specific to New York, it could be used effectively elsewhere.

▲ For Ordering Information, see p. 229

HEALTH CARE PROFESSIONALS

❶ AIDS Home Care And Hospice Manual

Visiting Nurses and Hospice of San Francisco
196 pages; 1987; $95.00; English.

This comprehensive manual for home and hospice care provides educational guidelines and resources for administrators, staff, and volunteers responsible for the care of persons with AIDS. It contains information about AIDS/HIV, epidemiology, pathophysiology and medical management, planning services for persons with AIDS, infection control, nursing intervention, psychosocial assessment, psychological issues of the care givers, assessment health history, and physical examination guidelines. Organized into modules, the manual contains objectives, text, and post-test exercises for self-assessment.

Reviewers' Comments: This systematic, problem-oriented manual is a comprehensive presentation of the major AIDS/HIV issues. It provides highly practical solutions to home and hospice care problems, using actual or hypothetical models. However, the readability is appropriate primarily for health care professionals.

▲ For Ordering Information, see p. 231

◯ Sexually Transmitted Diseases - A Handbook Of Protection, Prevention And Treatment

R & E Research, Inc.

❷ Stress Management Leaders Guide - A Facilitator's Manual For People At Risk For AIDS

UCSF AIDS Health Project
102 pages; looseleaf; 1987; $15.00; special rates / discounts; English.

This manual offers guidelines for organizing stress management workshops for people with HIV infection. It provides outlines for conducting eight weekly sessions with specific topics for each session, instructions for relaxation exercises, and sample handouts for members of the workshop. It intends to decrease unnecessary anxiety about AIDS/HIV, to encourage changes in behavior through peer support, and to strengthen immune responses by using stress management skills.

Reviewers' Comments: This typed, xeroxed guide is a general stress management program that has been adapted for persons with HIV infection. The acompanying tape is an audio relaxation piece for general use.

▲ For Ordering Information, see p. 230

❶ Advice About AIDS For Public Safety, Health And Emergency Personnel

Seattle-King County Department of Public Health
4 panels; illustrations; $.15; May 1986; English.

▲ For Ordering Information, see p. 228

◯ AIDS

Texas Commission on Alcohol and Drug Abuse

◯ AIDS: A Guide For Healthcare Workers And Service Providers

NO/AIDS Task Force

◯ AIDS And The Dental Professional

South Carolina Dept. of Health and Environmental Control Bureau of Preventive Health Services

❶ 1ST EDITION RECOMMENDED   ❷ 2ND EDITION RECOMMENDED   ◯ NOT RECOMMENDED

❷ AIDS And The Health Care Worker

Virginia Department of Health - AIDS Program
3 panels; illustrations; free; 1988; English.

This pamphlet provides information to health care workers about how to address more safely the problems and needs of those with HIV infection. It lists precautions for healthcare workers, noting that these precaution also protect patients whose immune systems are weakened by AIDS/HIV. The observation is made that, "taking unnecessary precautions damages the patient's ability to cope psychologically with the situation." Health care workers are encouraged to get the facts and to dispel myths and fears by discussing their concerns openly with other professionals. Virginia hotline numbers are given.

▲ For Ordering Information, see p. 231

❶ AIDS And The Health Care Worker, 5th Edition

Service Employees International, AFL-CIO, CLC
4 panels; illustrations; $.25; special rates / discounts; Mar 1988; English/Spanish.

▲ For Ordering Information, see p. 228

❷ AIDS Education & The Drug Treatment Professional

Los Angeles Centers for Alcohol & Drug Abuse
3 panels; illustrations; special rates / discounts; 1988; English.

This brochure addresses AIDS/HIV educators responsible for developing educational programs for intravenous drug users (IVDUs). It covers such topics as understanding the needs of IVDUs, the particular fears of IVDUs regarding AIDS/HIV, and strategies for intervention and education. Information about the Los Angeles Centers for Alcohol and Drug Abuse is included, and California State AIDS/HIV information hotline numbers for English and Spanish speaking callers are given.

▲ For Ordering Information, see p. 222

◯ AIDS - Good Nursing Care For The AIDS Patient

AIDS Action Committee of Massachusetts, Inc.

❶ AIDS Precautions For The First Responder

Health Education Resource Organization (HERO)
3 panels; illustrations; $.30, limited copies; 1987; English.

▲ For Ordering Information, see p. 220

◯ Be Safe - Prevent Needlesticks

AIDS Administration for the State of Maryland Maryland C.A.R.E.S.

◯ A Clinician's Guide To AIDS And HIV In Wisconsin

Wisconsin Division of Health, AIDS/HIV Program

❶ Health Care Providers And AIDS

AIDS Action Committee of Massachusetts, Inc.
4 panels; illustrations; 1987; English.

▲ For Ordering Information, see p. 213

◯ Infection Control Guideline For Health Care And Related Workers - AIDS

Philadelphia AIDS Task Force

◯ Infection Precaution Cards

California Nurses Association

◯ Precauciones Para El Personal Que Presta Servicios

Sexually Transmitted Diseases Control Program

❷ Preventing Bloodborne Infection At Work

San Diego Department of Health Services
2 panels; free, limited copies; 1988; English/Spanish.

This leaflet includes guidelines on washing hands, using gloves and masks, cleaning spills, disposing of needles, and sterilizing equipment.

▲ For Ordering Information, see p. 227

❶ Skin Conditions Related To AIDS And Human Immunodeficiency Virus (HIV) Infection

American Academy of Dermatology
11 pages; illustrations; free, limited copies; Jan 1988; English.

▲ For Ordering Information, see p. 214

◯ Universal Infection Precautions

California Nurses Association

❷ Worker Exposure To AIDS And Hepatitis B

U.S. Department of Labor/OSHA
4 panels; 1989; free; English/Spanish.

This brochure covers worker exposure to both HIV and HBV. It offers a brief history of AIDS/HIV in the United States and describes AIDS and other HIV-related illnesses. A list of recommended practices to prevent exposure to HIV and HBV is given with information on the enforcement of these practices by the Occupational Safety and Health Administration.

▲ For Ordering Information, see p. 230

❶ AIDS And Substance Abuse - A Training Manual For Health Care Professionals

UCSF AIDS Health Project
75 pages; looseleaf; 1987; $25.00; special rates / discounts; English.

This manual, designed as a training guide and self-paced text, covers the nature of substance abuse and its relationship to AIDS/HIV. Other topics include attitudes about AIDS/HIV and susbstance abuse, and barriers to substance abuse treatment. The manual includes four case histories and eight comprehensive nursing care plans, including "The Worried Well," "Patients with an AIDS Diagnosis," and the "Need of Ethnic Minority Patients."

Reviewers' Comments: The manual is very supportive of trainees with no IV drug abuse experience. Although they contain a few technical contradictions, the materials focus on the health care worker's values and feelings and could be a useful tool for counselors.

▲ For Ordering Information, see p. 230

◯ AIDS Curriculum Unit For Nurses And Nurse Midwives In Family Planning

Development Associates

❷ AIDS Educator Training Manual

Illinois Department of Public Health AIDS Facts for Life
98 pages; looseleaf; 1988; free, limited copies; English.

This manual is designed to train AIDS/HIV educators. Topics include: virology, immunology, HIV-related disorders, monitering the course of the disease, transmission, abstracts of relevant scientific reports, interrupting the further transmission of HIV, a study guide, and an examination.

Reviewers' Comments: The organization and presentation of this manual are limited. The content is accurate, but the language alternates between very simple and very complex. There are no stated or apparent objectives, and psychosocial issues are not addressed.

▲ For Ordering Information, see p. 221

---

❶ 1ST EDITION RECOMMENDED   ❷ 2ND EDITION RECOMMENDED   ◯ NOT RECOMMENDED

❶ AIDS - Facts For Life - A Train The Trainer Manual For AIDS Educators And AIDS Prevention Specialists

Illinois Department of Public Health AIDS Facts for Life
charts; 1987; free, limited copies; English.

This manual, primarily intended for health educators, addresses the topics of AIDS/HIV: its relationship to virology and immunology, viral transmission, and HIV-related disorders.

Reviewers' Comments: This curriculum provides an excellent medical review of epidemiology, retrovirology, and immunology for the non-scientist. This is a very complex task, effectively executed. It provides minimal instructions for risk reduction, however, and does not address the psychosocial aspects of AIDS/HIV. This publication should be used only for training of medical and health care professionals.

▲ For Ordering Information, see p. 221

❶ Aware Scorecard - An HIV Risk Assessment, Risk Reduction, and Health Education Tool

Health Education Resource Organization (HERO)
10 pages; charts; 1987; $15.00; English.

This multi-colored, plexiglass stand-alone chart/scorecard lists, ranks, and assesses currently known risk factors associated with HIV transmission and recommended risk reduction practices. This training tool is for professionals and volunteers who work with persons with AIDS/HIV infection, or those at risk of infection. The scorecard packet contains a 10-page General User's Guide and a marking pencil. The user may order additional companion teaching materials, including two-color paper copies of the Scorecard, a Trainer's Guide, with a 35mm slide of the Scorecard for use in training large audiences, and a Couselor's Guide. The curriculum will be available in Spanish.

Reviewers' Comments: This teaching tool and accompanying guide discuss complex subjects in highly technical language. This product is probably best used with highly motivated, well-educated trainees/clients.

▲ For Ordering Information, see p. 220

❷ Counseling & Education For The Prevention Of AIDS: A Training Course For Health And Social Service Workers

Center for Community Action to Prevent AIDS Hunter College
161 pages; spiral; 1988; $20.00; special rates / discounts; English.

This curriculum describes a five day, comprehensive training course designed to educate and prepare health and social service professionals working in a variety of settings to provide risk reduction information to their clients and patients. It includes information on training techniques, risk reduction counseling, pre- and post-HIV antibody test counseling, AIDS/HIV-related discrimination, sexuality, reproduction, counseling IV drug users and their sex partners, homophobia, and racial and cultural issues.

Reviewers' Comments: The curriculum is presented in a way that is not easy to read. The sessions are not clearly delineated and the reader may be confused by the lack of distinction between outlines, notes, and activities. The level of information is targeted toward workers with little or no AIDS/HIV knowledge, but a high level of knowledge is assumed for the trainer. The text is somewhat wordy and contains many typographical errors and omitted references.

▲ For Ordering Information, see p. 216

❷ A Model AIDS Curriculum For Home Health Aides

Southeastern Massachusetts University
40 pages; spiral; 1988; $25.00; special rates / discounts; English.

The goal of this training curriculum and resource manual is to adequately prepare home health aide agencies to respond to the AIDS/HIV epidemic. The basic information is divided into five sections with training objectives preceeding each section. They include basic definitions of AIDS related terms; a brief overview of the syndrome; proper daily procedural methods of infection control and housekeeping for aides working with patients; psychosocial aspects of AIDS; regional social services; guidelines; and home health aide concerns/problems. The manual is also available on MacIntosh format. A thirty minute video tape, currently in production will accompany this manual.

Reviewers' Comments: This manual is a very basic treatment of the issues for home health aides. Some inaccuracies exist in the material. For example, the definition of AIDS is outdated (they do not use the four-phase definition), and microphages are not discussed as part of the immune system. However, this piece is adequate as part of an overall training program.

▲ For Ordering Information, see p. 228

❷ **Prostitutes Prevent AIDS: A Manual For Health Educators**

California Prostitutes Education Project (CAL-PEP)
74 pages; spiral; 1988; $27.00; English.

This manual is aimed at public health departments, AIDS/HIV projects, and community-based agencies that want to develop an AIDS/HIV prevention project to help prostitutes protect themselves, their intimate sex partners, and their clients from HIV infection. The contents include a project description with goals and objectives, a proposed model of working with this population in terms of outreach, support groups and workshops; the addenda include information on how prostitution is organized in the United States, statistics on the prevalence of infection among North American prostitutes, what prostitutes can and are doing to prevent AIDS/HIV, safe sex guidelines, a discussion of education versus mandatory testing and quarantine, prostitution laws, and a bibliography. Also included are some materials used by CAL-PEP's outreach program in San Francisco.

Reviewers' Comments: This manual is highly comprehensive and gives a factual overview of the prevalence of HIV infection in the prostitute community. It is particularly helpful to instructors because it includes strategies for reaching prostitutes on the streets and for presenting information to them using a language and format which are acceptable to their community.

▲ For Ordering Information, see p. 216

❷ **A Self-Instructional Manual, AIDS-HIV: Information And Counseling In Family Planning Practice**

Planned Parenthood of Metropolitan Washington D.C.
68 pages; spiral; ilustrations; Mar 1988; $14.38; English.

Written primarily for family planning counselors, this self-instruction manual reviews facts about AIDS/HIV infection and symptoms, suggesting measures counselors may use to cope with their own fears and anxieties. It focuses on AIDS/HIV counseling, discussing client resistance, and providing sample responses to clients' questions regarding condom use, HIV antiboy testing, and homosexuality. It offers advice on how to explore and support a client's behavior change and unresolved feelings or lack of closure regarding the disease. A supplement includes a list of general resources and a reprint of the January 4, 1988 AIDS Weekly Surveillance Report.

Reviewers' Comments: This is a nicely organized and attractively presented self-instruction manual. It assumes that the counselor begins with a knowledge of AIDS/HIV transmission. The highly effective values clarification exercises could benefit anyone who has contact with HIV antiboy positive persons or persons at-risk.

▲ For Ordering Information, see p. 226

MULTICOMPONENT PROGRAMS

❷ **AIDS Education For Family Planning Clinic Service Providers**

• **Counseling With Family Planning Clients About AIDS**
42 pages; stapled; illustrations; 1988; $10.00; English

• **Facts And Feelings About AIDS**
53 pages; stapled; illustrations; 1988; $10.00; special rates / discounts; English.

• **Finding Out About AIDS In Your Community**
39 pages; stapled; illustrations; 1988; $10.00; English

• **A Review Of Infection Control For Family Planning Clinics**
89 pages; stapled; illustrations; 1988; $10.00; English

Institute For Development Training

This instructional manual addresses the general training needs of family planning service providers for AIDS/HIV education and is intended for multinational use. The manual contains basic medical information as well as core information on how to integrate AIDS/HIV education into family planning programs such as counseling, community outreach, and clinic infection control. Each module in this set contains directions for using the module, an introduction, lessons, and a glossary. Problem-solving activities encourage trainees to think about and apply this information in ways relevant to their work and community. The topics covered include an assessment of thoughts, concerns, and AIDS/HIV knowledge needs in module 1; an assessment of community needs for AIDS/HIV education and intervention in module 2; guidelines for helping clients to make health choices and for creating individualized AIDS/HIV education programs in module 3; and, in module 4, a guide to the control of the transmission of HIV and other infections in the family planning clinic setting.

Reviewers' Comments: The organization of this instructional program is good and the modular approach is satisfactory. However, difficulties arise out of the attempt to make the program applicable to all countries. The content is very simplistic for most family planning workers in the U.S., and there are a few misleading segments including vague descriptions of opportunistic infections and the encouragement of breast feeding for all mothers.

▲ For Ordering Information, see p. 221

❶ 1ST EDITION RECOMMENDED   ❷ 2ND EDITION RECOMMENDED   ○ NOT RECOMMENDED

❷ AIDS Module

- **Attitudes And Sexual Interviewing**
  1988; $50.00; English.
- **Ethical Dilemmas In AIDS**
  1988; $50.00; English.
- **Helping Patients To Cope With AIDS**
  1988; $125.00; English.
- **Job-Related Stress And Burnout**
  1988; $125.00; English.
- **Neuropsychiatric Complications Of AIDS**
  1988; $75.00; English.
- **Sexual Counseling About AIDS**
  1988; $125.00; English.
- **Sexual History Taking**
  1988; $125.00; English.

CIRID at UCLA

The AIDS Training Modules are instructional tools for health care professionals and community health educators. Each module consists of audiovisual and written instructional materials designed to teach skills that are necessary for the diagnosis and prevention of AIDS and HIV infection; to increase awareness of issues surrounding AIDS; and to address the personal emotional needs of health professionals. Each module also uses a particular format: panel discussion, dramatized case study, or interview. Titles include: Sexual History Taking; Sexual Counseling About AIDS; Attitudes and Sexual Interviewing; Ethical Dilemmas in AIDS; Coping; Job-Related Stress and Burnout; and Neuropsychiatric Complications of AIDS.

Reviewers' Comments: "*Attitudes and Sexual Interviewing*": This realistic video can serve as an effective trigger for open-ended discussion among practicing physicians.

"*Ethical Dilemmas in AIDS*": This module contains a number of realisitic and pertinent case studies. These studies are open-ended and effective for triggering discussion.

"*Helping Patients to Cope with AIDS*": The content of this module is accurate and geared for nurses and student nurses. The lecture/interview format of the video is tedious and moves slowly.

"*Job-Related Stress and Burnout*": The format of this module, using roundtable discussion with a group of staff nurses, makes the presentation slow and dull. This otherwise useful module is oriented for nurses and nursing students.

"*Neuropsychiatric Complications of AIDS*": The content of this module is probably most appropriate for practicing physicians. The format of the video is like grand rounds without the visuals and is somewhat monotonous.

"*Sexual Counseling about AIDS / Sexual History Taking*": These modules may appeal to clinicians who have limited experience with gay males and human sexuality practice. Clinicians who have broader experience in these areas may find the modules to be very basic. They may be best used with medical students. Busy urban clinicians may find them unrealistic and less useful when dealing with clients who have many problems surrounding issues of sexuality.

▲ For Ordering Information, see p. 217

❶ Preventing Transmission Of Infectious Diseases In The Workplace

Resource Technical Services, Inc.
20 min.; 1/2 in, VHS; 1987; $129.50; special rates / discounts; English/Spanish.

This multi-component educational course, composed of a slide/audio cassette tape or videotape, a master script, evaluation form, and summary of the Centers for Disease Control guidelines, instructs health care professionals and service providers in workplace safety techniques. A Spanish version of this program is available.

Reviewers' Comments: The content and coverage of this package are generally excellent. It comprehensively depicts the use of Universal Body Substance Precautions, and includes a good discussion on appropriate use of antibody testing. One caveat - since the theory of African origins of HIV has been debated, its use in this video is less than desirable. Overall, however, this package is well designed and technically produced for instructional purposes.

▲ For Ordering Information, see p. 227

PAMPHLETS

❷ AIDS And Emergency Care

Wisconsin Division of Health, AIDS/HIV Program
12 pages; 1988; free; English.

This booklet provides the recommended precautions for emergency care providers (ECP) to minimize their risk of occupational exposure to HIV. It describes AIDS/HIV, modes of transmission and the occupational risk of transmission for ECP. Universal blood and body fluid precautions that should be followed during contact with any patients are described in detail. Procedures for the cleaning and decontaminating soiled materials and accidental exposure to blood or body fluids are included. Wisconsin state laws related to AIDS/HIV are explained. Commonly asked questions, a list of resources, and a glossary are provided.

Reviewers' Comments: The discussion of precautions and transmission concerns is comprehensive. The recommendations are made with good use of support material. The reading level varies throughout the document, however, and the format is poor, offering little or no distinction of important topics.

▲ For Ordering Information, see p. 231

❶ AIDS Information For Physicians

Pennsylvania Medical Society Educational and Scientific Trust
32 pages; charts; Dec 1987; $1.00; English.

This concise information guide for physicians discusses AIDS/HIV policy guidelines, HIV testing procedures, counseling those infected with HIV, disclosure of test results, safe sex practices, pathogenesis, high risk "groups," and treatments for AIDS and HIV-related diseases. It also lists testing and counseling sites. It uses slang to discuss sexual practices.

Reviewers' Comments: Although this physicians' manual provides some good, easily accessed, basic information about HIV antibody testing, it does not deal with the affective dimensions of the testing process. In a few sections (e.g. treatment) the information is readily accessible but too limited to be useful.

▲ For Ordering Information, see p. 226

◯ Good Nursing Care For The Patient Infected With The Human Immunodeficiency Virus (HIV)

Health Education Resource Organization (HERO)

❷ Protecting America's Health Care Professionals: How To Minimize The Risk Of Transmission Of AIDS And Hepatitis B...

American Federation of Teachers
15 pages; illustrations; 1988; $.30; special rates / discounts; English.

This pamphlet provides information to workers whose jobs involve exposure to blood and body fluids. It explains the obligations of employers to maintain safer work areas and describes the implementation of safe work practices. It also details the rights of workers who become infected with HIV (and HBV) regarding their continued employment. A list of Federal OSHA offices by region is included as is a summary of the policy statement regarding workplace transmission risk published by the Federation of Nurses and Health Professionals/AFT.

Reviewers' Comments: This pamphlet provides a good basic overview of the issues of health and safety with information on employers' responsibilty in ensuring a safe work environment. The policy statement is straightforward, but there is not much information on the practical applications of these issues for employers.

▲ For Ordering Information, see p. 214

❷ Why You Should Be Informed About AIDS

Channing L. Bete Co., Inc.
16 pages; illustrations; 1988; special rates / discounts; English/Spanish.

This pamphlet uses a combination of words and cartoons to encourage health-care personnel and other care providers to learn about AIDS/HIV--both to dispel myths and fears and to protect themselves and others from contracting HIV. Topics covered include: HIV transmission routes; who can get AIDS/HIV; and precautions such as wearing gloves, avoiding needle sticks, and disposing of contaminated articles carefully. Specific recommendations are listed for practitioners of dental care, eye care, and postmortem care. Police officers, firefighters, prison personnel, and emergency medical technicians are cautioned to wear gloves when there is the possibility of coming into contact with body fluids.

Reviewers' Comments: This pamphlet is too simple for health care professionals but is useful for other health care workers.

▲ For Ordering Information, see p. 217

❶ 1ST EDITION RECOMMENDED   ❷ 2ND EDITION RECOMMENDED   ◯ NOT RECOMMENDED

POSTERS

❷ Be Safe Prevent Needlesticks

AIDS Administration for the State of Maryland Maryland C.A.R.E.S.
17 x 23; illustrations; color; 1987; free; English.

This poster details proper and improper handling and discard of needles to reduce risks of accidental needlesticks. It is directed toward health professionals and direct-care service providers.

Reviewers' Comments: The text and pictures offer a clear and specific message, but are small and therefore must be viewed from a short distance.

▲ For Ordering Information, see p. 213

❶ Linking The Science And Policy Of AIDS

The Johns Hopkins Health System Office of Public Affairs
11 x 14; charts; color; 1987; English.

This two-color poster for health care workers displays a checklist of the universal precautions to be taken when caring for patients. It specifically addresses concerns about AIDS/HIV contagion.

Reviewers' Comments: This poster is an appropriate reminder for health care workers.

▲ For Ordering Information, see p. 229

◯ We Practice Protection...Gloves, Masks, Protective Eyewear

National Institute of Dental Research, NIH

VIDEOS / FILMS

❶ AIDS

Carolina Biological Supply Company
28 min.; VHS; 1986; $49.95; English.

This videotape explains the nature of AIDS/HIV, how it attacks the immune system, and how it spreads. It shows the most common opportunistic diseases which attack people with the virus. It describes risky sexual behavior in general terms.

Reviewers' Comments: This video is primarily suitable for health profession or biology students. It needs updating and does not provide information about the means of preventing AIDS/HIV.

▲ For Ordering Information, see p. 216

❷ AIDS: A Working Definition

Video Services, University of Maryland
16:35 min.; VHS; 1988; $300.00; rental fee: $100.00/2 weeks; English.

This video offers a definition of AIDS/HIV, a description of populations at risk, and an overview of the current and projected incidence in a question and answer format. It provides factual information aimed at nursing assistants and others who provide responsive care for AIDS/HIV patients.

Reviewers' Comments: This video is too elementary for health care professionals, but may be useful for the general public and high risk groups.

▲ For Ordering Information, see p. 231

◯ AIDS: Alcohol And Drugs - Perceptions Versus Realities

Healthcare Network, Inc.

❷ AIDS And Hepatitis-B Precautions

Medfilms, Inc.
8 min.; 1988; $190.00; special rates / discounts; English.

This video targets laboratory, housekeeping, food service and maintenance staff. It addresses infection control training problems such as emloyees with unreasonable fear of infection and employees who take needless risks. It describes how AIDS/HIV & Hepatitis-B affect the body; how the viruses are transmitted; the risk associated with needlestick; and the absence of risk from casual contact, offering four precautions for protecting against infection. An instruction guide is included.

Reviewers' Comments: With clarity, logical organization, and an effective animated cartoon presentation of needed precautions, this video makes a good introduction to a hospital instruction program.

▲ For Ordering Information, see p. 222

◯ AIDS And The Health Care Provider

Advanced Imaging, Inc.

❶ AIDS And The Health Care Worker

AMI Television c/o Coronet/MTI Film & Video
28 min.; VHS; 1985; $425.00; English.

This program addresses the special fears and concerns of health care personnel regarding AIDS/HIV. It addresses several major concerns of health care workers, ranging from CPR to psychological impact, which can affect the quality of care provided. A discussion guide accompanies the video.

Reviewers' Comments: This video, using credible and knowledgable professionals in a talk show format, provides factual and practical information and advice for health care professionals. One technical production problem is the use of graphics which are difficult to see in large audience settings. The participants use the term and concept "risk groups" rather than "risk behaviors."

▲ For Ordering Information, see p. 215

❶ AIDS And The Health Care Worker

The Johns Hopkins Health System Office of Public Affairs
60 min.; VHS; 1987; $250.00; English.

This videotape consists of a series of three lectures by medical staff members of The John Hopkins University. It is designed to help the university staff deal effectively with AIDS/HIV. Citing the Centers for Disease Control's latest recommendations, it aims at allaying health workers' fears about contracting HIV from patient contact. There are question and answer segments in the film. No discussion guide is available.

Reviewers' Comments: This is a standard, videotaped, university medical center lecture and discussion. The presentations are good, but the length and lecture-style presentation may discourage some viewers.

▲ For Ordering Information, see p. 229

❶ AIDS Carriers In My Practice?

Medical Video Productions
28 min.; Jun 1987; $59.00; rental fee: $25.00/2 weeks; special rates / discounts; English.

This videotape contains a series of physician/patient interviews in an office setting. The interviews demonstrate how to elicit AIDS/HIV-related information in taking a medical history without expressing judgement about lifestyles. There is a discussion guide for this video.

Reviewers' Comments: This video, recommended for physicians and other health care providers outside of AIDS/HIV endemic areas, effectively uses dramatized doctor-patient vignettes to model discussion about AIDS/HIV risk. It demonstrates good interviewing and elicitation skills.

▲ For Ordering Information, see p. 223

❷ AIDS: Emotional Needs Of The Patient And Family

Video Services, University of Maryland
31:15 min.; VHS; 1988; $300.00; rental fee: $100.00/2 weeks; English.

This video explores psychosocial problems associated with persons with AIDS/HIV and their families. Topics addressed include developing professional confidence and emphathy, establishing therapeutic rapport, understanding the unique need of a particular patient, appreciating and responding to the patient's emotional states relating to impending death, and providing family members with necessary support.

Reviewers' Comments: This product highlights an AIDS/HIV experience that is more representative of the east coast. A broad range of psychosocial issues are highlighted, but the video does not deal with more advanced issues.

▲ For Ordering Information, see p. 231

❶ AIDS Encounters: Can the Doctor Make A Difference?

Kaiser Permanente Audio Visual Services
25 min.; VHS; 1986; special rates / discounts; English.

This video attempts to sensitize doctors to the concerns of clients in their practice, specifically gay men and Asians. The script notes that differences in language may hinder direct translation of cultural terms, such as safer sex, and thus may impact doctor - patient communications. A role play also demonstrates how to take a medical/sexual history of a patient in a non-judgemental fashion and how to counsel about safer sex practices. It uses HTLV-III terminology. There is no discussion guide available.

---

❶ 1ST EDITION RECOMMENDED   ❷ 2ND EDITION RECOMMENDED   ◯ NOT RECOMMENDED

Reviewers' Comments: The role play is poorly done. The video does not provide adequate instruction for developing communication skills, and the role play presented is not a good educational model of such skills.

▲ For Ordering Information, see p. 221

❷ AIDS, Herpes, And Hepatitis: Preventive Measures For Infection Control

National Health Publishing
35 min. (appx); VHS; 1988; $99.00; English.

Herpes, hepatitis, and AIDS/HIV infection control for health care workers is the subject of this video. The symptoms and modes of transmission for each type of herpes and hepatitis as well as AIDS/HIV are outlined and the seriousness of each discussed. Prevention methods are then described and demonstrated, such as effective methods for hand scrubbing, use of gloves, aprons, goggles, and masks, disposal of infected waste, use of needles and other medical sharps.

Reviewers' Comments: The objectives of this video are specific and clearly stated. It is very narrow in scope and addresses precautions only. It makes a good attempt to include HIV with other blood-borne infections, but it does not stress that HIV is more difficult to contract.

▲ For Ordering Information, see p. 224

❷ AIDS - Issues For Health Care Workers

Churchill Films
23 min.; VHS 16mm; 1988; $295.00; rental fee: $60.00/3 days; special rates / discounts; English.

Narrated from the point of view of hospital workers, this film provides information on how to guard against infection from HIV. Fears about AIDS/HIV are addressed by detailing the universal body fluids precautions as they apply to common patient care situations. Correct needle and waste disposal procedures, skin protection, cleaning and disinfection techniques are illustrated. Emphasis is placed on treating the AIDS/HIV patient with courtesy, compassion and respect, and protecting against HIV infection.

Reviewers' Comments: The video starts with basic concepts that can be helpful to non-health professionals, but may be too simple for RNs or physicians. It provides basic information on infection control and may be helpful to workers with little prior education about AIDS/HIV.

▲ For Ordering Information, see p. 217

❶ AIDS, Part I: The Diagnosis

Medcom, Inc.
41:15 min.; VHS; Apr 1987; $165.00; English.

This videotape covers our current knowledge of AIDS/HIV for a professional audience. It uses charts, graphs, photomicrographs of pathogenic organisms, electron micrographs of HIV, and photographs of lesions on AIDS patients to illustrate the narration. It discusses the epidemiology of AIDS/HIV in the United States, "at-risk" populations, modes of transmission, infection characteristics of HIV, and immunological responses to HIV infection. It explains the HIV antibody test and the meaning of positive or negative test results. The videotape covers the symptoms of AIDS/HIV, opportunistic infections, and the U.S. Centers fo Disease Control classifications of HIV infections in adults and children. The videotape ends with a brief discussion of azidothymidine and other investigational drugs. The package contains a frame-by-frame script booklet with a self-evaluation quiz and discussion questions and answers. This program is available in slide or videotransfer format.

Reviewers' Comments: Primarily for professional audiences, this video states and meets its objectives in a well-organized manner.

▲ For Ordering Information, see p. 222

◯ AIDS, Part II: Infection Control

Medcom, Inc.

❶ AIDS: Precautions For Lab Workers

The Johns Hopkins Health System Office of Public Affairs
60 min.; VHS; 1987; $250.00; English.

Produced in-house for The Johns Hopkins University medical staff, this videotape presents lectures by hospital staff members and the biosafety officer. It informs health care workers about ways of protecting themselves against exposure to HIV. It discusses safety protocols developed by the National Institutes of Health and Centers for Disease Control. There is no discussion guide available.

Reviewers' Comments: This video is excellent in content, but average in instructional design and technical production. It presents information specific to The Johns Hopkins Health System.

▲ For Ordering Information, see p. 229

❷ AIDS: Preventing Infection

Video Services, University of Maryland
17:30 min.; VHS; 1988; $300.00; rental fee: $100.00/2
weeks; English.

This video suggests measures on how to avoid exposure to
HIV and outlines steps to prevent infection. Guidelines are
detailed using examples of common accidental exposures
to potentially infected body fluids. Topics include what is
or is not an exposure, accidental needlesticks, blood splash,
and other environmental considerations. The program is
aimed at staff and employees working in health care environments.

*Reviewers' Comments: This well-done video uses clearly
implied objectives and summaries, with good illustrations
of how to engage in counseling health care workers. It's approach is humane and the technical quality is good.*

▲ For Ordering Information, see p. 231

◯ AIDS - The Legacy

Educational Productions

◯ AIDS - The Legacy - The Nurse

Educational Productions

◯ AIDS - The Legacy - The Physician

Educational Productions

◯ AIDS - The Legacy - The Social Worker

Educational Productions

❷ Beyond The Labels: The Human Side Of AIDS

Catholic Health Association of the United States
24 min.; VHS; 1988; $125.00; rental fee: $50.00/5
days; English.

The theme of this video is that, once a person has a serious,
probably fatal illness, the means by which the illness was
contracted becomes irrelevant to caregiving. The video
shows a wide spectrum of people with AIDS/HIV, revealing the ways in which they cope with their illness. The effect on family members, lovers, and caregivers is also
recorded. The need for education to reduce fear of those
with AIDS/HIV is emphasized. A pertinent quote from the
tape is, "You ask what a typical AIDS patient is like, and I
have to ask, what is a typical person like?" A discussion
guide is included.

*Reviewers' Comments: This video is well executed but
too long. Its main focus is on psychosocial aspects of
AIDS/HIV. It successfully shows that persons with
AIDS/HIV are individuals. The video has a strong
religious, primarily Catholic, orientation. Though the target audience is listed as health care providers, it is also useful for educators, church groups and community
organizations. The discussion guide adds to the video by
providing factual information for discussion, giving concrete learning objectives, and listing a variety of questions.*

▲ For Ordering Information, see p. 216

◯ Caring For The Latino AIDS Patient: Lessons From A Case History

Novela Health Foundation

❶ The Clinical Story Of AIDS

Carolina Biological Supply Company
28 min.; VHS; 1986; $149.95; English.

Featuring Dr. Paul Volberding, chief of the AIDS clinic at
San Francisco General Hospital, this videotape describes
the rapid progression of the AIDS epidemic from its early
appearances. Volberding explains how HIV attacks the immune system, and the symptoms that result. The video
describes the HIV antibody test and what it reveals. Dr.
Volberding also talks about some of the latest drugs used in
treatment.

*Reviewers' Comments: The video's computer-generated
graphics are distracting; however, Dr. Volberding's clear
and succinct presentation of clinical issues is excellent. No
discussion guide is provided. The video is appropriate
primarily for health care providers or those interested in the
medical dimensions of AIDS/HIV.*

▲ For Ordering Information, see p. 216

◯ Diagnosis: Life

Howard Brown Memorial Clinic

❶ Discussing Health Care And AIDS

The Exodus Trust
25 min.; VHS; 1986; $125.00; English.

In this video, several health care workers discuss how the
AIDS epidemic has affected their work with patients. A
role play between a health worker and a woman with a
negative HIV antibody test result demonstrates how to discuss AIDS/HIV, health, human sexuality, and safer sex
practices. The language is frank.

❶ 1ST EDITION RECOMMENDED   ❷ 2ND EDITION RECOMMENDED   ◯ NOT RECOMMENDED

Reviewers' Comments: This video is most suitable for health profession students to provide them with a framework for sexual issues discussions with patients or clients. It provides some helpful, practical suggestions to students. However, the role play is not effective since it portrays inappropriate rather thant appropriate practice.

▲ For Ordering Information, see p. 229

○ Facing Our Fears: Mental Health Professionals Speak

UCSF AIDS Health Project

○ Fear Of Caring

American Hospital Association

❷ HIV Test Counseling: Avoiding The Pitfalls

Novela Health Foundation
20 min.; VHS; 1988; $80.00; special rates / discounts; English.

Intended for health care practitioners, this video deals with pre- and post-HIV-test counseling. Issues covered include detecting HIV infection in an apparently low-risk patient and counseling a patient who has tested positive for the virus. A series of four dramatic dialogues between doctor and patient demonstrate counseling pitfalls and how to avoid them.

Reviewers' Comments: This is a good teaching tool that focuses on HIV counseling and interviewing techniques. The approach to HIV counseling is positive and realistic.

▲ For Ordering Information, see p. 225

❶ Infection Control: An AIDS Update

Carle Medical Communications
15 min.; VHS; 1987; $350.00; rental fee: $65.00/3 days; English.

This video attempts to relieve the fears of hospital workers who care for people with AIDS. It uses narration by a physician and an infection control practitioner along with scenes of AIDS patients and hospital workers to provide instruction on safe and effective care of people with AIDS. It includes information on the epidemiology of AIDS, routes of transmission, and proper blood/body fluid precautions for clinical and laboratory settings. It discusses and depicts procedures, such as handwashing, cleaning spills, disinfection or disposal of contaminated materials, as well as personal care of AIDS patients. No discussion guide is provided.

Reviewers' Comments: This informative video is well designed but does not include the current recommendations for the "Universal Precautions" of the U.S. Centers for Disease Control guidelines for infection control.

▲ For Ordering Information, see p. 216

❶ Is It Worth The Risk? Safe Handling Of Blood And Body Fluids

American Hospital Association
20 min.; VHS; Oct 1987; special rates / discounts; English.

This documentary addresses the need for health care employees to wear protective gear whenever there is a chance of exposure to blood or other body fluids. It uses simulated hospital situations to illustrate the universal precautions. The biosafety officer takes and emergency room nurse on a tour of the hospital to show how other sections deal with measures for protecting themselves from AIDS and other infectious diseases. There is no discussion guide available.

Reviewers' Comments: This is a visually excellent comprehensive video appropriate for the full spectrum of hospital workers. The video shows a multi-cultural sensitivity through its selection of actors/participants from various ethnic groups.

▲ For Ordering Information, see p. 214

❷ Needlestick

Medfilms, Inc.
8 min.; VHS; 1986; $170.00; special rates / discounts; English.

This video describes the dangers of infection including AIDS/HIV transmission from accidental puncture injuries from needles and other sharps. It encourages safe practices and behaviors, and strongly emphasizes that employees should assume responsibility for their own safety.

Reviewers' Comments: This is an infection control film, and it should be presented in the context of AIDS/HIV education.

▲ For Ordering Information, see p. 222

○ Nursing And AIDS: Professional And Personal Concerns

Video Services, University of Maryland

❷ Of Critical Importance: AIDS Precautions In Radiology

Carle Medical Communications
13 min.; VHS; 1988; $325.00; rental fee: $65.00/3 days; special rates / discounts; English.

This video, directed to an audience of radiologists, emphasizes the seriousness of the AIDS epidemic and outlines precautions radiologists should take to minimize their risk of becoming infected while working with patients. Noting that all blood should be considered potentially contaminated, the narrator describes the "universal precautions" to be taken: these may include using gloves, gowns, masks, and goggles, washing hands even after gloves are worn, disposing of needles and other "sharps" immediately in a protective container, and reporting any needle sticks or prolonged exposure to body fluids immediately so potential danger of contagion can be evaluated.

Reviewers' Comments: This is a credible presentation with up-to-date OSHA and universal precaution information. Review is used to emphasize main points. The technical quality of the film is good, although it is a little heavy on head shots. An excellent tool for radiology personnel.

▲ For Ordering Information, see p. 216

❷ Oral Manifestation Of AIDS

Office Sterilization and Asepsis Procedures Research Found. U. of Texas Health Science Ctr. Dental School at San Antonio
34 min.; VHS; 1988; $20.00; special rates / discounts; English.

This video provides an overview of the diagnosis and management of HIV-associated oral infections, as well as interviews with several of the speakers from the international symposium on AIDS/HIV, January, 1988, San Diego, CA.

Reviewers' Comments: While good for dentists, hygienists, and dental staff, this video is too long. The visuals are well-done and the production quality is excellent.

▲ For Ordering Information, see p. 225

❶ The Other Crisis: AIDS Mental Health

UCSF AIDS Health Project
45 min.; VHS; 1987; $100.00; rental fee: $25.00 / week; English.

In an informal interview format, this film explores the professional and personal concerns of mental health practitioners of various ethnic and minority background who work with people with AIDS/HIV. It gives particular attention to issues surrounding HIV antibody test counseling.

The six professionals interviewed offer factual knowledge about AIDS/HIV, their opinions, attitudes, experiences, personal trials, frustrations, suggestions, and advice to the viewer. Collectively, they dispel irrational fears about people with AIDS/HIV and offer helpful suggestions to their colleagues.

Reviewers' Comments: Although this presentation does not quite achieve its stated intention, it does provide the viewer insight into concerns and expectations of this acticulate, diverse group of mental health professionals.

▲ For Ordering Information, see p. 230

❶ Overcoming Irrational Fear Of AIDS

Carle Medical Communications
22 min.; VHS; 1987; $385.00; rental fee: $65.00 / 3 days; special rates / discounts; English.

In the video, psychologist Dr. Arthur Lange discusses with a group of health care providers how their feelings and fears about AIDS/HIV adversely affect their professional performance. Dr. Lange offers a training model to assist health care workers in overcoming negative, counterproductive thinking. In a question-and-answer format, Dr. Lange gives examples of issues and conflicts of people who treat AIDS patients and listens to comments of group members. A "Discussion Leaders' Guide", accompanying the video, presents written supporting material, selected bibliography, and suggested discussion questions.

Reviewers' Comments: This video provides a good training model for health care workers. The message is clear and concise and provides health care workers with guidelines for dealing with emotions arising from their care and support of persons with AIDS.

▲ For Ordering Information, see p. 216

❷ Pediatric AIDS

Video Services, University of Maryland
19:10 min.; VHS; 1988; $300.00; rental fee: $100.00/2 weeks; English.

John Johnson, MD, a specialist in perinatal care, discusses the increase in the number of children with HIV infection. Specific strategies are detailed to help these children with their complex medical needs. Guidance is provided on diagnosis and treatment for these infants.

Reviewers' Comments: Geared mainly to physicians and medical students, this basically is an illustrated lecture. Technically, the integration of words and visuals is poor. There is no mention of the emotional or psychosocial needs of infants and children.

▲ For Ordering Information, see p. 231

❶ 1ST EDITION RECOMMENDED　　❷ 2ND EDITION RECOMMENDED　　○ NOT RECOMMENDED

② Prevention Of Occupational Exposure To The AIDS Virus

Professional Training Systems, Inc.
60 minute laser disc; 1988; $1600.00; rental fee: $150.00/month; special rates / discounts; English.

This course was developed to reduce unrealistic fears of health care workers, and specify ways to prevent exposure to HIV on the job. It was developed in conjunction with Centers for Disease Control, community programs, and infection control specialists. It instructs workers on what causes AIDS/HIV, its effect on the body, and how the virus is and is not transmitted. It discusses the risk of occupational exposure and the need to follow specified universal precautions recommended by the Centers for Disease Control. It recommends types of protective attire to wear and when; preventive job practices; and proper environmental procedures. The course is approved by the American Nurses Association.

Reviewers' Comments: This is a good instructional tool, but the technical operation of the video disk was often clumsy - the viewer must cue each section. The purchase of the equipment may be prohibitive, but the rental is reasonable.

▲ For Ordering Information, see p. 227

❶ Psychosocial Interventions In AIDS

Carle Medical Communications
25 min.; VHS; 1987; $385.00; rental fee: $65.00/3 days; special rates / discounts; English.

This video is a composite of personal interviews with persons with AIDS/HIV and remarks by Dr. Susan Tross, a clinical assistant, attending-psychologist at Memorial Sloan-Kettering Cancer Center, and Rodger McFarland, former director of the Gay Men's Health Crisis of New York. The video defines AIDS/HIV and identifies the various stages in the AIDS/HIV process in which an individual may experience emotional problems. The stages are: suspected high-risk contact, HIV antibody testing, development of "ARC" or other HIV symptoms, AIDS diagnosis, symptom progression, and acute terminal illness. The video describes each stage in a physical/medical context and discusses the emotional consequences. People with AIDS share their feelings and discuss their emotional problems. There is no discussion guide available.

Reviewers' Comments: This is a quietly moving video that offers sensitive insight into the catastrophic nature of AIDS/HIV. It effectively balances the scientific/medical issues with the affective dimensions of the disease. Although the psychosocial spectrum concept used in the video may be slightly overstated, nothing detracts from the articulate presentations of the health professionals and the people with AIDS.

▲ For Ordering Information, see p. 216

○ Recognition And Prevention Of AIDS For Medical/Dental Offices - Plus Hepatitis B And Office Infection Control

American Technavision, Inc.

② Universal Precautions

Medfilms, Inc.
10:30 min.; VHS; 1988; $190.00; special rates / discounts; English.

Directed primarily at nurses, this video explains the CDC's Universal Precautions recommendations. It encourages professional judgement regarding the use of protective garments and equipment, advising that "over dressing" may adversely affect the patient, family, and guests and needlessly increase the hospital's expense for disposables such as gloves and masks. This videotape encourages viewers to assess the risk associated with each patient contact and take appropriate action. It also describes how Universal Precautions are similar to Blood and Body Fluid Precautions, which body fluids are and are not included in Universal Precautions, and four precautions to prevent transmission of infection. An instructional guide is inclued.

Reviewers' Comments: The video is simple and to the point with clear objectives and recommendations. It does a very good job of describing universal precautions.

▲ For Ordering Information, see p. 222

❶ Viruses, Retroviruses, And AIDS: An Interview With Dr. Luc Montagnier

Carolina Biological Supply Company
28 min.; Apr 1988; English.

This videotape features an interview with Dr. Luc Montagnier, the French researcher who is one of the discoverers of HIV. He describes his earlier work in virology and the events that led to his pursuit of the causes of AIDS. He explains how HIV attacks the immune system and considers possible directions of research in the future. No discussion guide is available.

Reviewers' Comments: This highly technical documentary is best suited for a high school or college science program. Persons unaccustomed to listening to a French accent may find this video difficult to understand.

▲ For Ordering Information, see p. 216

HIV POSITIVE INDIVIDUALS

BOOKS / MANUALS

❶ AIDS: A Self-Care Manual

AIDS Project Los Angeles
306 pages; Jun 1987; $8.25; English/Spanish.

This manual covers many of the concerns and needs of people with AIDS/HIV, those worried about the disease, and those caring or grieving for a person with AIDS. It discusses the various perspectives of self-care that people with AIDS/HIV need: socio-psychological, medical, therapeutic, socio-sexual, and spiritual. It also provides a compilation of self-care resources.

Reviewers' Comments: Comprehensive and up-to-date, this book covers the major AIDS/HIV medical, emotional and practical problems. It does not provide sufficient skill-building information, however.

▲ For Ordering Information, see p. 213

BROCHURES

❶ AIDS - If Your Antibody Test Results Are Positive

Maine Department of Human Services Office on AIDS
5 panels; illustrations; Jun 1987; English.

▲ For Ordering Information, see p. 222

❶ AIDS, The Law And You

AIDS Action Committee of Massachusetts, Inc.
4 panels; $.15; Feb 1987; English.

▲ For Ordering Information, see p. 213

◯ Alternative Health Care Approaches To AIDS & ARC

AIDS Action Committee of Massachusetts, Inc.

◯ Are You Being Discriminated Against Because Of AIDS/ARC?

San Francisco Human Rights Commission AIDS Discrimination Unit

❶ Coping With AIDS

San Francisco AIDS Foundation
4 panels; $.30; special rates / discounts; 1987; English.

▲ For Ordering Information, see p. 227

❶ Eating Right And AIDS

New York City Department of Health AIDS Education Training Unit
3 panels; illustrations; free, limited copies; May 1987; English/Spanish.

▲ For Ordering Information, see p. 225

◯ Fact Sheet No. 15 - Legal Status Of Persons With AIDS

Gay Community AIDS Project

◯ Fact Sheet No. 3 - Physical Symptoms Of AIDS

Gay Community AIDS Project

◯ For Health Care Professionals And AIDS Virus (HIV) Counselors - Information For The Individual With A Positive AIDS Virus (HIV) Antibody Test

Montana Department of Health & Environmental Sciences Montana AIDS Program

❶ 1ST EDITION RECOMMENDED   ❷ 2ND EDITION RECOMMENDED   ◯ NOT RECOMMENDED

○ **Guidelines For Persons Who Have Developed Antibody To HTLV-III**

Wellness Networks, Inc. - Flint

❶ **HIV Antibody - Information For Individuals With A Positive Test Result For Antibody Against The HIV Virus**

American Red Cross National Headquarters
3 panels; illustrations; Feb 1988; English.

▲ For Ordering Information, see p. 215

○ **Housing For People With AIDS - We're All In This Together**

Whitman-Walker Clinic

❷ **If You Are HIV Positive**

Being Alive
4 panels; free; 1989; English/Spanish.

This brochure urges individuals who are HIV positive to get help. It offers encouraging news that there are now treatments that can slow down or stop the virus from developing into AIDS. It suggests specific action: take the "test" and, if positive, find an experienced physician, offering Being Alive's Physician Referral Service as a resource. For those who test positive, three other tests are listed that can help determine the type of treatment. Three types of treatment are described. Advertising for other programs is included.

▲ For Ordering Information, see p. 215

❷ **Information For Persons With A Positive HIV Antibody Test Result**

North Carolina AIDS Control Program
4 panels; free; 1988; English.

Using a question and answer format, this brochure provides information for people whose HIV antibody test is positive. Topics covered include: the meaning of a positive test result; what to do to decrease the chance of developing AIDS; how to avoid transmitting the virus to others; who to tell and not tell about test results; considerations regarding sexual activity; and where to learn more. Local and national hotline numbers are given.

▲ For Ordering Information, see p. 225

○ **It's Not The Kind of Thing That You Tell Everyone...**

Maryland Department of Health and Mental Hygiene AIDS Administration

❶ **Latest Facts About AIDS - If Your Test For Antibody To The AIDS Virus Is Positive...**

American Red Cross National Headquarters
4 panels; Oct 1986; English/Spanish.

▲ For Ordering Information, see p. 215

❷ **Living With HIV**

NO/AIDS Task Force
4 panels; $.10; special rates / discounts; 1988; English.

This brochure provides detailed information about HIV infection and the ramifications of being HIV antibody positive. It defines AIDS, describes T-4 helper cells, and explains what it means to be "HIV positive." General symptoms of HIV infection, AIDS, and ARC are listed. Statistics regarding the probabilities of developing ARC or AIDS after HIV infection are presented and discussed. Confidentiality issues surrounding diagnosis are raised, and readers are encouraged to be discrete when disclosing a diagnosis to others. Suggestions regarding diet, sleep, and attitude encourage the reader to maintain health after diagnosis, and information is presented regarding local availability of drugs and studies, health precautions, and resources and support groups. Local and statewide hotline numbers are included.

▲ For Ordering Information, see p. 225

❶ **My Plan To Better Health**

Riverside County Department of Health AIDS Activities Program
2 panels; illustrations; free, limited copies; May 1987; English.

▲ For Ordering Information, see p. 227

○ **Recommendations For A Person With A Positive HIV Antibody Test**

Colorado Department of Health AIDS Education & Risk Reduction Program

❷ Special Immunology Service AIDS Information Pamphlet

Children's Hospital of Philadelphia
3 panels; free, limited copies; Dec 1988; English.

This brochure is designed to be given to and discussed with parents who have just been told their child is HIV positive. It is intended to stimulate discussion between parents and a social worker. Basic information on HIV and AIDS is provided along with an explanation of the ELISA test.

▲ For Ordering Information, see p. 217

❶ While You Are Waiting

Mississippi State Department of Health
2 panels; free, limited copies; Oct 1987; English.

▲ For Ordering Information, see p. 223

❶ Who To Tell...When You Are Positive On The HIV Antibody Test & How To Tell Them!

Wellness Networks, Inc. - Flint
4 panels; free; 1987; English.

▲ For Ordering Information, see p. 231

MULTICOMPONENT PROGRAMS

❷ Coping With AIDS

- **Diagnosis Of Symptoms**
- **Living With AIDS**
- **Treatment And Management Of Opportunistic Infections**
- **Treatment Of The HIV Virus**
- **What Is AIDS?**
  Various; VHS 3/4; 1989; $250.00; rental fee: $60.00/3 days; special rates / discounts; English.

Churchill Films

This five-part series from the Hospital Satellite Network is a primer for persons with AIDS and those involved with them. Resources are listed at the close of each program.

(1) "What is AIDS?": (19 minutes) reviews how AIDS/HIV disables the immune system, rendering persons with AIDS/HIV susceptible to opportunistic infections and explains the difference between AIDS and AIDS-Related Complex (ARC). It tells how AIDS/HIV is transmitted, dispels the myth that it is a "gay" disease, and discusses the symptoms which may signal the onset of AIDS. This video also emphasizes the importance of support groups for persons with AIDS and those close to them, and outlines some of the common coping stategies.

(2) "Diagnosis of Symptoms": (17 minutes) explains in detail many of the symptoms associated with the development of AIDS, discusses the four stages of the onset of AIDS, and tells how the diagnosis is made. The varying length of the incubation period is discussed, as is the mystery of why AIDS develops very quickly in some, relatively slowly in others. Some of the possible emotional consequences of a diagnosis of AIDS are raised.

(3) "Treatment and Management of Opportunistic Infections": (17 1/2 minutes) lists common opportunistic infections due to AIDS and how they can be cured, how others can be managed medically, and how survival can be prolonged. It states that having AIDS/HIV doesn't have to cause the end of an intimate relationship and outlines precautions necessary to avoid transmitting the virus. It discusses briefly the importance of non-medical factors for good survival.

(4) "Treatment of the HIV Virus": (17 1/2 minutes) discusses AZT as a treatment which interrupts reproduction of HIV, thus slowing down the progress of the disease. Other treatments currently under study are discussed. The film emphasizes the importance of attitude and of persons with AIDS taking responsibility for their own treatment and lives. It warns against falling prey to people who sell expensive, ineffective and sometimes dangerous remedies. It also emphasizes the importance of support groups.

(5) "Living with AIDS": (17 1/2 minutes) presents a person with AIDS and his family who discuss how AIDS has affected their lives. It lists precautions to avoid bringing on opportunistic infections and transmitting the virus. A number of long-term survivors of AIDS/ARC and their families discuss the importance of attitude and other non-medical factors contributing to survival. Some of the issues involved in accepting a diagnosis of AIDS are raised.

Reviewers' Comments: While this series provides an overview of the various issues surrounding AIDS and its treatment, there are some weaknesses. Inappropriate terms, for example, are used throughout (AIDS "patient, HIV "virus"), the content of some of the programs is not sufficiently focused or organized; and some viewers may infer bias in comments like, children with HIV infection or AIDS are "the most tragic cases."

▲ For Ordering Information, see p. 217

---

❶ 1ST EDITION RECOMMENDED   ❷ 2ND EDITION RECOMMENDED   ○ NOT RECOMMENDED

PAMPHLETS

❶ AIDS Medical Guide

San Francisco AIDS Foundation
   38 pages; charts; 1986; free, limited copies; English.

The AIDS Medical Guide provides information about the range of infections caused by HIV, including AIDS and AIDS dementia, and discusses the cancers and opportunistic infections that can occur in AIDS patients. The diagnosis, transmission, and prevention of HIV infections are discussed. The cancers and opportunistic infections that individuals with AIDS may develop are described in terms of the course of the disease, causative agents, diagnostic tests, and treatments. The following diseases are included: Kaposi's sarcoma, lymphoma, Pneumocystis Carinii pneumonia, toxoplasmosis, cryptosporidiosis, progressive multifocal leukoencephalopathy and infections caused by Candida Crytoccoccus, Mycobacterium avium intracellulare, Cytomegalovirus, and Herpes. A short glossary is included as an appendix.

Reviewers' Comments: Although it needs some updating, this handbook is informative and thorough. The language is technical and difficult.

▲ For Ordering Information, see p. 227

❶ Coping With ARC

San Francisco AIDS Foundation
   18 pages; Dec 1987; free, limited copies; English.

This booklet discusses many aspects of ARC: methods of diagnosis, possible treatments, the effects of drugs and alcohol on the immune system, confidentiality, employment, sexual practices, stress, and whom should be told of the diagnosis. It includes a list of symptoms, where to get financial help, and counseling services in the San Francisco area.

Reviewers' Comments: This comprehensive medical and psychological discussion of ARC is appropriate though difficult reading for people with ARC, their social network, and health care professionals. Some of the resource information is specific to the San Francisco area. Some of the medical information presented in the pamphlet requires a high reading level. The content of the pamphlet is excellent, covering many issues of concern to persons with ARC. The guide to financial assistance resources is notably helpful.

▲ For Ordering Information, see p. 227

❷ HIVIES Manual, Guidelines, And 12 Steps

Illinois Alcoholism and Drug Dependence Association
   12-16 pp. each; 1987; $7.50; English.

This three-booklet set is for facilitators and group members (substance abusers who are, or think they might be, HIV positive). The manual provides leaders with a model for empowering the support/self-help group, brief information about HIV infection, resource ideas, and suggested topics for discussion. The booklet of guidelines for starting and running a support group is addressed to facilitators. It includes suggestions on number and attitude of facilitators, meeting place, guidelines for facilitators, rules of order, introduction to HIV infection, and "HIVIES 12 Steps," which are based on the 12-step program of Alcoholics Anonymous. The third booklet, addressed to group members, details the process of change required in each of the 12 steps such as admitting one's own infection; believing that a higher power can guide one to healthy behavior; taking a moral inventory; admitting problems to others; and seeking through prayer, medication, nutrition, and exercise to move towards healthy behavior and spiritual awakening.

Reviewers' Comments: This program is recommended only for those who are twelve-step true believers and who have a professional facilitator. The facilitator's guide is too brief for use by anyone other than an experienced facilitator. This package differs from the traditional Alcoholics Anonymous twelve-step process in that a facilitator is used and there is a stronger emphasis on God and prayer.

▲ For Ordering Information, see p. 221

◯ Infection Precautions For People With AIDS And ARC Living In The Community

San Mateo County AIDS Project

❶ Legal Answers About AIDS

Gay Men's Health Crisis, Inc.
   16 pages; 1988; $1.00; special rates / discounts; English.

In a question-and-answer format, this pamphlet addresses the legal issues that concern people with AIDS, particularly gay male PWAs. Section One discusses making a will, will contests, and life insurance proceeds and wills. The remaining sections describe the use of living wills and power of attorney, discrimination, sexual orientation and refusal to submit to the HIV antibody test, insurance issues, and landlord/tenant relations. It also answers questions about deportation issues that might concern undocumented HIV infected workers.

Reviewers' Comments: This booklet is a concise legal guide for people with AIDS/HIV who live in the New York area. It would be a useful model for groups considering developing a similar publication for their regions. This guide is clearly written, with a minimum of legal jargon.

▲ For Ordering Information, see p. 219

◯ Living With AIDS

Lambda Legal Defense and Education Fund, Inc.

❷ The Next Step

Greenwich Department of Health
20 pages; Jan 1989; free; English/Spanish.

This pamphlet answers some of the questions posed by people who have recently learned of their positive HIV antibody status. It introduces some of the issues that face HIV positive persons and provides references to other resources. Although some of the resources listed are particular to the State of Connecticut, the main body of information is not location-specific. "The Next Step" is also available in Spanish and in a shortened, simplified English edition.

Reviewers' Comments: This pamphlet has very good prevention information and excellent, much needed discussions of the physician-patient relationship, choosing a physician, alternative treatments, managing one's post-test sex life, and informing parents about HIV antibody status. It is very comprehensive and positive in attitude. The reading level is too high for low-literacy populations, but it is nevertheless a worthwhile resource for HIV antibody positive individuals. The Spanish version meets the minimum acceptance criteria.

▲ For Ordering Information, see p. 220

❷ Positive Images

Minnesota AIDS Project
8 pages; 1987; $.20; English.

This pamphlet addresses the issues of people who have been informed that they have tested positive for the HIV antibody. It advises them not to panic and to learn more about the disease. In a question and answer format, the following issues are addressed: when to see a doctor; whether the test could be wrong, what sexual activities are safer, how to use a condom, whether having sex with others who are HIV positive or negative is safe, how HIV affects pregnancy, and ways to stay healthy. The "Positive Images" support group for those who have tested positive is described and Minnesota hotlines are listed.

Reviewers' Comments: This is a good pamphlet for someone who has just received HIV antibody test results. Overall it is a useful resource, although the reading level is high and it needs to be used with counseling or other publications to address fully all of the issues raised.

▲ For Ordering Information, see p. 223

◯ So...You Tested Positive...Now What?

Columbus AIDS Task Force

POSTERS

❷ If You Are HIV Positive

Being Alive
12 x 22; color; 1988; free; English/Spanish.

This poster encourages intervention to prolong health for those who are HIV positive. Against a deep blue background, yellow, chalk-like lettering says, "If you are HIV positive...Don't get AIDS. Get help." The Being Alive phone number in Los Angeles is included.

Reviewers' Comments: The message gives hope to HIV positive people and tells them where to get help. Although the phone number is too small, the graphic presentation is excellent.

▲ For Ordering Information, see p. 215

VIDEOS / FILMS

❷ AIDS Alive - A Portrait Of Hope

New Focus Films, Inc. Division of Northern Lights Alternatives
60 min.; VHS; Feb 1989; special rates / discounts; English/Spanish.

This video illustrates the importance of a determination to live for persons with AIDS/HIV, focusing on maintaining hope. It profiles the lives of seven long term survivors of AIDS who have taken responsibility for saving their own lives and explores the ways in which they have been accomplishing this task. These profiles are interwoven with interviews and consultations with healing practitioners such as Dr. Bernie Siegel, Louise Hay, Sally Fisher, Dr. Laurence Badgley, and Dr. Alan Levin. Information is presented on medical treatments and holistic methods, and

❶ 1ST EDITION RECOMMENDED   ❷ 2ND EDITION RECOMMENDED   ◯ NOT RECOMMENDED

includes demonstrations of such methods as acupuncture, nutrition, visualization, and herbs and vitamins.

Reviewers' Comments: This video presents refreshing examples of people with AIDS with self-empowerment. It raises points about alternative therapies and presents a variety of holistic approaches and spiritual views on surviving with HIV infection. The approach of self-help is as a complement to traditional medicine. This is a controversial subject within the medical and general communities.

▲ For Ordering Information, see p. 224

◯ Living With AIDS Related Condition (ARC)

The Exodus Trust

❷ PWA Power

Gay Men's Health Crisis, Inc.
28 min.; VHS; 1988; $79.95; special rates / discounts; English.

In this tape, a diverse group of people with AIDS/HIV talk about their experiences, offering insight to those recently diagnosed with AIDS. First person accounts about the birth of the PWA self-empowerment movement are included.

Reviewers' Comments: Although the video has poor production quality, the messages presented are accurate and valid for HIV positive individuals. It includes both men and women with AIDS/HIV who openly discuss living with HIV infection. There is helpful information regarding positive aspects of diagnosis; the video provides positive role models for PWAs.

▲ For Ordering Information, see p. 219

◯ Work Your Body

Gay Men's Health Crisis, Inc.

HIV TEST RECIPIENTS

❷ After The Test / Despues El Examen

AIDS Project Los Angeles
4 panels; $.25; special rates / discounts; 1988; English/Spanish.

This brochure discusses the implications of positive and negative antibody test results. It answers commonly-raised questions on what to do next, and how to prevent infection and transmission. It includes a wallet-sized tearout portion with California hotline numbers and basic information on the prevention of HIV transmission.

▲ For Ordering Information, see p. 213

❶ AIDS And HIV Counseling And Testing

New York State Department of Health
3 panels; free; Aug 1987; English.

▲ For Ordering Information, see p. 225

❷ AIDS And The HIV Antibody Test

Howard Brown Memorial Clinic
3 panels; special rates / discounts; 1988; English.

This brochure provides basic descriptions of AIDS/HIV, its affect on the immune system, and how HIV is spread. Also included is information on the ELISA and Western Blot tests for HIV, with descriptions of test results and issues of to be aware of when considering taking a test. General tips on health and attitudes are also given.

▲ For Ordering Information, see p. 221

❶ AIDS Counseling And Testing For HIV Antibody: The Facts

Rhode Island Department of Health AIDS Program
3 panels; free, limited copies; Dec 1987; English.

▲ For Ordering Information, see p. 227

❶ AIDS - Information About HIV Antibody Testing

Maine Department of Human Services Office on AIDS
4 panels; illustrations; Jun 1987; English.

▲ For Ordering Information, see p. 222

❶ AIDS - Information For The Individual With A Negative AIDS Virus (HIV) Antibody Test

Denver Disease Control Service
3 panels; illustrations; free, limited copies; Sep 1986; English.

▲ For Ordering Information, see p. 218

❶ AIDS - Information For the Individual With A Positive AIDS Virus (HIV) Antibody Test

Denver Disease Control Service
3 panels; illustrations; free, limited copies; Feb 1987; English.

▲ For Ordering Information, see p. 218

◯ AIDS Test Results

Cristo AIDS Ministry

❶ AIDS: The Antibody Test

New York City Department of Health AIDS Education Training Unit
3 panels; illustrations; free, limited copies; Feb 1987; English/Spanish.

▲ For Ordering Information, see p. 225

◯ AIDS Virus Antibody Test

Seattle-King County Department of Public Health

---

❶ 1ST EDITION RECOMMENDED   ❷ 2ND EDITION RECOMMENDED   ◯ NOT RECOMMENDED

❶ The AIDS Virus Antibody Test - Pro And Con

Cascade AIDS Project
3 panels; 1987; English.

▲ For Ordering Information, see p. 216

❶ AIDS: What You Should Know About The Antibody Test

Virginia Department of Health - AIDS Program
3 panels; illustrations & photographs; 1987.

▲ For Ordering Information, see p. 231

❶ AIDS - Why Should I Take The AIDS Virus (HIV) Antibody Test?

Denver Disease Control Service
3 panels; illustrations; free, limited copies; Sep 1986; English.

▲ For Ordering Information, see p. 218

❷ Fact Sheet No. 4 - The HIV Antibody Test - Should I Take It?

Gay Community AIDS Project
4 panels; $.10; 1988; English.

This brochure is designed to provide information to help one make the decision whether to take the HIV antibody test. The information provided includes what the test reveals, "groups" at risk for infection; possible concerns related to taking the HIV antibody test; what it means to receive a negative or positive result; whom to inform of a positive result, and common symptoms of AIDS, ARC, and/or HIV infection. Further information about preventing transmission is included.

▲ For Ordering Information, see p. 219

◯ For Health Care Professionals And AIDS Virus (HIV) Counselors - Why Should I Take AIDS Virus (HIV) Antibody Test?

Montana Department of Health & Environmental Sciences Montana AIDS Program

❶ The HIV Antibody Test

Cook County Hospital AIDS Service
5 pages; free, limited copies; 1987; English.

▲ For Ordering Information, see p. 218

❷ The HIV Antibody Test

American College Health Association
4 panels; $.50; special rates / discounts; 1988; English.

This brochure offers a frank discussion of the HIV antibody test. It analyzes the pros and cons, describes the tests, discusses what the results mean and how they will be used, and urges that individuals be tested only at sites that offer pre- and post-test counseling.

▲ For Ordering Information, see p. 214

◯ The HIV Antibody Test: What's The Deal?

D.C. Commission of Public Health

❶ HIV Antibody Testing

AIDS Foundation Houston, Inc.
4 panels; free, limited copies; 1987; English.

▲ For Ordering Information, see p. 213

❶ HIV Antibody - Information For Individuals Interested In Being Tested For Antibody Against HIV Virus

American Red Cross National Headquarters
3 panels; illustrations; Feb 1988; English.

▲ For Ordering Information, see p. 215

◯ If Your HIV Antibody Test Is Negative

Fenway Community Health Center

❷ Information For Persons Who have Taken HIV Antibody Test

Hawaii State Department of Health STD/AIDS Prevention Program
4 panels; free; 1988; English.

This brochure explains the meaning of both positive and negative HIV antibody test results. It provides information about safer sex practices, the potential for transmitting the virus to others, when to see a doctor, special concerns for women, and how to keep healthy. Hawaii AIDS resource numbers are listed. The English version of this brochure meets the minimum acceptance criteria, as do the Chinese, Ilocano, Visayan, and Tagalog translations. The translations in Japanese, Thai, Korean, and Cambodian do not meet acceptance criteria. The language reviewers were unable to assess translations in Vietnamese, Laotion, Samoan, Tongan, and Hawaiian.

▲ For Ordering Information, see p. 220

○ **Information For Persons With A Negative HIV Antibody Test Result**

North Carolina AIDS Control Program

❶ **Informational Guide-HIV Antibody Testing Program /**
Guia De Información - Programas De Pruebas Para La Detección Del Anticuerpo HIV

Los Angeles County Dept. of Health Services AIDS Program Office
3 panels; graphs; free; 1987; English/Spanish.

▲ For Ordering Information, see p. 222

❷ **La Prueba De Anticuerpos Al Virus Del SIDA**

Sexually Transmitted Diseases Control Program
7 panels; free; 1988; Spanish.

This brochure explains the acronyms "SIDA" and "HIV." It discusses the HIV antibody test and explains the significance of positive and negative test results. It contains a list of test locations in Puerto Rico.

▲ For Ordering Information, see p. 228

○ **La Prueba De Anticuerpos Al Virus No Diagnostica El SIDA**

Sexually Transmitted Diseases Control Program

○ **Questions & Answers - HIV Antibody Testing**

Colorado Department of Health AIDS Education & Risk Reduction Program

○ **Recommendations For A Person Not At Risk For AIDS With A Negative HIV Antibody Test**

Colorado Department of Health AIDS Education & Risk Reduction Program

○ **Recommendations For A Person At Risk For AIDS With A Negative HIV Antibody Test**

Colorado Department of Health AIDS Education & Risk Reduction Program

❶ **Should I Have The Test?**

Mississippi State Department of Health
2 panels; free, limited copies; Oct 1987; English.

▲ For Ordering Information, see p. 223

○ **Should I Have The Test?**

Wellness Networks, Inc. - Flint

❷ **Should I Take The Test? /**
Debo Tomar El Examen?

AIDS Project Los Angeles
4 panels; illustrations; $25.00; special rates / discounts; 1988; English/Spanish.

Using a question and answer format, this brochure provides a brief explanation of the AIDS/HIV antibody test, a description of how the test is administered, and definitions of AIDS and HIV. It discusses implications of test results and instances where testing may be advisable (ie. pregnancy, IV needle-sharing, unprotected high-risk sex). It explains confidential vs. anonymous tests, and refers readers to California alternative test sites. A wallet-sized tearout portion with California hotline numbers is included as is basic information on the prevention of HIV transmission.

▲ For Ordering Information, see p. 213

❶ **Should I Take the Test?**

Bay Area Physicians for Human Rights
3 panels; illustrations; free, limited copies; Jun 1986; English.

▲ For Ordering Information, see p. 215

○ **Should You Be Tested For Infection With The AIDS Virus Prior To Marriage?**

Idaho Department of Health and Welfare AIDS Program

---

❶ 1ST EDITION RECOMMENDED   ❷ 2ND EDITION RECOMMENDED   ○ NOT RECOMMENDED

❷ Should You Be Tested?

Georgia Department of Human Resources
4 panels; free, limited copies; 1988; English.

This brochure for those considering HIV antibody testing, describes the HIV antibody test and discusses how to interpret the results, patients' rights, and issues raised by the decision to have or not to have the test. It provides basic information on HIV transmission, encourages sharing the results with current and past sex and needle sharing partners, and recommends safe sex practices and precautions for IV drug users. It lists additional Georia resources for more information.

▲ For Ordering Information, see p. 220

◯ Should You Be Tested?

Massachusetts Department of Public Health

❷ The Test

AIDS Prevention Project Dallas County Health Department
3 panels; free; 1987; English.

This brochure briefly describes HIV, its modes of transmission, and high-risk behavior. It also notes that persons infected with the virus may never develop AIDS and may pass the virus on for years, not knowing they are infected. The blood test for HIV antibodies is described, with the warning that the choice to take the test should not be made lightly, since there is neither a cure nor a vaccine. Those who are tested are encouraged to be very careful whom they tell, since they may have problems with insurance, housing, or employment simply because they've been tested. A list of precautions is given for everyone to follow, regardless of testing status.

▲ For Ordering Information, see p. 213

❷ What Do HIV Test Results Really Mean?

Illinois Alcoholism and Drug Dependence Association
Card; illustrations; special rates / discounts; 1987; English.

This wallet card briefly explains the implications of negative and positive HIV antibody test results. It also recommends transmission prevention behaviors such as condom use and drug avoidance. Phone numbers for general AIDS/HIV information and drug treatment referral are included. It contains information specific to Illinois; however, camera-ready art is available for agencies in other states who wish to reprint the materials.

▲ For Ordering Information, see p. 221

❷ What Do Your Test Results Mean?

Georgia Department of Human Resources
4 panels; free, limited copies; 1988; English.

This brochure provides an overview of what the HIV antibody test does and does not indicate. It briefly describes the implications of positive and negative test results including the possibility of false results. Suggestions are offered for preventive measures and safer sex guidelines and high-risk behaviors that are illegal in Georgia for HIV positive individuals are summarized. It lists toll-free AIDS information phone numbers within Georgia only.

▲ For Ordering Information, see p. 220

◯ What Everyone Should Know About AIDS And HIV Antibody Testing

Riverside County Department of Health AIDS Activities Program

❶ What Is "The Test"?

AID Atlanta, Inc.
4 panels; free, limited copies; May 1987; English.

▲ For Ordering Information, see p. 213

❶ Your Test Is Negative

Mississippi State Department of Health
2 panels; free, limited copies; Sep 1987; English.

▲ For Ordering Information, see p. 223

PAMPHLETS

◯ About The HIV Antibody Test

Planned Parenthood of New York City

◯ The Pros And Cons Of The HTLV-III Antibody Test And The National Gay Rights Advocates

Bay Area Physicians for Human Rights

❶ Questions And Answers About The HIV Antibody Test

Health Education Resource Organization (HERO)
8 pages; Apr 1987; $.50, limited copies; English.

This pamphlet provides a thorough discussion of HIV antibody testing in a question-and-answer format. It addresses the reasons for taking the test and what negative and postive results mean. It also describes a number of coping strategies for those who test positive.

Reviewers' Comments: This pamplet uses the question-and-answer format effectively to present a thorough discussion of the scientific aspects of HIV antibody testing. It does not adequately emphasize, however, the psychological, counseling, and confidentiality issues surrounding testing.

▲ For Ordering Information, see p. 220

◯ What You Should Know About HIV Antibody Testing (AIDS Virus Antibody)

Connecticut Department of Health Services AIDS Program

POSTERS

❷ Confused? Counseling Helps

Illinois Alcoholism and Drug Dependence Association
15 x 18; illustrations; color; 1987; special rates / discounts; English.

This poster encourages counseling to those considering antibody testing for HIV. It identifies many of the complex issues involved with testing and informs viewers that anonymous, confidential testing can be found through their local health departments. It contains information specific to Illinois; however, camera-ready art is available for agencies in other states who wish to reprint the materials.

Reviewers' Comments: The main message of this poster is conveyed accurately, and it's emphasis on HIV antibody test and related counseling is positive. It would be very good for a clinic setting, however, the print is too small.

▲ For Ordering Information, see p. 221

VIDEOS / FILMS

❶ The AIDS Antibody Test

San Francisco AIDS Foundation
15:30 min.; VHS; 1987; $45.00; English.

Belva Davis and Dr. Paul Volberding narrate this videotape on the HIV antibody test. Animated sequences illustrate explanations of the role of T-cells in immunity and transmission of HIV. It explains what negative and positive HIV antibody tests mean and advises persons with positive test results to practice safer sex, not to share needles, and to talk to physicians. It urges persons contemplating taking the antibody test to consider their feelings if the results are positive, to select a trusted friend that can be told of the results, and to have the test performed at a center that offers anonymity and counseling. There is no discussion guide available.

Reviewers' Comments: The visual display effectively explains the function of the immune system and modes of transmission. The videotape does not adequately discuss the specific HIV antibody testing procedures and related issues.

▲ For Ordering Information, see p. 227

◯ AIDS - HIV Antibody Test Counseling

The Exodus Trust

❶ Counseling The HIV Antibody Positive Patient

Los Angeles County Medical Association
15.26 min.; VHS; Dec 1987; $35.00; English/Spanish.

This docudrama opens with a bisexual man expressing his fears and concerns about his job after testing HIV antibody positive. His physician explains the meaning of the test results to him, offers to omit the results from his medical records, and questions him about his sexual practices and possible ARC symptoms. The doctor gives him a physical examination and then counsels him on safe sex practices. He advises him to use condoms and spermicides and to avoid high risk behaviors. The doctor mentions that the man may have symptoms of depression, and he suggests counseling for him and his wife. The doctor gives the man frank information, but leaves him with hope for the future. A Spanish language dubbed version of this video is available, but was not reviewed.

Reviewers' Comments: This is a well-produced dramatization of a physician-patient interaction, highlighting key issues in the counseling and treatment of newly-diagnosed HIV antibody positive individuals.

▲ For Ordering Information, see p. 222

❶ 1ST EDITION RECOMMENDED   ❷ 2ND EDITION RECOMMENDED   ◯ NOT RECOMMENDED

○ **Cybil - Personal Perspectives On AIDS
   And Related Disorders**

**Health Education Resource Organization
   (HERO)**

❶ **What's Next? After The Test**

UCSF AIDS Health Project
   15 min.; VHS; Aug 1985; $100.00; rental fee: $25.00/1
   week; English.

This videotape helps people understand the HIV antibody
test and its results, psychologically and medically. A sub-
stantial portion of the film focuses on the reactions of
people receiving test results. It stresses that a positive test
does not mean "AIDS," and a negative result does not
mean the test recipient is free of HIV infection. The film
addresses possible ways for counselors to help recipients
deal with the information, including advice for discussion
with past, present, or future sexual partners. Some of the
discussion includes sexually explicit language.

*Reviewers' Comments: This cleverly animated video for
educated, white, gay or bisexual men is excellent for use at
HIV testing centers.*

▲ For Ordering Information, see p. 230

IV DRUG USERS

BOOKS / MANUALS

❶ What Every Drug Counselor Should Know About AIDS

Manisses Communications Group, Inc.
73 pages; Dec 1987; $24.95; English.

This manual targets the drug counselor whose clients risk infection with HIV. It covers the following topics: basic AIDS/HIV facts, AIDS awareness and risk assessments, HIV antibody testing, risk reduction and health counseling, client treatment planning, and special issues--volunteers, support groups, prevention education, and women and AIDS. This publication includes a glossary and resource section.

Reviewers' Comments: The small print and the volume of information may overwhelm the average reader, thereby limiting the usefulness of this otherwise excellent manual.

▲ For Ordering Information, see p. 222

BROCHURES

❶ The Adventures Of Bleachman / Las Aventuras De Bleachman

San Francisco AIDS Foundation
5 panels; illustrations; 1988; English/Spanish.

▲ For Ordering Information, see p. 227

❶ AIDS

Hispanos Unidos Contra SIDA/AIDS
3 panels; illustrations; special rates / discounts; 1987; English/Spanish.

▲ For Ordering Information, see p. 221

○ AIDS, Alcohol, Drugs And Your Health

Whitman-Walker Clinic

○ AIDS And Drug Abuse

Montefiore Medical Center Department of Social Medicine, AIDS Education Project

❶ AIDS And Drug Use - If You Shoot Drugs, Here's What You Should Know

Cook County Hospital AIDS Service
3 panels; free, limited copies; 1987; English/Spanish.

▲ For Ordering Information, see p. 218

❶ AIDS And Drugs

Good Samaritan Project
3 panels; illustrations; free; Mar 1987; English.

▲ For Ordering Information, see p. 220

❶ AIDS And Drugs

North Central Florida AIDS Network
3 panels; illustrations; free, limited copies; Sep 1987; English.

▲ For Ordering Information, see p. 225

❶ AIDS And Drugs - The Best Prevention Is No Injection

New York City Department of Health AIDS Education Training Unit
3 panels; illustrations; May 1987; English/Spanish.

▲ For Ordering Information, see p. 225

❶ AIDS And Drugs - The Best Protection Is No Injection

Tampa AIDS Network
3 panels; illustrations; free, limited copies; Sep 1987; English.

▲ For Ordering Information, see p. 229

❶ 1ST EDITION RECOMMENDED   ❷ 2ND EDITION RECOMMENDED   ○ NOT RECOMMENDED

**❶ AIDS And IV Drug Users /
AIDS Y Las Drogas Intravenosas**

Connecticut Department of Health Services AIDS Program
3 panels; illustrations; free, limited copies; Feb 1987; English/Spanish.

▲ For Ordering Information, see p. 218

**○ AIDS And Needle Use /
AIDS Y El Uso De Agujas**

Haight Asbury Free Medical Clinic

**○ AIDS And Needle Use /
AIDS Y La Aguja**

San Mateo County AIDS Project

**❶ AIDS And Other Dangers Of
Shooting Drugs /
SIDA-AIDS Y Otros Peligros
Relacionadas Con Drogas**

**Los Angeles County Dept. of Health Services
AIDS Program Office**
3 panels; 1986; English/Spanish.

▲ For Ordering Information, see p. 222

○ AIDS And The IV Drug User

**Dimension Communications Network
(DCN)/RAMSCO Publishing Co.**

**❶ AIDS And The IV Drug User /
AIDS Y El Consumidor De Drogas
Por Via Intravenosa (IV)**

**Texas Department of Health Bureau of AIDS and
STD Control**
3 panels; illustrations; free, limited copies; Feb 1987; English/Spanish.

▲ For Ordering Information, see p. 229

○ AIDS And The Legal System

**Association for Drug Abuse Prevention and
Treatment (ADAPT)**

**○ AIDS Information You Need To Stay
Alive**

Massachusetts Department of Public Health

○ AIDS Is Killing Drug Users

San Diego Department of Health Services

❷ AIDS Kills (Bleach Decontamination)

**Illinois Alcoholism and Drug Dependence
Association**
Card; illustrations; special rates / discounts; 1987; English/Spanish.

This card urges IV drug users to avoid infection with the AIDS virus. It gives illustrated directions for cleaning needles and states, "These simple steps only take a minute. Isn't it worth it?" Phone numbers are included for general AIDS/HIV information and drug treatment referral. It contains information specific to Illinois; however, camera-ready art is available for agencies in other states who wish to reprint the materials. The Spanish translation meets the minimum acceptance criteria although some grammatical/typographical errors were noted.

▲ For Ordering Information, see p. 221

○ AIDS Risk Reduction: Needles And AIDS

NO/AIDS Task Force

❶ AIDS - Shooting Up And Your Health

New Mexico AIDS Services, Inc.
3 panels; illustrations; 1987; English.

▲ For Ordering Information, see p. 225

**○ Alcohol Drugs And AIDS /
Alcohol Drogas Y SIDA**

San Francisco AIDS Foundation

❷ Anonymous Testing For HIV

**Illinois Alcoholism and Drug Dependence
Association**
Card; illustrations; special rates / discounts; 1987; English/Spanish.

This wallet-sized card provides phone numbers for HIV antibody testing, information about AIDS/HIV, and drug treatment counseling referral. It provides an illustrated step-by-step description of the antibody testing process. It contains information specific to Illinois; however, camera-ready art is available for agencies in other states who wish to reprint the materials. The Spanish translation meets the minimum acceptance criteria although some grammatical/typographical errors were noted.

▲ For Ordering Information, see p. 221

❷ Are You At Risk For AIDS?

Illinois Alcoholism and Drug Dependence Association
Card; illustrations; special rates / discounts; 1987; English/Spanish.

This wallet card contains a list of ten "Have you ever?" questions. It explains that a reader who answers even one of the questions in the affirmative is at risk for HIV infection and suggests that the risk behavior be avoided. Phone numbers in Illinois are included for general AIDS/HIV information and drug treatment referral. The card contains information specific to Illinois, though camera-ready art is available for agencies in other states who wish to reprint the materials. The Spanish translation meets the minimum acceptance criteria although some grammatical/typographical errors were noted.

▲ For Ordering Information, see p. 221

❶ Are You Hooked On IV Drugs? You Should Know about AIDS.

Beth Israel Medical Center
3 panels; illustrations; 1986; English/Spanish.

▲ For Ordering Information, see p. 215

◯ Cleaning Your Works / Limpiando Sus Agujas y Jeringas

Haight Asbury Free Medical Clinic

❶ Drug Users! Don't Share Needles! / A Todos Que Usan Drogas: ¡No Comparten Las Agujas!

AIDS Project of the East Bay
3 panels; illustrations; 1987; English/Spanish.

▲ For Ordering Information, see p. 213

❷ Drugs And AIDS

Hawaii State Department of Health STD/AIDS Prevention Program
3 panels; free; 1988; English.

This brochure suggests three ways alcohol and drug use may increase one's chances of contracting AIDS/HIV. Preventive measures are encouraged and Hawaii AIDS information resource numbers are listed. Also listed are prevention recommendations and statistics relating AIDS/HIV to drug and alcohol abuse. The English version of this brochure meets minimum acceptance criteria, as do the Chinese, Ilocano, Visayan, and Tagalog translations. Translations in Japanese, Thai, Korean, and Cambodian fail to meet minimum screening standards. The language reviewers were unable to assess translations in Vietnamese, Laotian, Samoan, Tongan, and Hawaiian.

▲ For Ordering Information, see p. 220

❷ Drugs, Sex, And AIDS

American Red Cross National Headquarters
7 panels; free; 1989; English.

This brochure discusses the dangers of IV drug use and also addresses HIV-related issues regarding other drugs like PCP, cocaine, and alcohol. Information is provided about sexual transmission, transmission prevention, talking to sexual partners about AIDS/HIV, condom use, children and pregnancy, and testing.

▲ For Ordering Information, see p. 215

◯ Fact Sheet No. 7 - Drugs, Alcohol And AIDS

Gay Community AIDS Project

❶ Free Dope!

Multicultural Prevention Resource Center (MPRC)
3 panels; illustrations; 1987.

▲ For Ordering Information, see p. 223

◯ Get Into Drug Treatment

Illinois Alcoholism and Drug Dependence Association

❶ 1ST EDITION RECOMMENDED   ❷ 2ND EDITION RECOMMENDED   ◯ NOT RECOMMENDED

② **Hey Man, Let Me Use Your Works**

People of Color Against AIDS Network
3 panels; photographs; free, limited copies; 1988; English.

The cover of this brochure is black with white letters reading "Hey, man, let me use your works," followed in red by the phrase "Famous last words." Inside is the warning, "Don't let bad blood come between you." Drug users are warned not to share needles, given instructions on how to clean the syringe with bleach, and left with the message, "Anyone can get AIDS." A Seattle AIDS information number is given.

▲ For Ordering Information, see p. 226

○ **The Mainline Message**

Association for Drug Abuse Prevention and Treatment (ADAPT)

❶ **Needles, Drugs And AIDS**

AIDS Task Force of Central New York
3 panels; Dec 1986; English.

▲ For Ordering Information, see p. 213

○ **Poppers - Your Health...And AIDS...Can You Afford The Risk?**

San Francisco AIDS Foundation

❶ **Pssst...Escuchen! Tecatos! / Don't Gamble With AIDS...It's a Stacked Deck!**

Multicultural Prevention Resource Center (MPRC)
3 panels; illustrations; $.25, limited copies; 1987; English/Spanish.

▲ For Ordering Information, see p. 223

❶ **Reach For The Bleach**

Health Education Resource Organization (HERO)
Card; illustrations; $.30, limited copies; 1987; English.

▲ For Ordering Information, see p. 220

❶ **STOP - AIDS Alert / ALTO - SIDA Alerta**

Illinois Alcoholism and Drug Dependence Association
4 panels; illustrations & photographs; 1987; English/Spanish.

▲ For Ordering Information, see p. 221

○ **Sex, Needles, AIDS: It Could Be You**

Wisconsin Division of Health, AIDS/HIV Program

❶ **Sharing Needles Can Give You AIDS / Tu Puedes Conraer El SIDA Al Compartir Agujas**

San Francisco AIDS Foundation
Card; illustrations; free, limited copies; 1987; English/Spanish.

▲ For Ordering Information, see p. 227

○ **Shooting AIDS: IV Drug Use And The Risk Of AIDS**

Howard Brown Memorial Clinic

❶ **Shooting Up And AIDS**

New York City Department of Health AIDS Education Training Unit
3 panels; illustrations; free, limited copies; Feb 1987; English/Spanish.

▲ For Ordering Information, see p. 225

❶ **Shooting Up And Your Health**

San Francisco AIDS Foundation
3 panels; illustrations; English/Spanish.

▲ For Ordering Information, see p. 227

○ **Shooting, Sharing And AIDS - What You Need To Know**

Colorado Department of Health AIDS Education & Risk Reduction Program

○ **Some Straight Answers About AIDS And IV Drugs /**
Peligro Grave: AIDS/SIDA Y Las Drogas

AIDS Foundation Houston, Inc.

❷ **Somethings You Don't Share With Anyone**

D.C. Commission of Public Health
3 panels; illustrations; special rates / discounts; 1988; English.

This brochure urges drug users not to share drug paraphernalia. It illustrates methods for cleaning needles and offers brief suggestions for safe sex. Washington, D.C. area phone numbers for treatment centers, AIDS/HIV facts, testing, and counseling are listed.

▲ For Ordering Information, see p. 218

❷ **Stop Sharing Needles**

Illinois Alcoholism and Drug Dependence Association
Card; illustrations; special rates / discounts; 1987; English/Spanish.

This wallet card uses images and slogans to urge IV drug users to stop sharing needles. Examples are, "You will feel good about yourself," "Sharing is not caring," and "There are better ways of showing friendship and trust." Phone numbers are included for AIDS/HIV information and drug treatment referral. It contains information specific to Illinois; however, camera-ready art is available for agencies in other states who wish to reprint the materials. The Spanish translation meets the minimum acceptance criteria although some grammatical/typographical errors were noted.

▲ For Ordering Information, see p. 221

❶ **Up Front - About Drug Use And AIDS**

Up Front Drug Information
3 panels; illustrations; free, limited copies; 1986; English/Spanish.

▲ For Ordering Information, see p. 231

○ **When The Party's Over**

Indiana State Board of Health

INSTRUCTIONAL PROGRAMS

○ **Addicts Helping Addicts Prevent AIDS**

Illinois Alcoholism and Drug Dependence Association

PAMPHLETS

○ **AIDS And Chemical Dependency**

Hazelden Educational Materials

○ **AIDS And Shooting Drugs**

Channing L. Bete Co., Inc.

❶ **The Works: Drugs, Sex And AIDS**

San Francisco AIDS Foundation
35 Pages; illustrations; 1987; $1.00; English.

This comic book targets all adult IV drug users. Using stories and factual explanations, the comic book discusses all aspects of AIDS transmission, risk behaviors, risk reduction, and facts about the disease. It confronts the fears some may have about casual transmission. It contains explicit discussions and illustrations of safe and unsafe sexual practices. It gives detailed instructions on cleaning needles with bleach and water.

Reviewers' Comments: This comic book presents information and suggestions in a non-judgmental, culturally-sensitive fashion. Although the comic book is a bit long, it provides enough humor and variety to hold one's attention.

▲ For Ordering Information, see p. 227

❶ 1ST EDITION RECOMMENDED   ❷ 2ND EDITION RECOMMENDED   ○ NOT RECOMMENDED

POSTERS

❶ AIDS Can Blow Your High

Health Education Resource Organization (HERO)
11 x 17; illustrations; color; 1987; $1.50, limited copies; English.

This white-on-black poster with bright red highlights states, "AIDS Can Blow Your High. If you're not going to stop, at least use clean needles." A large illustration of a syringe and a bright splash of blood dominate this poster. It also includes telephone numbers for more information.

Reviewers' Comments: This poster presents sharp graphics and suggests an alternative preventative measure for the user who won't quit drugs.

▲ For Ordering Information, see p. 220

◯ AIDS Kills People Who Shoot Drugs

Massachusetts Department of Public Health

◯ The AIDS Pyramid

Illinois Alcoholism and Drug Dependence Association

◯ AIDS, Sex And Drugs - Don't Pass It On!

New York City Department of Health AIDS Education Training Unit

❷ Are You Dying To Get High?

New Haven Health Department
14 x 20; illustrations; color; 1988; $3.00; English/Spanish.

This poster was conceived by recovering addicts at the Addiction Prevention Treatment Foundation (APT) treatment facility in New Haven with the aid of outreach staff. The messages conveyed are to get off drugs, stop sharing needles, and/or clean "works" with bleach. Graphics illustrate how to clean syringes effectively.

Reviewers' Comments: This presents clear messages to IV drug users in a nonjudgmental way. The print is small, especially on the Spanish version.

▲ For Ordering Information, see p. 224

❶ BleachMan

San Francisco AIDS Foundation
11 x 14; illustrations; color; 1987; English/Spanish.

"BleachMan" dominates this poster proclaiming, "Bleach-Man says: clean it with bleach." Step-by-step illustrations show how easy it is to clean "works" and to reduce the risk of contracting AIDS. The English and Spanish versions meet the selection criteria.

Reviewers' Comments: This poster may catch the eye of younger IV drug users, but the cleaning instruction pictures and captions are very small and require close-range viewing. Laundromats in high IV drug-use neighborhoods might be appropriate places to display this poster.

▲ For Ordering Information, see p. 227

❷ Compartiendo Agujas Es Jugando Con Su Vida

Association for Drug Abuse Prevention and Treatment (ADAPT)
1987; free; Spanish.

This poster contains an illustration of a pair of dice on which the words "Life," "Death," and "AIDS" replace the numbers. The message of the text is that sharing needles is the same as gambling your life away. The poster is recommended as an exception to the screening standards. It contains misspellings and incorrect grammatical constructions.

Reviewers' Comments: This poster is recommended as an exception because of the need for this kind of information among IV drug users. The Spanish translation contains grammatical errors.

▲ For Ordering Information, see p. 215

◯ Cuando Se Infecta Con El SIDA

Association for Drug Abuse Prevention and Treatment (ADAPT)

◯ Don't Let AIDS Deal You A Losing Hand - Know The Facts

New York City Department of Health AIDS Education Training Unit

❶ Don't Share

San Francisco AIDS Foundation
   28 x 11; photographs; color; English.

In giant red block letters, running the length of an enlarged syringe, this poster warns IV drug users, "Don't Share."

Reviewers' Comments: The effectiveness of the ominous warning of this poster is diminished by the lack of follow-up information or referrals.

▲ For Ordering Information, see p. 227

❶ Drug Addicts: Stop AIDS! Clean Your Works!

Multicultural Prevention Resource Center (MPRC)
   17 x 22; illustrations; color; 1987; $2.50; English.

This lavender and orange poster depicts and explains a three-step procedure for cleaning needles with bleach and water. An illustration on the bottom of the poster shows a night street scene with one person leaning against a lamp post and another leaning against the wall of a shop.

Reviewers' Comments: This useful poster clearly and simply depicts the process of cleaning needles, which should encourage the practice. Bolder lettering and larger print would further enhance this poster.

▲ For Ordering Information, see p. 223

○ Hey Man, No Sharing

Brooklyn AIDS Task Force

❶ How To Get High

Long Island Association For AIDS Care, Inc.
   18 1/2 x 22 1/2; photographs; color; 1987; special rates / discounts; English.

This black-and-white photo poster focuses on the forearm of a man preparing to "shoot up." It also shows the hand of his companion passing him a dirty, loaded syringe. It warns, "How to get high and get AIDS in one shot. Don't share the works and you won't share AIDS."

Reviewers' Comments: In addition to warning IV drug users of the dangers of sharing "works," this poster effectively informs the partners and relatives of drug users, as well as the general community, of these dangers.

▲ For Ordering Information, see p. 222

○ If You Won't Kick An Old Habit, Start A New One

AIDS Administration for the State of Maryland Maryland C.A.R.E.S.

❶ Pssst...Escuchen! Tecatos! / Don't Gamble with AIDS...It's A Stacked Deck!

Multicultural Prevention Resource Center (MPRC)
   17 x 22; illustrations; color; 1987; $2.50; English/Spanish.

This poster shows four playing cards illustrated with a hand holding a syringe, a pirate's face, a skull, and a joker labeled AIDS. The poster depicts the three-step process of cleaning needles with bleach and water. The English and Spanish versions meet the minimum screening criteria. There is a coordinated brochure with the same title.

Reviewers' Comments: This poster is suitable for a methadone or drug treatment clinic. The Spanish version uses street language commonly understood by people who use hard drugs.

▲ For Ordering Information, see p. 223

❷ Somethings You Don't Share With Anyone

D.C. Commission of Public Health
   17 x 22; photographs; black & white; 1988; special rates / discounts; English.

This poster, targeted to drug users, displays a black and white photograph of drug paraphernalia and a red spot of blood at the end of a needle. The caption warns: don't share your works, your cooker, your cotton, your water jar.

Reviewers' Comments: This poster would be especially good for free clinics, STD clinics, and drug treatment centers. The message requires supplemental information like a brochure or pamphlet.

▲ For Ordering Information, see p. 218

○ Take Care, Don't Share. AIDS Kills

Massachusetts Department of Public Health

---

❶ 1ST EDITION RECOMMENDED   ❷ 2ND EDITION RECOMMENDED   ○ NOT RECOMMENDED

PUBLIC SERVICE ADS (TV, RADIO, PRINT)

❷ AIDS Radio Public Service Campaign - "Drug Users"

Connecticut State Department of Health
60 sec.; 1988; special rates / discounts; English.

In this radio ad, a woman describes her husband's use of IV drugs. The woman has learned that her baby has HIV, which means that she is also infected. The final message is that condom use is essential since IV drug users are 100 times more likely to get AIDS.

Reviewers' Comments: Though the general approach is good, this PSA contains some medical inaccuracies, e.g., "baby has AIDS, means the mother has AIDS too." There is no follow-up for further information - no hotline or resource number.

▲ For Ordering Information, see p. 218

❷ Drug Abuse And AIDS Public Education Program

- **Most Babies With AIDS**
  8 1/2 x 11; black & white; 1988; free; English.

- **Sharing Needles Can Get You More Than High**
  8 1/2 x 11; black & white; 1988; free; English.

- **When You Share Needles**
  8 1/2 x 11; black & white; 1988; free; English.

- **If You Ever Shoot Drugs**
  8 1/2 x 11; black & white; 1988; free; English.

- **A Man Who Shoots Up Can Be Very Giving**
  1988; free; English.

National Institute on Drug Abuse ORC

This series of five photographic posters addresses the risks of AIDS/HIV transmission to drug users, their partners, and their children.

"Most babies with AIDS are born to mothers or fathers who have shot drugs," shows a photograph of a baby carriage with an IV stand and hanging plastic bag. Additional text urges drug users to avoid pregnancy until they are sure they aren't infected, to protect themselves with condoms, and to get into a drug treatment program. A hotline number is listed.

"Sharing needles can get you more than high. It can get you AIDS," displays a photo of a syringe being passed from one person's hand to anothers. Beneath the photo is an explanation about how AIDS/HIV is contracted from needle-sharing and urges drug users to join a treatment program. A hotline number is listed.

"When you share needles you could be shooting up AIDS," shows a photograph of hands holding a syringe and "cooker." Further copy explains this point, and urges addicts to join a treatment program. A hotline number is listed.

Four babies of various ethnic backgrounds, sitting up laughing are the focus of the poster whose headline reads, "If you ever shot drugs, get tested before you get pregnant. Don't make them the AIDS generation." Further text includes information about how babies and their mothers contract AIDS/HIV. Condom use and drug treatment are urged. A hotline number is listed.

A poster whose caption reads: "A man who shoots up can be very giving; he can give you and your baby AIDS." shows a pregnant woman standing with her hands on her stomach, gazing at the viewer with a worried expression. Additional text explains how this can occur, and urges condom use and drug treatment. A national AIDS hotline number is given.

Reviewers' Comments: In general the messages in these posters are powerful emotionally and visually. Some of the visuals, such as the IV stand next to the baby carriage, may be strong for some audiences. Several of the poster photographs present multi-ethnic or multi-racial images, which is a positive step towards eliminating ethnic and racial stereotypes. The copy at the bottom of the posters that provides contacts or further information is often too small to be easily read.

▲ For Ordering Information, see p. 224

❷ Guess Who Else Can Get AIDS If You Shoot Drugs

National Institute on Drug Abuse ORC
8 1/2 x 11; print; black & white; 1988; free; English.

This poster reads, in large letters, "Guess who else can get AIDS if you shoot drugs," beneath which is a photograph of a baby bottle on its side, with the text, "Your baby can." Additional copy explains that AIDS/HIV is transferred through IV drug use and shared needles and encourages women to protect themselves with condoms, to enroll in a drug treatment program, and to take the HIV test before getting pregnant.

Reviewers' Comments: The message on this poster is clear and appealing, even though details on preventive measures are not complete. Information on cleaning needles, etc., would strengthen the presentation.

▲ For Ordering Information, see p. 224

❷ **If You're Dabbling In Drugs...You Could Be Dabbling With Your Life**

CDC National AIDS Information and Education Program
Multimedia; Oct 1988; free; English.

This America Responds To AIDS print ad is also available as a poster. With a photograph of an athletic black male and text, it conveys the message that sharing needles puts one at risk for infection with HIV. It provides the number of the National AIDS Hotline and is available in a variety of sizes. Government agencies and AIDS/HIV organizations are free to localize the ad according to need.

Reviewers' Comments: The reading level of this ad is too high and the language too formal to be effective with teenagers. It does dispel the myth that there is no risk of HIV infection through skin popping. It should show or explain how to clean "works."

▲ For Ordering Information, see p. 216

❶ **John Jackson**

Multicultural Prevention Resource Center (MPRC)
30 sec.; TV; color; 1987; $75.00; English/Spanish.

This public service announcement shows a young black person with AIDS who became infected by sharing needles. A narrator states that he died within nine months. During his illness, his buddies did not visit him; many of them are still sharing needles. It displays a telephone number for information on AIDS/HIV.

Reviewers' Comments: This television announcement provides a hard-hitting, powerful message dealing with AIDS/HIV and drugs.

▲ For Ordering Information, see p. 223

❷ **Stop Shooting Up AIDS**

National Institute on Drug Abuse ORC
Radio; 1988; free; English.

These thirteen PSA's cover many situations relevant to IV drug users. Through different scenarios, the three ways of transmitting AIDS/HIV are described and drug users are urged to assess their transmission risks and to protect themselves.

Reviewers' Comments: directly address their topic, discussing needle sharing and where to call to get into drug treatment programs. An important improvement would be for the PSAs to contain information on how to clean needles.

▲ For Ordering Information, see p. 224

VIDEOS / FILMS

○ **AIDS And Chemical Dependency**

Hazelden Educational Materials

❷ **The Best Defense**

Focal Point Productions
19 min.; VHS; 1988; $229.00; rental fee: $50.00/5 days; special rates / discounts; English/Spanish.

This video instructs sexually active and IV drug-using viewers and their partners in protecting themselves against HIV transmission. It opens with a scene of several IV drug users shooting up in someone's home; the "leader" of the group cleans the works they share with bleach despite peer pressure not to clean them. A second scene shows a black heterosexual couple "negotiating" safer sex. Each of these scenes is followed respectively by instruction in cleaning needles and condom use. The segments which describe putting a condom on and taking one off use extended metaphors of military combat to make their point. A third scene involves an Hispanic couple facing the possibility that one of them has AIDS/HIV. Each of the three scenes is left somewhat unresolved, and the resolutions are used to close the video.

Reviewers' Comments: This video is appropriate not only for IV drug users (IVDUs), but for their sexual partners and family members. Those who consider using this film should screen it carefully before deciding to use it with IVDUs and IVDUs in treatment since it shows people shooting up and getting high. The cast presents a good ethnic mix. Highly creative and humorous adaptations of 1940's/1950's newsreel clips were well-used to describe condom use.

▲ For Ordering Information, see p. 219

❷ **Drugs And AIDS: Getting The Message Out**

National Institute on Drug Abuse ORC
27:40 min.; VHS; 1988; free; English.

This video demonstrates how various resources in a community can be mobilized to convey the message about AIDS/HIV to IV drug users. Some examples include: a minister talking from the pulpit to his congregation about a young woman church member who recently died from AIDS and how church members had supported her; a woman who is an ex-addict talking to others on the street about using condoms and not sharing needles; and a moblie health unit going to a city housing project to discuss drug use and other health problems as well as AIDS/HIV. This and other documentary footage shows the challenges and successes this community is having in reaching IV drug users. An extensive program guide is also included, with

❶ 1ST EDITION RECOMMENDED   ❷ 2ND EDITION RECOMMENDED   ○ NOT RECOMMENDED

step-by-step ideas about how to use the video and how to mobilize the community. Additional education resources are also listed.

Reviewers' Comments: This video is most appropriate for use in areas of high-incidence drug use and would be more useful as a supplement to an instructional module. The video production is fair. It presents a clear message to drug users that help is available, and does so without being judgmental of the drug using communities. The instructional guide for the video is not recommended.

▲ For Ordering Information, see p. 224

❶ Needle Talk

New York City Department of Health AIDS Education Training Unit
27 min.; VHS; Dec 1987; free, limited copies; English/Spanish.

In this documentary-style videotape physicians and educators talk frankly about IV drug use, sex, and AIDS/HIV transmission. Scenes depict persons with AIDS in hospitals, men going in and out of an abandoned building (presumably a "shooting gallery"), and a demonstration of proper cleaning of needles and "works" with rubbing alcohol or bleach. An AIDS/HIV educator discusses "safer sex" and explains proper condom use to a group of young women. The cast includes blacks, Hispanics, and whites. There is no discussion guide available.

Reviewers' Comments: This video is a frank, streetwise presentation of HIV epidemiology and risk reduction behaviors. It provides an excellent demonstration on cleaning "works" and explicit descriptions of how to use condoms. The scenes of minority people with AIDS are compelling. The articulate physicians and educators present technical information clearly and simply.

▲ For Ordering Information, see p. 225

LATINO COMMUNITY

BROCHURES

**❶ AIDS/SIDA: Infórmese! /
AIDS: The Facts**

American Red Cross National Headquarters
3 panels; special rates / discounts; 1987;
English/Spanish.

▲ For Ordering Information, see p. 215

**◯ Alianza: Programa De Educación Sobre
El SIDA Para Latinos**

D.C. Commission of Public Health

**❶ Care For Your Health /
Cuida Tu Salud**

Hispanos Unidos Contra SIDA/AIDS
2 panels; illustrations; $.19; 1988; English/Spanish.

▲ For Ordering Information, see p. 221

◯ Datos Acerca Del SIDA

San Diego Department of Health Services

**◯ El SIDA No Discrimina /
AIDS Does Not Discriminate**

New York State Department of Health

❶ El SIDA Y El Lugar De Trabajo

AIDS Project Los Angeles
5 panels; illustrations; 1986; Spanish.

▲ For Ordering Information, see p. 213

**❶ Facts About AIDS /
Datos Sobre SIDA**

**Florida Department of Health and Rehabilitative
Services**
1 page; free, limited copies; 1988; English/Spanish.

▲ For Ordering Information, see p. 219

❷ Infórmate De Lo Que Es El SIDA

American Red Cross National Headquarters
4 panels; free; 1989; Spanish.

This brochure covers a range of basic AIDS/HIV information. It describes what it is, causes, and transmission.
Symptom information is briefly outlined. Aspects of HIV
antibody testing are covered: what the test actually indicates, what the implications are of a positive result, testing
availability, and what to do in the event of a positive result.
Simple transmission prevention guidelines are provided.

▲ For Ordering Information, see p. 215

❷ La Solución Es Prevención

D.C. Commission of Public Health
2 panels; special rates / discounts; 1987;
Spanish/Spanish.

This brochure asserts to readers that prevention is the solu-
tion to AIDS. It provides basic symptom information and
some statistics regarding the impact of AIDS on the Latino
community in the United States. The Alianza address and
phone number are included, along with a Washington, D.C.
AIDS hotline number. Similar brochures which are slightly
more specific are available for men, women, and young
people.

▲ For Ordering Information, see p. 218

**◯ La Vida De La Mujer Latina Y Su Bebe
Esta En Peligro - AIDS - SIDA**

Bebashi, Inc.

**◯ Las Mujeres Y SIDA /
Women And AIDS**

Gay and Lesbian Community Services Center

❶ 1ST EDITION RECOMMENDED   ❷ 2ND EDITION RECOMMENDED   ◯ NOT RECOMMENDED

**❶ Las Mujeres Y El SIDA /
Women And AIDS**

San Francisco AIDS Foundation
   4 panels; illustrations; $.30; special rates / discounts;
   1987; English/Spanish.

▲ For Ordering Information, see p. 227

❷ Man To Man

San Francisco AIDS Foundation
   3 panels; 1988; English.

The brochure explains simply how to prevent AIDS/HIV.
It gives specific instructions and illustrations for using a
condom. Men are encouraged to talk about safe sex and
stay informed. AIDS/HIV hotline numbers are provided.
There are four versions of the cover for this brochure, each
with a different man holding a personals ad. The contents
inside are identical.

▲ For Ordering Information, see p. 227

**❶ ¡ Protèjase Contra AIDS/SIDA! Tambien
Es Un Problema Hispano**

AIDS Foundation Houston, Inc.
   3 panels; free; Aug 1987; Spanish.

▲ For Ordering Information, see p. 213

**◯ Protect Yourself Against AIDS /
Protegete Contra El SIDA**

Los Angeles Centers for Alcohol & Drug Abuse

**❷ Recomendaciones Para Proteger La
Salud Mental Del Paciente**

Sexually Transmitted Diseases Control Program
   1 page; free; 1987; Spanish.

This leaflet provides skeletal guidance regarding caring for
the mental health of persons with AIDS. It addresses the
need for a compassionate, unbiased approach to caring for
people with AIDS.

▲ For Ordering Information, see p. 228

**❶ SIDA (AIDS) - Reducción De Riesgo /
AIDS Risk Reduction**

Gay and Lesbian Community Services Center
   1 panel; 1987; Spanish.

▲ For Ordering Information, see p. 219

**◯ SIDA: Enfermedad Que Los Latinos
Podemos Evitar**

**Los Angeles County Dept. of Health Services
AIDS Program Office**

**◯ SIDA (AIDS) Se Puede Prevenir /
AIDS Can Be Prevented**

Gay Men's Health Crisis, Inc.

❷ SIDA: Lo Que Usted Necesita Saber

Seattle-King County Department of Public Health
   3 panels; $.20; 1988; Spanish/Spanish.

This brochure defines the Spanish acronym "SIDA" and
presents facts about the transmission of AIDS virus. It contains the phone number of a local SIDA hotline in Seattle.

▲ For Ordering Information, see p. 228

**◯ Spanish Point Of Purchase Materials -
Los Hispanos Tambien Adquieren El
SIDA (AIDS)**

**CDC National AIDS Information and Education
Program**

**❶ Stop AIDS - If You Care...Don't Share /
Usarios De Drogas... Detengan el SIDA
(AIDS) - Si Te Importa...No Lo
Compartas**

AIDS Action Committee of Massachusetts, Inc.
   3 panels; illustrations & photographs; 1987;
   English/Spanish.

▲ For Ordering Information, see p. 213

PAMPHLETS

❶ AIDS - What A Woman Needs To Know / El SIDA - Lo Que Toda Mujer Necesita Saber

Hispanic AIDS Committee for Education and Resources, Inc. (HACER)
27 pages; illustrations; $1.25; English/Spanish.

This bilingual booklet provides Latina and English speaking women with the basic information about AIDS/HIV. The simple language is supplemented by charcoal-like sketches. Questions and answers cover how HIV is transmitted, the risks to women and their children, symptoms, the HIV antibody test, treatment, and protective measures. Both the English and Spanish versions meet the selection standards.

Reviewers' Comments: The length and reading level of this pamphlet may discourage some readers. It is simply and attractively formated.

▲ For Ordering Information, see p. 220

❷ AIDS Can Attack Anyone

Vida Latina
23 cards; Apr 1988; free; English/Spanish.

This pamphlet, targeted mainly to the Hispanic community, consists of an outer folder with 23 brightly color-coded cards inside. The cards, each containing a discrete topic, provide individualized information for men, women, IV drug users, homosexuals, and the general public. Cards that identify risk behavior can be modified by the individual counselor who gives out the pamphlet. Topics cover the general aspects of HIV, including: HIV and how it is transmitted, who can get infected, and how to protect against infection.

Reviewers' Comments: This is appropriate for individuals who are shy, unknowledgable, or anxious about questions relating to AIDS/HIV. The translation could be improved.

▲ For Ordering Information, see p. 231

❶ Chicos Modernos

Community Outreach Risk Reduction Education Program (CORE)
17 pages; illustrations; 1987; free; Spanish.

For young gay or bisexual Latinos, "Chicos Modernos" tells the story of two gay friends in comic book form. The younger of the two, Carlos, is being recklessly promis-

cuous in the eyes of his friend Juan. Juan warns Carlos that his behavior puts him at risk of contracting AIDS/HIV. The story develops around Juan's concern for Carlos as he explains safer sex. When the topic of condom use comes up, a footnote explains in detail the proper use of condoms. Similarly, footnotes expand on other references. These include a basic summary of AIDS/HIV medical facts, a list of high risk "groups," and the fact that having numerous sex partners increases one's risk. Carlos sees the light and, although he experiences embarrassment, buys condoms. He meets another young man who also practices safer sex, and they end up going steady. This is available only in Spanish.

Reviewers' Comments: Although this comic book is for the gay or bisexual Latino man, it includes information that is useful for everyone. However, the slang used may be too frank for the general Latino audience. The comic book format is entertaining and easy to read.

▲ For Ordering Information, see p. 217

❷ El Despertar De Ramón

Novela Health Foundation
4 pages; 1988; $.30; special rates / discounts; Spanish/Spanish.

This photographic soap opera depicts a middle class Latino father's struggle to understand and accept the fact that his son has AIDS.

Reviewers' Comments: This is a visually appealing and sensitive treatment of a father's reaction to his son's diagnosis. It addresses common myths about AIDS. The text contains minor grammatical errors.

▲ For Ordering Information, see p. 225

❶ El SIDA No Descrimina / AIDS Does Not Discriminate

Orange County Health Care Agency AIDS Community Education Project
20 pages; photographs; 1987; Spanish.

Using the story of a fictional Latino family, this photographic comic book presents facts about AIDS/HIV transmission, antibody testing, risk behaviors, and risk reduction. A heterosexual "macho" man discovers he has contracted the disease he thought affected only homosexuals. The pamphlet addresses this and other misconceptions about AIDS/HIV and concludes with the Latino man learning of his wife's pregnancy.

Reviewers' Comments: The presentation and simple language make this appropriate for Latinos at any level of reading ability.

▲ For Ordering Information, see p. 225

❶ 1ST EDITION RECOMMENDED   ❷ 2ND EDITION RECOMMENDED   ○ NOT RECOMMENDED

❷ El SIDA: Lo Que Debe Saber

AIDS Project Los Angeles
20 pages; 1988; $.50; special rates / discounts; Spanish.

This photographic soap opera targets sexually active Latino men. It explains the transmission risks of AIDS to heterosexual and bisexual men.

Reviewers' Comments: This photographic comic book is visually appealing and concise. It is an appropriate educational piece for sexually active men.

▲ For Ordering Information, see p. 213

❷ Fotonovela: Ojos Que No Ven

Instituto Familiar De La Raza - Latino AIDS Project
30 pages; 1988; $2.00; special rates / discounts; English.

This comic book is a photographic soap opera version of the Spanish language film of the same title. The story explores and addresses common myths about AIDS.

Reviewers' Comments: This is a culturally sensitive and visually appealing comic book that holds the reader's interest. It's a good companion to the video.

▲ For Ordering Information, see p. 221

❷ La Gran Decisión De Marta Y Jose / Marta & Jose's Big Decision

Hispanic Health Council
7 pages; illustrations; 1988; special rates / discounts; English/Spanish.

This comic book, illustrated with computer graphics, was created by and for Hispanic teenagers. It focuses on a teenage couple who decide not to have premarital sex. Parents' attitudes, AIDS/HIV, unwanted pregnancy, and future goals are all considered in their decision-making process. Their discussion dispels myths about "risk groups" while directing attention to risk behavior. AIDS/HIV is addressed within a broad context of health, social, and personal concerns.

Reviewers' Comments: Though targeted toward teenagers, this cartoon/comic is appropriate for any young adult. It can be a good resource for teachers and useful for inspiring questions. There is a strong message of abstinence and a good model for problem solving through discussion. Both the Spanish and English versions meet the minimum acceptance criteria.

▲ For Ordering Information, see p. 221

◯ Lo Que Debería Saber Acerca De SIDA...Un Cuento Que Podría Ser Verdad

National Safety Council

POSTERS

❷ Comparte La Vida, No Agujas

Association for Drug Abuse Prevention and Treatment (ADAPT)
1987; free; Spanish.

This poster shows a needle dripping blood next to a death certificate. The text reads, in Spanish, "Share life, not needles. AIDS is forever."

Reviewers' Comments: This poster has an effective visual impact. It uses death to motivate IV drug users to protect themselves.

▲ For Ordering Information, see p. 215

❷ Compartiendo No Es Queriendo

Association for Drug Abuse Prevention and Treatment (ADAPT)
1987; free; Spanish.

This poster presents an illustration of a needle dripping blood on two tombstones which have the word "AIDS" written on them. The message of the text is that sharing needles isn't loving.

Reviewers' Comments: This poster is visually impactful. Its message, "Compartiendo no es queriendo," is somewhat ambiguous.

▲ For Ordering Information, see p. 215

❶ Drugs And AIDS: Don't Play Lottery With Your Life / Drogas y SIDA: No Juegues Lotería Con Tu Vida

Instituto Familiar De La Raza - Latino AIDS Project
17 x 24; illustrations; color; 1986; $3.18; special rates / discounts; English/Spanish.

This brightly colored poster is in Spanish and English. Pictured on a lottery board are various cards such as La Botella, PCP--El Diablito, La Corazon (heart) and La Familia. The death card (a skeleton) is about to be played. The Latino AIDS Project phone number is listed.

Reviewers' Comments: This poster is culturally relevant and has good production and visual impact. It is specifically intended for regions with high concentrations of Mexican or Mexican-American populations; it may offend other Latino or Hispanic populations.

▲ For Ordering Information, see p. 221

❷ Hand With Syringe Poster

AIDS Research and Education Project, Psychology Department California State University at Long Beach
1987; $1.25; Spanish.

The Spanish text of this poster reads "Those who share needles risk contracting AIDS and losing their lives!!" It speaks to Latino IV drug users and is geographically targeted to the Los Angeles area.

Reviewers' Comments: This poster is visually appealing. It does contain grammatical errors.

▲ For Ordering Information, see p. 213

❷ Life / Death Latino Face Poster

AIDS Research and Education Project, Psychology Department California State University at Long Beach
1988; $1.25; Spanish.

This Spanish language poster makes the point the AIDS also affects heterosexual Latino men. It reads "AIDS also attacks macho men. Inform and protect yourself." The text is superimposed on an illustration of a man's face, half of which is skull only.

Reviewers' Comments: This poster is visually appealing and straightforward.

▲ For Ordering Information, see p. 213

❶ Los Niños Tambien Tienen SIDA / Children Have AIDS, Too

Albert Einstein College of Medicine AIDS Family Care Center
14 x 17; color; Spanish.

Printed in bold red and blue letters on heavy white stock, this poster, in Spanish, addresses pregnant Latino women. It states: "If you are pregnant and concerned about AIDS, please call me," and lists a hotline number below. It urges Latinos to request brochures for additional information.

Reviewers' Comments: The poster's message is clear, but may not attract attention. It is one of a limited number of Spanish language posters.

▲ For Ordering Information, see p. 214

◯ Los Tres Amigos / The Three Friends

Los Angeles Centers for Alcohol & Drug Abuse

❷ Menudo Says: Learn About AIDS

New York State Department of Health
1988; special rates / discounts; Spanish.

The group Menudo is presented in a photograph on this poster. The short text encourages the viewer to become informed about AIDS. The New York State SIDA hotline number is included.

Reviewers' Comments: This attractive poster may motivate young Latinos to become more knowledgeable about AIDS. It contains no information about AIDS, but provides a means for the viewer to find information.

▲ For Ordering Information, see p. 225

❷ Menudo Says: Protect Yourself From AIDS

New York State Department of Health
1988; special rates / discounts; Spanish.

This poster presents an album cover-type photograph of the singing group Menudo. The short text urges the viewer to talk about AIDS. The New York State SIDA hotline number is given in both the English and Spanish versions.

Reviewers' Comments: Although the poster contains no medical information about AIDS it is very attractive and piques the readers interest, and it provides a means of accessing further information.

▲ For Ordering Information, see p. 225

❷ SIDA /AIDS Es Un Peligro Para Todos

D.C. Commission of Public Health
19 x 23; photographs; black & white; 1987; special rates / discounts; Spanish.

The text of this poster urges the viewer not to become a victim of ignorance, but to inform him or herself about AIDS/HIV. The photograph presented is of several "ordinary" Latinos who are representative of various groups within the Latino community: men, women, blacks, and various age groups. The poster is meant to have wide appeal and includes two numbers for more information (in Spanish) in the Washington, DC, area.

Reviewers' Comments: This is a good eye-catching poster, but the Spanish mixes formal and informal usage.

▲ For Ordering Information, see p. 218

❶ 1ST EDITION RECOMMENDED   ❷ 2ND EDITION RECOMMENDED   ◯ NOT RECOMMENDED

❷ Vida Vs. SIDA

Sexually Transmitted Diseases Control Program
1987; free; Spanish.

In a question and answer format this highly textual poster explains what AIDS/SIDA is, how it is and is not transmitted, and some transmission prevention facts.

Reviewers' Comments: The information in this poster is medically accurate. However, the poster presents some information in a biased manner.

▲ For Ordering Information, see p. 228

PUBLIC SERVICE ADS (TV, RADIO, PRINT)

❶ Chui And Maria Elena

Multicultural Prevention Resource Center (MPRC)
30 sec.; TV; color; 1987; $75.00; English/Spanish.

This public service video announcement shows a wedding picture of a Latino couple. The narrator states that the man was a junkie, got AIDS, and died within nine months without knowing he had transmitted AIDS/HIV to his pregnant wife. It gives a telephone number for information on AIDS.

Reviewers' Comments: This announcement is excellent for male Latino IV drug users.

▲ For Ordering Information, see p. 223

❷ Menudo

New York State Department of Health
30 sec. each; TV; color; 1988; $50.00;
English/Spanish/Spanish.

This PSA addresses Hispanic youth and emphasizes how fun and exciting it is to be a teenager. It explains that in the "age of AIDS" teenagers need to take responsibility for the continuing enjoyment of their youth, urging them to learn protective measures against the sexual transmission of HIV.

Reviewers' Comments: An innovative, unusually appealing, culturally appropriate video that uses a popular rock group, Menudo, to get its message across. It encourages young people to talk with family members about AIDS/HIV. The production and the message are excellent.

▲ For Ordering Information, see p. 225

❷ On The Wrong Track / Huellas Peligrosas

CDC National AIDS Information and Education Program
Multimedia; Oct 1988; free; English/Spanish.

This America Responds To AIDS print ad contains a photograph of a couple's held hands. The narration explains that "Anna" is making a mistake by going out with an IV drug user and that she has choices to make if she wants to protect herself from AIDS/HIV: get him to stop, leave him, or make sure he wears a condom when they have sex. Both the English and Spanish versions provide the number of the National AIDS Hotline. The ad is available in a variety of sizes, and government agencies and AIDS organizations are free to localize it according to need.

Reviewers' Comments: This ad raises the reader's interest and provides solid options to readers in "Anna's" situation. However, the text inaccurately implies that stopping drug use or drug counseling alone will alleviate the danger of AIDS/HIV infection.

▲ For Ordering Information, see p. 216

❷ Spanish Language AIDS Public Service Announcements

Hispanic Health Alliance
TV; 1988; $13.00; Spanish/Spanish.

The first of these three TV PSA's, "Rumores," presents individuals whispering AIDS/HIV-related rumors into each other's ears. The final person in this grapevine is an informed woman who breaks the pattern and tells the viewer not to believe rumors about AIDS/HIV; learning the facts is the way to prevention. "Conozca a su pareja" has a man and a woman sitting next to each other on a sofa, thinking about the possibility that the other may be HIV-infected. They turn to each other and say, "May I ask you something?" The "informed woman" reappears to tell the viewer that it is important to know, to ask, and to protect yourself. "Conoce su nivel de reisgo?" has a young man who asks the viewer whether he or she has engaged in any of various risky behaviors, such as unprotected sex or drug use. He suggests that any viewer who has should find out more about AIDS/HIV. All three give an Illinois AIDS/HIV information phone number.

Reviewers' Comments: These well thought out PSAs accomplish the goals of promoting AIDS/HIV awareness: dealing with fear, getting people to think about risks and learning ways to protect themselves. They are good examples for groups who want to put together their own public service announcements.

▲ For Ordering Information, see p. 221

VIDEOS / FILMS

○ Gente Como Nosotros / People Like Us

State of New Mexico AIDS Prevention Program Health & Environment Department

❷ Images: Crisis On AIDS

New Jersey Network
30 min.; VHS 3/4; 1987; $95.00; rental fee: $50.00/2 weeks; English.

This edition of the program "Images" presents interviews in English with Spanish subtitles and vice versa. New Jersey's Commissioner of Health discusses programs to combat the AIDS/HIV virus in the community of IV drug users. A person with AIDS relates his history of drug use. Also interviewed are health educators, a New York City councilman, and representatives of organizations that organize AIDS fundraising events. Some topics discussed are: the impact of the AIDS/HIV epidemic in New Jersey; manditory and confidential testing for HIV infection; and how to reach target groups with AIDS education programs.

Reviewers' Comments: This is a good, general overview of the impact of the AIDS/HIV epidemic on New Jersey. It is appropriate for both Latino and general audiences.

▲ For Ordering Information, see p. 225

❷ No Nos Engañemos

Los Angeles County Dept. of Health Services AIDS Program Office
22 min.; VHS; 1987; $24.95; Spanish.

This video contains a narrative voice-over and a series of still photographs which together form a documentary-type presentation of basic AIDS/HIV information. The main figure is a Latino doctor in Los Angeles who is shown in the office and giving a seminar for the lay Latino community. In these settings he interacts with patients and community members, presents information, answers questions, and dispels myths. Topics covered include casual contact, how HIV impairs the immune system, how a person can be infected and not show signs or symptoms of infection, how HIV affects individuals differently, and how HIV is transmitted through unprotected sex and needle sharing, among others.

Reviewers' Comments: This is a good introduction to basic information on AIDS/HIV, and it is appropriate for general Latino audiences. Pleasant narration and a successful use of case studies convey this information well.

▲ For Ordering Information, see p. 222

❶ Ojos Que No Ven / Eyes That Fail To See

Instituto Familiar De La Raza - Latino AIDS Project
51:34 min.; VHS; 1988; $356.00; rental fee: $75.00/2 weeks; special rates / discounts; Spanish.

In this video, actors portray people in the Latino community who are affected by the AIDS/HIV epidemic. They enact scenes in which a mother who discovers her son is homosexual speaks to a counselor who helps her come to terms with the news and explains HIV transmission so she can talk to her son and daughter; an employee who visits a fellow employee dying of AIDS in a hospital; a young woman who has trouble accepting her brother's homosexuality; a former drug dealer whose former accomplice comes to see him after getting out of jail and tries to lure him back into using IV drugs, but a drugs and AIDS/HIV counselor helps him resist the temptation; and a pregnant woman whose husband is sleeping with a prostitute, among others. The storylines are interwoven to show how complicated the process of HIV transmission can be, but the overall message is one of compassion and hope. The original video is in Spanish; the English version is dubbed.

Reviewers' Comments: Although targeted at Mexican-Americans, this video is equally appropriate to other Hispanic sub-groups. It is an excellent, clever, and culturally sensitive video about the impact of AIDS/HIV on the Latino family. The dubbing of the English version is distracting, but does not prevent the viewer from being engaged by the film. It is highly recommended.

▲ For Ordering Information, see p. 221

❷ SIDA Y Su Familia

AIDS Prevention Project Dallas County Health Department
11:30 min.; 1988; $8.22; special rates / discounts; Spanish.

This video uses a "talking head" format to inform the general Latino community about AIDS/HIV. The narrator discusses basic aspects of HIV: how it is transmitted through needle sharing and unprotected sex, what HIV does to the immune system once it infects someone and how to protect against sexual transmission. Condom use is suggested for all types of sexual relations. The video does not explain how to clean IV drug needles. Dallas phone numbers are provided where the viewer can obtain further information.

Reviewers' Comments: This is an effective video for the entire family, since the language is simple. Though one person does most of the talking, making the presentation somewhat boring, the information is factual. The explanations of transmission and prevention measures (including condom use) are clear and complete. The hotline appearing at the end of the video is a regional contact for the state of Texas.

▲ For Ordering Information, see p. 213

❶ 1ST EDITION RECOMMENDED   ❷ 2ND EDITION RECOMMENDED   ○ NOT RECOMMENDED

❷ Una Cuestión De Vida O Muerte: Una Historia Sobre El SIDA

New York State Department of Health
> 20 min.; VHS; 1988; $20.00, limited copies; special rates / discounts; Spanish.

This video uses a soap opera format to present AIDS/HIV information. The story centers around one family and its attempt to cope with the reality of AIDS/HIV. A young woman teaches her sister about condoms and she and her boyfriend talk about safer sex. Other scenes inform the viewer about casual contact, transmission through needle sharing and unprotected sex, and transmission prevention. The video is highly emotional and is targeted at sexually active young people.

Reviewers' Comments: It would be advisable to use this video with the assistance of a health educator. Fear is used as a technique to get adolescents to change behavior, and the video is very powerful. It is sensitive to both cultural and religious values, and peer counseling among adolescents is used to good effect.

▲ For Ordering Information, see p. 225

❷ Una Perspectiva Latina

Los Angeles County Dept. of Health Services AIDS Program Office
> 25 min.; VHS; 1987; $24.00; special rates / discounts; Spanish.

This video uses a question-answer format to provide basic information on AIDS/HIV. "People in the street" ask questions about HIV, transmission, and other basic aspects of HIV and HIV-infection, and the questions are answered by a physician in non-technical language.

Reviewers' Comments: The question and answer format of this video is appealing and the questions are interesting. It promotes credibility by using health care and medical personnel as well as a representative of the religious community. It is particularly recommended for health care educators to engage Latinos in discussion of the issues.

▲ For Ordering Information, see p. 222

PARENTS, EDUCATORS, AND ADMINISTRATORS

BOOKS / MANUALS

○ **How To Protect Your Family From AIDS**

National AIDS Prevention Institute

❷ **Lynda Madaras Talks To Teens About AIDS**

Newmarket Press
106 pages; hardcover; illustrations; 1988; $5.95; special rates / discounts; English.

Written for parents, teachers, and young adults aged 14 through 19, this book serves as a guide for talking to teens about AIDS. In the preface, Madaras discusses her approach to prevention education and gives six tips for talking to teens about AIDS. Madaras addresses the myths and the facts about the disease, the symptoms, the modes of transmission, high-risk groups, information on abstinence and safe-sex practices (e.g. proper use of condoms; "outercourse" or dry sex), blood-to-blood transmission (e.g. how AIDS is transmitted through IV drug use and transfusions) and preventive measures. A final chapter encourages teens to fight against AIDS through awareness, fundraising and education. This chapter also provides a listing of AIDS hotline numbers by state, along with additional resource information.

Reviewers' Comments: This product requires at least a tenth grade reading level and may be most appropriate for educated middle class readers. While it provides comprehensive coverage of AIDS-related issues for teens, it shows less familiarity with teenage drug use and inner-city issues. It provides frank, matter-of-fact discussions and illustrations of condom usage, sexual issues and offers good examples of how to handle difficult situations with peers.

▲ For Ordering Information, see p. 225

BROCHURES

❷ **AIDS, Adolescents, And The Human Immunodeficiency Virus**

Center for Population Options
1 page; special rates / discounts; Oct 1988; English.

This fact sheet is designed to create an awareness of the increasing high risk of HIV infection in teenagers because of their experimentation with sex and drugs. The information is presented as bulleted points covering the following topics: the status of HIV infection in the United States; HIV infection among teenagers and young adults; sexual intercourse and sexually transmitted diseases; drug and alcohol use; runaways and prostitution among the teenage population; and knowledge and attitudes about HIV infection and prevention. Statistics are presented which illustrate the high risk of transmission of HIV among teenagers. A list of references is provided.

▲ For Ordering Information, see p. 217

○ **AIDS In The Workplace - A Supervisory Guide**

National Safety Council

○ **AIDS: What Parents Need To Know**

Seattle-King County Department of Public Health

❶ **AIDS, Your Child And You - Answers About Children And AIDS**

AID Atlanta, Inc.
3 panels; free, limited copies; May 1987; English.

▲ For Ordering Information, see p. 213

❶ **Children And AIDS**

Rhode Island Department of Health AIDS Program
3 panels; illustrations; free, limited copies; Apr 1987; English.

▲ For Ordering Information, see p. 227

❶ 1ST EDITION RECOMMENDED   ❷ 2ND EDITION RECOMMENDED   ○ NOT RECOMMENDED

○ **Children And AIDS: What Should Parents Know?**

Ohio Department of Health - AIDS Unit

❶ **Children Can Get AIDS, Too - Questions And Answers / Los Niños Tambien Pueden Contraer SIDA- Preguntas / Respuestas**

Albert Einstein College of Medicine AIDS Family Care Center
3 panels; illustrations; free; Jun 1987; English/Spanish.

▲ For Ordering Information, see p. 214

❷ **Children, Parents, And AIDS**

American Red Cross National Headquarters
6 panels; free; 1989; English.

This brochure addresses parents' concerns regarding potential HIV infection of their children. It gives some basic information, and discusses such issues as AIDS/HIV in school, how children become infected, casual contact, talking with children about AIDS/HIV, and talking with teenagers about sexual transmission and condom use.

▲ For Ordering Information, see p. 215

❶ **How To Talk To Your Children About AIDS**

Sex Information And Education Council Of The United States
6 panels; free, limited copies; 1986; English.

▲ For Ordering Information, see p. 228

❶ **How To Talk To Your Teens And Children About AIDS**

National PTA
6 panels; $.20; special rates / discounts; 1988; English.

▲ For Ordering Information, see p. 224

❷ **Ideas For Talking To Your Child About AIDS**

Seattle-King County Department of Public Health
1 page; $.20; 1988; English.

This leaflet provides ideas and information for talking about the AIDS/HIV virus to children from ages five to seventeen. It provides a roster of topics to be covered by particular ages so that information on HIV can be conveyed in an appropriate context of health care knowledge and a system of family values. The body of the leaflet informs parents and educators of the kinds of AIDS/HIV-related questions to expect from young people and suggests responses appropriate to the child's age and knowledge level.

▲ For Ordering Information, see p. 228

○ **Latest Facts About AIDS - AIDS And Children - Information For Parents Of School-Age Children**

American Red Cross National Headquarters

○ **Latest Facts About AIDS - AIDS And Children - Information For Teachers And School Officials**

American Red Cross National Headquarters

○ **Questions And Answers On AIDS**

American Federation of Teachers

❷ **School Systems And AIDS: Information For Teachers And School Officials**

American Red Cross National Headquarters
7 panels; free; 1989; English.

Besides covering basic AIDS/HIV information, this brochure discusses such issues as protecting children from HIV infection in the school setting, first aid and CPR in schools, how safe schools are for a child with HIV infection, who should be informed of such a student, and school employees with HIV infection. Criteria are presented for an effective school health education program on AIDS/HIV.

▲ For Ordering Information, see p. 215

❶ Talking With Your Child About AIDS

ETR Associates/Network Publications
3 panels; illustrations; special rates / discounts; 1988; English.

▲ For Ordering Information, see p. 219

❶ Talking With Your Teenager About AIDS

ETR Associates/Network Publications
4 panels; illustrations; special rates / discounts; 1988; English.

▲ For Ordering Information, see p. 219

❷ Talking With Your Teenager About AIDS

AIDS Prevention Project Dallas County Health Department
3 panels; free; 1988; English.

This brochure encourages adults to talk with teens about AIDS, even though both adults and teens may feel uncomfortable speaking frankly about drugs and sex. It emphasizes the importance of these discussions because hearing about AIDS can make adolescents fearful, and because they need to know how to protect themselves. Before talking with teens, adults are encouraged to prepare themselves; facts are listed as well as hints for helping the conversation go smoothly. The Dallas, Texas and National AIDS Hotline numbers are listed.

▲ For Ordering Information, see p. 213

◯ Teachers And Parents: The ABC's - Talking About HIV With Children

Special Immunology Service, Children's Hospital

◯ What Every Parent Should Know About AIDS

American Red Cross National Headquarters

❷ When A Child's Test Is HIV Positive

Special Immunology Service, Children's Hospital
3 panels; free, limited copies; 1988; English.

This brochure is designed to help parents cope with the news that a child has tested positive for the HIV virus. Using question and answer format, it covers the issues such as what the test means; whether or not to tell the child, caregivers, family, and friends; what happens next; and how to protect those who come in contact with the child from potential infection. The overall message of the Children's Hospital staff is one of support--"Our goal is to take one step at a time with you and your child."

▲ For Ordering Information, see p. 228

◯ Will My Child Get AIDS?

NO/AIDS Task Force

❶ You And Your Family - You Can Protect Yourselves From AIDS. It's Easy

Massachusetts Department of Public Health
2 panels; illustrations; free, limited copies; Dec 1987; English/Spanish.

▲ For Ordering Information, see p. 222

❷ Your Child And AIDS

Hawaii State Department of Health STD/AIDS Prevention Program
3 panels; illustrations; free; 1988; English.

This brochure provides information to parents whose children are in a daycare center or school where another child may have AIDS or HIV infection. The difficulty of transmitting the virus through casual contact in this setting are explained as are Hawaii's guidelines for dealing with AIDS/HIV cases in the schools.

▲ For Ordering Information, see p. 220

❶ Your Child And AIDS - A Simple Guide For Parents With Children In Daycare And Public Schools

San Francisco AIDS Foundation
3 panels; illustrations & photographs; $.30; special rates / discounts; 1988; English/Spanish.

▲ For Ordering Information, see p. 227

❶ 1ST EDITION RECOMMENDED   ❷ 2ND EDITION RECOMMENDED   ◯ NOT RECOMMENDED

INSTRUCTIONAL PROGRAMS

❶ An AIDS Curriculum For Adult Audiences

Arizona Department of Health Services Office of Health Promotion and Education
108 pages; paperback; graphs; Nov 1987; English.

This curriculum, designed for training professionals giving AIDS/HIV presentations in the community or at worksites, contains six sections. Section One states the goal and objectives of the program and includes a list of needed materials. Section Two provides a detailed guide for standard AIDS/HIV presentation which covers cause, diagnosis, risk behaviors, transmission, HIV antibody testing, symptoms, and prevention of AIDS/HIV. Section Three contains background materials, including key articles about AIDS/HIV, summaries of available videotapes, and an Arizona general population survey. Section Four provides teaching tools: 12 overhead transparency masters, local and national surveillance reports, and information on the rights of persons with AIDS/HIV. Section Five lists brochures and fact sheets for trainees and Section Six includes evaluation tools.

Reviewers' Comments: Although the curriculum content is good, the resource materials need to be updated and the assessment instruments improved. Sample lesson plans would be helpful.

▲ For Ordering Information, see p. 215

❷ Dealing With AIDS

American Association of School Administrators
30 pages; stapled; charts; Mar 1988; $5.00; special rates / discounts; English.

This pamphlet is designed as a guide for developing AIDS/HIV education programs consistant with local needs and standards for early elementary through high school students. Concerned school administrators and parents are encouraged to start by getting approval from the superintendent and the school board. The next step recommended is establishing a task force including a broad spectrum of concerned citizens from within the school and the community. Also included are: evaluation criteria for any program developed; sample learner outcomes; age-based sample lesson plans; a glossary and a resources section of organizations, curricula, literature, parent materials, film and video, data bases, and hotline numbers.

Reviewers' Comments: This pamphlet makes the assumption that the reader is already knowledgeable about AIDS/HIV. While some of the sample exercises are good, leadership that is needed for developing skills and changing behavior is not outlined.

▲ For Ordering Information, see p. 214

❷ Does AIDS Hurt?

ETR Associates/Network Publications
149 pages; paperback; 1988; $14.95; special rates / discounts; English.

This book gives teachers, parents, and administrators who spend time with children under 10, basic information and suggested guidelines for addressing the issues surrounding AIDS/HIV. It emphasizes the use of age-appropriate responses to children's questions. Maintaining that children do not need explicit information about AIDS/HIV, the book underscores the importance of a solid general health education in giving children the tools to understand concepts about disease transmission. Classroom examples demonstrate effective ways of providing relevant and appropriate AIDS/HIV education to young students.

Reviewers' Comments: This is an excellent resource book for teachers, educators, and social service workers. It is well-organized, comprehensive, and highly recommended.

▲ For Ordering Information, see p. 219

○ Preventing AIDS - Health Education Curriculum Supplement For Middle Level Schools

North Carolina AIDS Control Program

○ What Kids Need To Know About AIDS

Planned Parenthood of N.E. Pennsylvania

MULTICOMPONENT PROGRAMS

❷ Parent-Teen AIDS Education Project

- **Manual**
  127 pages; 3 ring binder; charts; 1988; special rates / discounts; English.
- **Talking With Teens With Jane Curtin**
  27:20 min.; VHS; 1988; English.
- **Talking With Your Teen About AIDS**
  3 panels; photographs; $.30; special rates / discounts; 1988; English/Spanish.

San Francisco AIDS Foundation

This multi-component package is directed primarily at parents, encouraging them to discuss AIDS/HIV with their teens. It provides information and advice on establishing community-based parent organizations to promote AIDS/HIV education among parents, and to develop better dialogues between parents and adolescents.

The manual includes outlines of programs to educate parents of teens and guidelines for implementing these programs. It includes sections on cultural and ethnic considerations, working with the local media, and guidelines for writing an AIDS/HIV policy. One section on parent meeting guides is also included in Spanish. The appendices contain basic AIDS/HIV information, a summary of resources for educators, a listing of AIDS Lifeline television stations, and sample AIDS/HIV policies.

The video suggests that parents face the possibility that their teens are sexually active or use drugs. It shows a peer counseling group discussion with teens. There is a brief discussion of the facts about AIDS/HIV, and the parents of a teenager who died of the disease tell their story. The video ends with three parent/teen scenarios that illustrate ways to discuss AIDS/HIV openly and honestly.

The brochure invites parents not only to talk to their teens, but to learn the facts, share feelings, and listen. It states briefly how AIDS/HIV is contracted and how it can be prevented.

Reviewers' Comments: This is a complete, well thought out, and clearly written program. It provides a realistic time frame, empowers parents, and is a non-threatening way of educating parents along with their teenaged children. The brochure is brief and should be used only as part of the program.

This video is a good icebreaker for parents. The role-playing vignettes between parents and children are believable and well done. Parents are characterized as human, not all-knowing. Ideally, a resource person should be present at the screening to answer questions raised by the video.

▲ For Ordering Information, see p. 227

PAMPHLETS

◯ A.I.D.S. - Your Child & The School

R & E Research, Inc.

◯ AIDS And Children

Washington State Office on HIV\AIDS

◯ AIDS And The Education Of Our Children: A Guide For Parents And Teachers

U.S. Government, Department of Education

❶ Carolina Tips - AIDS: Education Against Fear

Carolina Biological Supply Company
4 pages; photographs; Feb 1986; special rates / discounts; English.

This pamphlet, primarily for science teachers, describes the history of AIDS, and HIV, modes of transmission and prevention, and evidence of infection. It includes electron micrographs of HIV and color photographs of the manifestations of some of the diseases associated with HIV infection.

Reviewers' Comments: Although somewhat outdated (e.g. the pamphlet uses "HTLV-III" instead of "HIV"), this pamphlet is a useful resource for science teachers.

▲ For Ordering Information, see p. 216

❷ From Parent To Parent: Talking To Our Kids About AIDS

Minnesota AIDS Project
8 pages; 1987; $.20; English/Spanish.

This pamphlet, produced by a group of concerned Minnesota parents, encourages other parents to talk to their children about AIDS/HIV. Very basic information is provided in simple language about what AIDS/HIV is, how it is and is not contracted, and what teens need to know. It also contains parent-to-parent suggestions on how to talk about AIDS/HIV with children and why discussing it with them is vital.

Reviewers' Comments: This is a concise piece which can serve as an introductory guide to AIDS/HIV for parents.

❶ 1ST EDITION RECOMMENDED ❷ 2ND EDITION RECOMMENDED ◯ NOT RECOMMENDED

Its information is not comprehensive, but it is encouraging and helpful for parents. Because its information is limited it should be followed-up by more in-depth "AIDS 101" education. This would be a great "hand-out" at supermarkets, doctors' offices, and PTA meetings.

▲ For Ordering Information, see p. 223

❷ How To Talk With Your Child About AIDS

Planned Parenthood Federation of America
17 pages; illustrations; May 1988; $.75; English.

This pamphlet serves as a guide for parents on how to communicate with their children about AIDS/HIV. It provides facts about HIV and prevention, safer sex practices, IV drug use, and ways to enhance a child's ability to make informed responsible choices. Parents are given age-appropriate guidelines for approaching this issue, as well as a list of resources to aid children in coping with death and dying.

Reviewers' Comments: The pamphlet is well written and factual. It has a high reading level and is probably best suited for distribution to parents who have an education of high-school level or above. The information presented is age-specific and offers useful "how to" steps.

▲ For Ordering Information, see p. 226

❷ Steps To Help Your School Set Up An AIDS Education Program

National Coalition of Advocates for Students
19 pages; illustrations; 1987; $4.00; English/Spanish.

This pamphlet targets parents, educators, and administrators using statistics on teen sexual activity and drug use to demonstrate the urgent need for AIDS/HIV education and broader sex education in the schools. A brief outline of basic facts about AIDS/HIV and prevention is followed by ideas on how to help the school set up a good AIDS/HIV education program. A checklist for picking a good AIDS/HIV curriculum and a brief list of other resources are also included.

Reviewers' Comments: This is a rare document for parents and has a reading level which is appropriate for a broad audience. The checklists are outstanding. The statistics on teen sex are on the low side, but the information is important for parents to have. This is a good background resource for parents.

▲ For Ordering Information, see p. 223

❶ What Parents Need To Tell Children About AIDS / Lo Que Los Padres Deben Decir A Sus Niños Sobre El SIDA

New York State Department of Health
6 pages; photographs; Aug 1987; free, limited copies; English/Spanish.

This pamphlet encourages parents to talk with their teen and preteen children about AIDS/HIV. It presents clear, concise answers to the essential questions that parents should address with their children (e.g., "How Don't You Get AIDS? How Do You Get AIDS?"). Although it urges young people to postpone sex, it provides safer sex information for those who are already sexually active. Both the English and Spanish versions meet the selection standards.

Reviewers' Comments: The language and tone of this pamphlet are direct, but reassuring. Although addressed to parents, it could be read by teens with high school reading skills. The colorful photographs provide a good visual modeling of parent/teen communication. It encourages frankness in the discussion of AIDS/HIV and compassion for people with AIDS/HIV.

▲ For Ordering Information, see p. 225

POSTERS

❶ Talk About AIDS Before It Hits Home / Hable Del AIDS Antes De Que Toque A Su Puerta

New York City Department of Health AIDS Education Training Unit
14 x 23; photographs; color; free, limited copies; English/Spanish.

This poster emphasizes the need for parents to discuss the facts of AIDS/HIV with their teenage children. The text also encourages abstinence, while urging sexually active adolescents to use condoms. Both English and Spanish versions meet the selection criteria.

Reviewers' Comments: This poster delivers an appropriate and important message to parents. The text of the poster, however, is somewhat lengthy.

▲ For Ordering Information, see p. 225

PUBLIC SERVICE ADS (TV, RADIO, PRINT)

❷ Your Daughter Worries About AIDS.

CDC National AIDS Information and Education Program
Multimedia; black & white; Oct 1988; free; English.

In this America Responds To AIDS print ad the dialogue reveals to a father that AIDS/HIV is a concern to his daughter. In the course of conversation he learns that he needs to initiate a conversation about AIDS/HIV with his daughter because she isn't likely to bring it up with him. The ad provides the number for the National AIDS Hotline and is available in a variety of sizes. Government agencies and AIDS/HIV organizations are free to localize it to meet their needs.

Reviewers' Comments: The print ad addresses how parents are unrealistic about their children's sex lives and encourages parents to take the first step toward discussing AIDS/HIV with their children. The headline successfully grabs the reader's attention.

▲ For Ordering Information, see p. 216

VIDEOS / FILMS

❷ AIDS And The Schools

Indiana State Board of Health
23:17 min.; VHS; Sep 1988; $6.00; English.

This video discusses the planning steps needed to deal with AIDS/HIV in the school setting. Topics include training of school personnel, admissions policies, and discrimination. Discussions are targeted for school administrators and personnel, as well as concerned parents.

Reviewers' Comments: This video explains the Indiana State Senate Bill 9 (Indiana AIDS Bill) mandating AIDS/HIV education in schools and might be useful to other states that are contemplating similar legislation. However, it is unclear to which audience this video would be most appropriate. Abrupt transitions from scene to scene make it difficult to follow.

▲ For Ordering Information, see p. 221

◯ AIDS - Men And Sexuality

The Exodus Trust

❶ AIDS: On The Front Line

Harris County Medical Society Houston Academy of Medicine
22.25 min.; VHS; 1987; $30.00; rental fee: $8.00/14 days; English.

This videotape gives teachers basic information about the nature of AIDS/HIV, how and why it has spread, and how to alert adolescent students to its dangers. It emphasizes risk behaviors, rather than risk groups, and discusses sexual behavior in general terms. It encourages teachers to communicate to students the importance of saying no to sex and intravenous drug use. No discussion guide is available.

Reviewers' Comments: This videotape makes good use of TV techniques and will hold teachers' interest. Its approach to the topic is scientific; however, the video does include some value-laden emphasis on abstinence and has dated statistics.

▲ For Ordering Information, see p. 220

❶ AIDS: The Surgeon General's Update

Future Vision
32 min.; VHS; 1988; $95.00; English.

This video opens with a personal message from U.S.Surgeon General Koop stressing the need for education as our best defense against AIDS/HIV. Other narrators discuss the disease, AIDS related infections and malignancies, signs and symptoms of ARC and AIDS, how the virus is and is not transmitted, safety procedures for handling body fluids, and protective measures for individuals. They advise on safer sex behaviors and on pregnancy for high risk women. Other topics include confidentiality in testing and treatment; responsibilities of local and state AIDS task forces; and the impact of AIDS/HIV on schools, the health care system, government, and business. There is no discussion guide available.

Reviewers' Comments: This video provides the latest scientific information on the incidence of AIDS and preventive measures. However, it omits sexual and drug use partners of hemophiliacs in the discussion of people at risk and shows overuse of protective gear by a person cleaning up a spill. Some of the visual cuts do not relate to the text and narrative.

▲ For Ordering Information, see p. 219

---

❶ 1ST EDITION RECOMMENDED   ❷ 2ND EDITION RECOMMENDED   ◯ NOT RECOMMENDED

❶ AIDS: What Do We Tell Our Children?

Walt Disney Educational Media Company c/o Coronet/MTI Film & Video
22 min.; VHS; 1987; $345.00; English.

This videotape provides comprehensive information on AIDS/HIV: how it is transmitted, why our children are at risk, and what can be done to prevent infection. The narrator, Carol Burnett, asks several physicians and AIDS/HIV health educators for specific recommendations on how to teach children about AIDS/HIV. Answers provide viewers with strategies to promote risk-reduction behavior for young people. A discussion guide is available.

Reviewers' Comments: This well-paced, non-controversial video provides parents with good basic information on AIDS/HIV. This video is most suitable for white, middle-class audiences.

▲ For Ordering Information, see p. 231

❷ AIDS: What Every Teacher Must Know

Instructional Media Institute
76 min.; VHS; 1988; $259.00; special rates / discounts; English.

This video and accompanying educator's manual provides teachers with the facts about AIDS/HIV and helps them develop strategies and the skills to teach prevention in across grade levels. An AIDS/HIV training workshop is conducted for teachers, who are encouraged to obtain parental, community, and school administration support for an AIDS/HIV prevention program and clear guidelines on the appropriate questions to handle that are within the values of their specific community. The first half of the video provides factual information on HIV, AIDS, HIV diseases, modes of transmission, blood tests for HIV, and prevention of infection. In the second half of the program, a nine-step method to help teachers handle difficult questions is introduced. The teachers practice answering difficult questions by role-playing situations with the moderator. The educator's manual provided with the video reiterates the information presented, provides guidelines for teaching AIDS/HIV in grades K-12, and includes overhead projection masters with a commentary. A teacher's guide is included.

Reviewers' Comments: The quality of this video is good, and the trainer in it is very capable. Where a school district can not identify a well-qualified trainer for AIDS/HIV education, this film provides and excellent alternative. Some "ice-breaker" activities to establish comfort in dealing with issues of sex and sexuality should be used if this is presented as a total package.

▲ For Ordering Information, see p. 221

❷ Focus On Education: AIDS In The Classroom

American Federation of Teachers
30 min.; VHS; 1987; special rates / discounts; English.

This video helps educators understand the issues that surround AIDS/HIV education in the classroom. It opens with a news-like report that introduces the topic, highlighting issues of controversy such as sex education for very young students. The body of the video is a discussion hosted by Gwen Kelly addressing these issues more directly. Among the panelists is Surgeon General C. Everett Koop.

Reviewers' Comments: The excellent discussion of opposing views on sex education may raise the anxiety level of some educators. There is very little discussion of AIDS/HIV education per se.

▲ For Ordering Information, see p. 214

❷ Mark And Joey

Planned Parenthood of San Diego and Riverside Counties
30 min.; VHS 3/4; 1989; $100.00; English.

This video is an informative drama about the family process which occurs when a son reveals that he has AIDS. Mark arrives home from college during Thanksgiving and tells his family he has AIDS. His brother Joey has the hardest time facing the new reality, although the video illustrates the tensions and perspectives of all members of the family. Some AIDS/HIV information is presented in the conversations that take place, but the focus of the video is the family system and how it copes first with the acceptance of the diagnosis and the fact that a member is dying. In particular the video emphasizes the need "to come to terms" with the situation and "to let go" of the dying member. The video was written and directed by local talent from San Diego.

Reviewers' Comments: This is a well-done video that deals with the difficult subjects of homosexuality, bisexuality, IV drug use, death, and dying. Risk behaviors are portrayed rather than risk groups. The messages about death are somber, but the family support message is positive.

▲ For Ordering Information, see p. 226

PASTORAL COUNSELORS

BROCHURES

❶ AIDS: A Christian Response

Universal Fellowship of Metropolitan Community Churches
3 panels; $.30; 1987; English.

▲ For Ordering Information, see p. 230

❶ AIDS: Is It God's Judgment?

Universal Fellowship of Metropolitan Community Churches
3 panels; $.30; 1987; English.

▲ For Ordering Information, see p. 230

◯ Homosexuality - What The Bible Does...And Does Not Say

Universal Fellowship of Metropolitan Community Churches

INSTRUCTIONAL PROGRAMS

❷ Educational Program on AIDS

AIDS Ministries Program
33 pages; stapled; illustrations; Nov 1988; $10.00; special rates / discounts; English.

This instructional program offers a model AIDS/HIV education format for the Christian community. The first two sections contain a curriculum focusing on AIDS/HIV information and increasing awareness through discussion, role playing, reading, and writing exercises. The next section provides an agenda for mobilizing the ministry to provide educational and support services. The final sections contain the text of a service whose theme is responding to AIDS/HIV as Christians, and suggested formats for the application and implementation of the curriculum in diverse congregational settings.

Reviewers' Comments: This guide offers a step-by-step, non-judgmental approach. A high level of AIDS/HIV literacy is required of the user. A resource chapter would be a helpful addition.

▲ For Ordering Information, see p. 213

PAMPHLETS

❷ Confronting The AIDS Crisis: A Manual For Synagogue Leaders

Union of American Hebrew Congregations
25 pages; 1988; $5.00, limited copies; English.

This package provides information and guidelines to rabbis for discussions on AIDS/HIV virus with congregations. Support materials include resolutions from the Union of American Hebrew Congregations, Illinois State legislation on AIDS, the Surgeon General's Report on AIDS, and an annotated bibliography. Guidelines for counseling people with AIDS/HIV and family members, and a collection of essays based on biblical concepts are provided. The CDC pamphlet, "What You Should Know About AIDS," is included.

Reviewers' Comments: This comprehensive product offers extensive guidelines and stresses a non-judgemental approach to caring for people with AIDS/HIV. Although directed at synagogue leaders, it may be used by individuals of any religion.

▲ For Ordering Information, see p. 230

❷ Worship In A Troubling Time: An AIDS-Related Resource For The United Church Of Christ

United Church Board for Homeland Ministries AIDS Program
8 pages; 1988; $.45, limited copies; English.

This pamphlet contains suggestions to the members of the United Church of Christ for formal worship in the era of AIDS/HIV. Sample prayers are included relating to petition, confession, reconciliation, thanksgiving, and healing. There are also suggestions for an appropriate order of worship and pertinent hymns.

Reviewers' Comments: This is an excellent resource guide for congregations and pastors. It stresses the church's non-judgemental role in AIDS/HIV-related issues.

▲ For Ordering Information, see p. 230

---

❶ 1ST EDITION RECOMMENDED   ❷ 2ND EDITION RECOMMENDED   ◯ NOT RECOMMENDED

PEOPLE WHO CARE

BOOKS / MANUALS

❷ Buddy Programs TA Packet

National AIDS Network (NAN)
126 pages; stapled; 1988; $15.00; special rates / discounts; English.

This manual provides extensive materials on setting up and running a buddy program for those with HIV infection and AIDS. Buddies may provide services from simple companionship to grocery shopping to legal advocacy. Since each provider and client base is different, the focus is on setting up programs that are well-tailored to the cultural sensitivities of clients. Issues covered are: an overview of buddy programs; buddy recruitment, screening, training, assignments, follow-up, and burnout; and policies and guidelines. Included in appendices are samples of forms used by various AIDS organizations for applications, contracts, training schedules and client referral.

Reviewers' Comments: This packet is comprehensive and clearly written. It includes strategies for dealing with difficult issues such as sex, suicide and burnout.

▲ For Ordering Information, see p. 223

BROCHURES

❶ AIDS's Effects On The Brain

UCSF AIDS Health Project
2 panels; $.65; special rates / discounts; Apr 1987; English/Spanish.

▲ For Ordering Information, see p. 230

◯ AIDS: Guide For Family And Friends

NO/AIDS Task Force

◯ Edikasyon Nou Sou SIDA

Haitian & Caribbean Foundation for Education and Development

❶ Latest Facts About AIDS

American Red Cross National Headquarters
4 panels; Oct 1986; English/Spanish.

▲ For Ordering Information, see p. 215

◯ Medidas De Prevención Para Familiares, Amigos, Y Compañeros

Sexually Transmitted Diseases Control Program

◯ Precauciones Para El Control De Infecciones En Personas Con SIDA

Sexually Transmitted Diseases Control Program

❶ Recommended Precautions For Caregivers Of Children With AIDS

Albert Einstein College of Medicine AIDS Family Care Center
3 panels; free; Jul 1987; English/Spanish.

▲ For Ordering Information, see p. 214

❷ When A Friend Has AIDS

Hawaii State Department of Health STD/AIDS Prevention Program
3 panels; free; 1988; English.

This brochure encourages anyone who has a friend with AIDS to maintain contact and provide as much support as possible. Some of the suggestions are to call, visit, touch, share meals, go for a walk, offer to do chores, offer to answer mail, help with shopping, celebrate holidays, and ask about the illness. Hawaii hotline numbers are listed.

▲ For Ordering Information, see p. 220

❶ When A Friend Has AIDS... / Cuando Un Amigo Tiene AIDS...

Chelsea Psychotherapy Associates
3 panels; $.30; special rates / discounts; 1987; English/Spanish.

▲ For Ordering Information, see p. 217

PAMPHLETS

❶ AIDS/HIV Infection In Children: A Guide For The Family

Los Angeles County Dept. of Health Services AIDS Program Office
12 pages; illustrations; 1988; free, limited copies; English.

This guide provides the parents of HIV-infected children with answers for many of their questions: What is AIDS? How did my child become infected with HIV? Do all children with HIV have AIDS? What are the symptoms? Does it spread and in what manner?

Reviewers' Comments: This is a short well-written pamphlet appropriate for parents of HIV antibody positive children. It does not, however, meet adolescent needs or interests. The pamphlet erroneously cites persons who have lived in areas where HIV is prevalent as being at "high risk."

▲ For Ordering Information, see p. 222

❶ The Child With AIDS: A Guide For The Family

Children's Hospital of New Jersey Children's Hospital AIDS Program (CHAP)
32 pages; illustrations; 1986; free, limited copies; English.

This pamphlet gives comprehensive coverage of the medical, psychological, and practical complications posed by pediatric AIDS. It focuses on common, real-life situations facing parents of children with AIDS.

Reviewers' Comments: This pamphlet has a compassionate, sensitive tone, but may be too medically technical in some sections. The assistance of a health professional in reviewing this information with parents may enhance the pamphlet's effectiveness.

▲ For Ordering Information, see p. 217

❶ Children With AIDS: Guidelines For Parents And Caregivers

AIDS Task Force of Central New York
7 pages; photographs; 1987; $.10; English.

This pamphlet presents "how-to" guidelines for dealing with the daily problems of caring for children with AIDS. The author, a child psychologist, discusses physical exercise, diet, household chores, affection, illness, medication and immunizations, and accidents and injuries. A final section explains how to tell a child and family members of the condition.

Reviewers' Comments: This pamphlet provides practical and helpful information for parents and caretakers. However, the print is small and the photographs of children's artworks are not used to advantage. The language is somewhat formal and does not reflect a multicultural sensitivity.

▲ For Ordering Information, see p. 213

◯ Family Information And Resource Guide

Illinois Alcoholism and Drug Dependence Association

❶ The Family's Guide To AIDS

San Francisco AIDS Foundation
9 pages; 1987; free, limited copies; English.

This booklet, addressing friends and family, discusses patient advocacy, insurance forms, living with someone with AIDS/HIV, emotional stress, and sharing medical information. It concludes with local referrals and a booklist. It is part of the series entitled "A series of Handbooks for People with AIDS."

Reviewers' Comments: This publication is more appropriate for the families of gay and bisexual men with AIDS (particularly in the San Francisco area). Sensitively written and informal in tone, it confronts issues and problems and discusses practical solutions and approaches to dealing with them.

▲ For Ordering Information, see p. 227

POSTERS

❶ I Have AIDS - Please Hug Me - I Can't Make You Sick

The Center for Attitudinal Healing
11 x 15; illustrations; color; Aug 1987; free, limited copies; English.

This poster seeks to arouse compassion for people with AIDS, especially children. A sad child-like figure drawn in crayon and shown with arms outstretched says, "I have AIDS, please hug me, I can't make you sick." It conveys the message that AIDS does not discriminate and that hostility and fear toward those whom it infects is undeserved.

❶ 1ST EDITION RECOMMENDED   ❷ 2ND EDITION RECOMMENDED   ◯ NOT RECOMMENDED

Reviewers' Comments: This poster effectively states that we should give support and compassion to people with AIDS.

▲ For Ordering Information, see p. 229

PUBLIC SERVICE ADS (TV, RADIO, PRINT)

❷ What Do You Do When Your Best Friend Has AIDS?

CDC National AIDS Information and Education Program
Multimedia; black & white; Oct 1988; free; English.

This America Responds To AIDS print ad is also available as a poster. The photograph is of "Susan," who discusses how hard it is for her to be there for someone she loves who is dying of AIDS. She asserts that she will "hang in there," and the message encourages readers to learn about AIDS/HIV. The ad provides the number for the National AIDS Hotline and is available in a variety of sizes; radio PSA version of this ad is also available. Government agencies and AIDS organizations are free to localize it according to need.

Reviewers' Comments: Although the ad may be thought-provoking for those who will take the time to read it all the way through, its objectives are unclear, and some of its implications are inaccurate. For example, it implies that if you know a PWA, you have only two options: to abandon that person or to stay with him/her, in which case both of you will fall apart. However, the ad accurately implies that there is no danger of contracting HIV through being a caretaker of a PWA.

▲ For Ordering Information, see p. 216

VIDEOS / FILMS

❷ AIDS: A Family Experience

Carle Medical Communications
33 min.; VHS; 1987; $395.00; rental fee: $75.00/3 days; special rates / discounts; English.

Don, a man with AIDS, and his mother, father, two sisters, and one brother share their experience of learning about and coping with Don's illness. Several health professionals' comments are interspersed with frank comments from each family member on various aspects of coping: learning of Don's illness and learning of his homosexuality at the same time; and figuring out where Don would live since he could no longer take care of him-

self. Each person also discusses coming to grips with fear of contagion; fear of stigma; the "roller coaster of Don's being near death several times and then improving significantly; his gradual loss of abilities; and the anger, denial, and recognition of Don's eventual death. The family's expressed hope is that their struggle will be of value for others in coping with AIDS/HIV in themselves or a family member.

Reviewers' Comments: A representation of the diverse relationships a family experiences is provided. Overall, positive support and compassion are portrayed, with the exception of the "brother," who is judgmental about homosexuals. The discussion of the problems families may encounter and the explanation of the death stages are handled well.

▲ For Ordering Information, see p. 216

◯ Bugsy's Last Stand

Medfilms, Inc.

❶ Chuck Solomon: Coming Of Age

Outsider Productions
57.16 min.; VHS; 1986; English.

This documentary-style videotape features Chuck Solomon, a well known gay member of the San Francisco Theater Community. It also focuses on his community and their collective strength in living with the disease. Using his 40th birthday as a backdrop, the film alternates party scenes with interviews and reminiscences with Solomon, his lover, and friends. The film describes the pain and personal trials of having AIDS or watching it claim a loved one. It also emphasizes the sense of community, love, and strength that the AIDS crisis engenders. There is no discussion guide available.

Reviewers' Comments: This is a good gay community-empowerment video appropriate for gay support service providers or families of persons with AIDS. It is a documentary, rather than an educational film.

▲ For Ordering Information, see p. 226

◯ Male Couples Facing AIDS

Mariposa Education And Research Foundation

◯ No Sad Songs

Filmakers Library, Inc.

❶ Too Little, Too Late

Fanlight Productions

48 min.; VHS; 1987; $198.00; rental fee:
$150.00/week; special rates / discounts; English.

This documentary enters the lives of families in which a loved one has died of AIDS. Despite fear and rejection from neighbors and co-workers, these family members and significant friends choose to love and support their dying loved one to a peaceful end. It also presents an inside view of an art therapy class in which persons with AIDS talk openly about their fears of death and dying and their conflicts with family members. In a Mothers of AIDS Patients (MAP) support group, mothers talk about their own journeys toward reconciliation with infected loved ones. The openness of those interviewed urges parents of persons with AIDS to reach out before it is too late. The film encourages viewers to empathize with the suffering of persons with AIDS and their families. The producer does not indicate the availability of a discussion guide.

Reviewers' Comments: This video effectively addresses the issues of homophobia, rejection, prejudice, and grief. It is an excellent video especially for families and friends of people with AIDS/HIV or ARC. The video is lengthy and the editing is sometimes abrupt.

▲ For Ordering Information, see p. 219

❶ 1ST EDITION RECOMMENDED   ❷ 2ND EDITION RECOMMENDED   ○ NOT RECOMMENDED

POLICY MAKERS AND LAWYERS

BROCHURES

❷ AIDS Fallacies

Health Issues Taskforce of Cleveland
   1 page; free; 1988; English.

Designed for public health educators, members of the media, policymakers, and other public officials, this flyer discusses five widely used terms which contribute to public misunderstanding about HIV transmission and infection, the possible results of HIV infection, and the meaning of the HIV antibody test. The flyer discusses the misinformation implied by each term, and suggests alternatives for use in educating the general community about AIDS/HIV.

▲ For Ordering Information, see p. 220

◯ AIDS - Information For North Carolina Legislators

North Carolina AIDS Control Program

PSYCHOLOGISTS AND SOCIAL WORKERS

BOOKS / MANUALS

❷ Volunteer Management TA Packet

National AIDS Network (NAN)
> 120 pages; stapled; 1988; $15.00; special rates / discounts; English.

This manual is designed to provide management skills to employees and volunteers involved in AIDS/HIV-related programs. Some of the topics covered include: who volunteers and why; volunteer recruitment, screening, training, deployment, maintenance, and recognition; policies and guidelines. Appendices provide sample forms and other resources.

Reviewers' Comments: This product is comprehensive and contains valuable information. However, it tends to be wordy and is sometimes unclear. The type is small and difficult to read and the technical presentation could be made more engaging by use of visuals.

▲ For Ordering Information, see p. 223

BROCHURES

◯ A Primer On Psychosocial Issues

Minnesota AIDS Project

INSTRUCTIONAL PROGRAMS

❶ AIDS Trainer's Guide

- **AIDS Trainer's Guide**
  > 92 pages; looseleaf; Apr 1987; $10.00; English.

- **AIDS Resource Manual**
  > Looseleaf; Apr 1987; $25.00; English.

New York State Department of Social Services, Office of Human Resource Development

This comprehensive AIDS/HIV education and information program is designed for New York State social service workers. It includes the AIDS Trainer's Guide, the AIDS Resource Manual, and the newsletter, AIDS Update.

The Guide provides a curriculum for a three-hour training session covering AIDS/HIV definitions, symptoms, methods of transmission, high risk behaviors, safety measures in the workplace, psychological impact of the illness, and service needs and resources. It includes pre- and post-tests, trainer's notes, content guides, student exercises, evaluation forms, and 20 handouts suitable for copying. The Guide summarizes state regulations regarding confidentiality and anonymity of HIV testing programs, and non-discriminatory health care delivery to persons with AIDS/HIV. The need for education, information, and counseling as the most effective means of changing behavior is strongly emphasized as a method of reducing the spread of the virus.

The Resource Manual includes supplementary material for use by social services staff and includes sections on medical and psychological aspects of AIDS/HIV; social and legal service implications; safety; infants, children, and adolescents; and general training. It also includes a bibliography, other resource publications and copies of the New York State directives on AIDS/HIV.

The newsletter is issued periodically to update and supplement information in the Guild and Manual.

Reviewers' Comments: This excellent educational package is effectively designed and organized. The Resource Guide and newsletter are useful companions to the training program. Though targeted specifically for New York State social service workers, these training tools serve as a good model for other similar agencies.

▲ For Ordering Information, see p. 225

❶ 1ST EDITION RECOMMENDED   ❷ 2ND EDITION RECOMMENDED   ◯ NOT RECOMMENDED

❷ Counseling On The Antibody Test

Center for AIDS and Substance Abuse Training
24 pages; looseleaf; charts; 1988; $3.50; English.

This in-service training program discusses the role of substance abuse treatment counselors in assisting clients making decisions on the HIV antibody test. HIV infection and the body's response to HIV are explained. The HIV antibody test is described and the interpretation of the negative, positive and equivocal results are reviewed. Methods of conveying the facts about HIV antibody tests are listed. The reasons why testing may and may not be advised for an individual and pre and post test counseling issues are presented with strategies to deal with these issues. Voluntary consent, informed decision making, and confidentiality are presented as three critical elements in HIV antibody test counseling. Role plays are included, and guidelines are provided for support to clients with positive results. A trainer's guide and a participant's manual are included.

Reviewers' Comments: This program provides a good overview of antibody test issues with well-designed outlines, objectives, and self-test guides. The sessions may be lengthy for HIV+ sypmtomatic individuals. The reading level may be too high for some users; however, since it is used as a teaching/training guide, instructors can simplify the presentation of materials according to need. The program is adaptable for use in all areas of HIV test counseling, not only substance abuse agencies. The three-ring binder format allows for easy additions, up-dates, and deletions.

▲ For Ordering Information, see p. 216

❷ Dysfunctional Families And HIV Infection

Center for AIDS and Substance Abuse Training
40 pages; looseleaf; 1988; $5.75; English.

This program introduces strategies for substance abuse treatment counselors helping families cope with the stressful situation of HIV infection and related illness. The structure and processes of the typical dysfunctional family are explored and applied to chemically dependent families with HIV infected members in treatment. The counseling issues raised when dealing with dysfunctinal families and HIV infection are examined and strategies to deal with these issues are presented. Involving the family in the treatment program and helping families to become supportive of the HIV infected client are among the goals of the counselor. The basic skills and strategies to achieve these goals are reviewed and practiced in role playing situations. Additional articles on this topic are included. A trainer's guide and a participant's manual are provided.

Reviewers' Comments: This program provides effective exercises and resource materials and a good breakdown of various family processes. It is comprehensive enough to be used by less experienced trainers with good clinical skills, but may not be appropriate for all types of health care professionals--it's geared more for those doing clinical work

with families. The participant manual is easy to read; it requires a fairly high literacy level, but is probably okay for the counselor population. The three-ring binder format allows for easy additions, up-dates, and deletions.

▲ For Ordering Information, see p. 216

❷ Focus On Women

Center for AIDS and Substance Abuse Training
1988; $7.75; English.

This in-service training program provides substance abuse treatment staff with an overview of women's AIDS/HIV-related needs and suggests ways to respond to these needs and promote risk reduction for female IV drug abusers and female sexual partners of IV drug abusers. The specific needs of these two groups for substance abuse treatment and AIDS/HIV prevention are described. Principles of empowerment and strategies to achieve it are discussed with regard to women's issues. This instructional program recommends theses strategies for risk reduciton counseling. Specific women's issues that may affect risk reduction counseling are explored. Participants identify priorities and develop plans to meet their needs. AIDS/HIV-related resources for women are listed and additional articles on the subject are included. A trainer's guide and participant's manual are provided.

Reviewers' Comments: This program offers good information appropriate to all lesbian and bisexual women and has examples of effective experiential exercises. It goes beyond risk reduction counseling in that it deals with the critical issue of empowerment for women. Furthermore, it involves the participants in program planning for improving services to women in their agencies and communities. More emphasis might be placed on the context of the women's issues addressed, particularly on the interaction between these issues and the working class, minority/ethnic community. The three-ring binder format allows for easy additions, up-dates, and deletions.

▲ For Ordering Information, see p. 216

❷ Issues For Gay, Lesbian, And Bisexual Clients

Center for AIDS and Substance Abuse Training
41 pages; looseleaf; charts; 1988; $5.75; English.

This program is designed to direct in-service training of substance abuse treatment center's staff on gay, lesbian and bisexual lifestyles and the counseling issues related to these groups when in treatment in the "Age of AIDS." Sexual minorities are defined, the basic elements of sexuality and the theories of the development of sexual orientation are presented. The sexual minority issues that clients may introduce in counseling and the AIDS/HIV issues that effect these groups are addressed. The counselors' beliefs and attitudes about these groups are examined in order to help them deal with these groups effectively. The program encourages an evaluation of each center's response to gay, lesbian and bisexual clients. Resources are provided to enable the treatment staff to develop a listing of referral services for these groups. Additional articles on the subjects are included. A trainer's guide and participant's manual are provided.

Reviewers' Comments: This program suffers a lack of visuals: graphics, comics, etc. However, it is informationally rich and contains good articles for participants. The three-ring binder format allows for easy additions, updates, and deletions.

▲ For Ordering Information, see p. 216

❷ Preventing AIDS Among Substance Abusers: A Training Program For Substance Abuse Treatment Counselors

Center for AIDS and Substance Abuse Training
90 pages; looseleaf; charts; 1988; $15.25; English.

The training program provides substance abuse treatment counselors with information on the relationship of AIDS and HIV to substance abuse and offers the counselors approaches for preventing AIDS/HIV among substance abusers, particularly in communities with lower incidences of AIDS/HIV. The important role of substance abuse counselors in AIDS/HIV prevention and the barriers to AIDS/HIV prevention are discussed. The "window for opportunity" for prevention programs in areas with lower incidences of AIDS/HIV is described. Information is presented on transmission, treatment, and prevention. The theories of prevention education and characteristics of successful prevention efforts are presented. Participants develop strategies for conducting targeted AIDS/HIV prevention. The HIV antibody tests and counseling clients about them are discussed. Counselors are trained to assist clients in assessing their personal risk of infection and in developing risk reduction and health promotion plans.

The trainer's guide provides detailed instructions for delivery of the two day training program. The program consists of eight units. The purpose of each unit, topics covered, and materials needed for the units are provided. A script of the program is provided as a guide for the trainer. Background information is included for certain units.

This manual is designed to promote active participation in this two day training program. An outline with objectives are provided for each unit. Reproductions of material presented in the program and case studies are included. Additional articles on the topic are also included.

Reviewers' Comments: The program provides a good timeline and outline of objectives, and the content of many articles is useful. The materials are lengthy and are organized poorly with regard to readability. No AIDS/HIV organizational resources are listed for referral. The program would benefit from personal accounts of HIV+ individuals, especially recovered or active IV drug users.

▲ For Ordering Information, see p. 216

❷ Preventing AIDS Among Substance Abusers: A Training Program In Administrative Planning For Substance Abuse Treatment Programs

Center for AIDS and Substance Abuse Training
40 pages; looseleaf; 1988; $16.50; English.

This program assists directors of out-patient substance abuse treatment programs in areas of lower incidences of AIDS/HIV to develop programs that prevent the spread of HIV in their communities. The program draws on the experiences of treatment centers in cities with high incidences of AIDS/HIV and stresses the "window of opportunity" for areas with lower incidences to prevent the development of AIDS/HIV in their substance abuse communities. The challenges of AIDS/HIV that are presented to substance abuse treatment center administrators are reviewed and goals are generated to address these challenges. Basic information on AIDS and HIV is reviewed and staff member concerns about HIV are discussed in case situations. Fundamental concepts of prevention education and some of the barriers to preventing HIV infection and AIDS among substance abusers are discussed. The benefits and limitations of antibody testing and the problems encountered in the development of policies on antibody testing are reviewed. The legal and ethical issues surrounding patient confidentiality and the "duty to warn" are included. Laws concerning AIDS/HIV-related problems of clients and their implications for the treatment centers are reviewed. Other AIDS/HIV related treatment issues including changes in counseling styles, community linkages, and medical care are presented. Funding for AIDS prevention and treatment services and the political and public relation issues that administrators may encounter are discussed. Participants develop a six month planning program for the development of AIDS/HIV related programs.

The trainer's guide provides detailed instructions for delivering the 2 1/2 day training program. The program consists of one introductory session and eight units. Each unit contains a perspective that describes the purpose, topics and material needed for the unit and a training outline. A "script" of the program is provided as a guide for the trainer and background information is provided for certain units.

The participant's manual supports the information presented in the program and serves as a reference resource for the participant. Outlines and objectives are presented for every unit and worksheets and reproductions of material presented in the program are included. Additional articles are included on this topic.

Reviewers' Comments: This is an extensive program with good resources. It contains reproduced materials, some of which are of very poor production quality. The program has a good timeline and outline of objectives, but is time consuming. It could be simplified for increased effectiveness in low incidence areas. The three-ring binder format allows for easy additions, up-dating, and deletions.

▲ For Ordering Information, see p. 216

❶ 1ST EDITION RECOMMENDED   ❷ 2ND EDITION RECOMMENDED   ○ NOT RECOMMENDED

② **Preventing AIDS In The IV Drug-Using Community: An Orientation To Community Health Outreach**

Center for AIDS and Substance Abuse Training
92 pages; looseleaf; charts; 1988; $20.00; English.

This training program is an orientation for community health outreach workers about AIDS/HIV and for skills development in bringing the messages of prevention and risk reduction to the IV drug user communities. An overview of community health outreach programs and barriers to their implementation are discussed. Basic information is presented on HIV, AIDS and other HIV-related illnesses, transmission, HIV antibody testing, epidemiologic information, treatment, and risk reduction strategies. Training is provided to assist clients in decisions about HIV antibody tests. The theories of prevention and the role of the outreach workers in counseling clients on risk reduction are included. Rules of conduct for outreach workers and ways to become accepted in a community are discussed. Future training needs and the skills learned in this workshop are assessed by the participants.

The trainer's guide provides detailed instructions for the delivery of the three-day training program. The program consists of 10 units. The purpose of each unit, topics covered, and materials needed for the units are provided. A "script" of the program is available as a guide for the trainer. Background information is included for some units.

The participant's manual serves as a reference resource for the participants. Outlines and objectives are presented for each unit. Worksheets and roleplaying information are also included. Additional articles are provided on the topic.

Reviewers' Comments: The organization of materials in this program is excellent with clearly defined objectives. The support materials allow for constructive participant involvement. This is one of the better manuals of its level. The language of the outreach worker text should be simpler, and the glossary expanded to include health education and street terms. Although the program provides a post-test instrument for attitudes regarding AIDS/HIV, there is none for AIDS/HIV knowledge and skills. The issues of homosexuality and substance abuse need to be addressed, and the role of the outreach worker in dealing with behavior maintenance on the street should also be added since this is where relapse occurs. The package requires an experienced trainer. The three-ring binder format allows for easy additions, up-dates, and deletions.

▲ For Ordering Information, see p. 216

② **Risk Reduction Counseling**

Center for AIDS and Substance Abuse Training
33 pages; looseleaf; 1988; $5.50; English.

This program is designed to direct in-service training of substance abuse treatment counselors for substance abusers about risk reduction for AIDS/HIV. Basic principles of health and prevention education are discussed. Information

on AIDS/HIV is presented and ways to communicate this information are suggested. The importance of clients personally assessing their risk of infection is stressed. Methods and skills for risk reduction counseling to change behavior and ways to help clients sustain changes in their behavior are discussed. Several articles on this topic are included. A trainer's guide and participant's manual are provided.

Reviewers' Comments: This is a comprehensive and easy-to-understand trainer's guide which provides useful and necessary instruction for the prospective trainer. The exercises and reading materials are useful. The issues of needle sharing and sanitation of "works" do not receive appropriate attention, which is important given that this program is targeted to counselors working with IV drug users. The three-ring binder format allows for easy additions, up-dates, and deletions.

▲ For Ordering Information, see p. 216

VIDEOS / FILMS

○ **Approaching The Topic Of AIDS**

The Exodus Trust

② **The Buffer Zone: The Mental Health Professional In The AIDS Epidemic 1989**

Carle Medical Communications
25 min.; VHS; 1989; $385.00; rental fee: $65.00/3 days; special rates / discounts; English.

In this video the mental health professionals, persons with AIDS/HIV, mental health professionals from New York's Gay Men's Health Crisis, and others with extensive experience working with persons with AIDS/HIV, outline coping issues. These include: reactions to the news of positive or negative results in HIV antibody tests; the uncertainty of when or whether HIV positivity will develop into full-blown AIDS; the emotional "roller-coaster" of bouts of serious illness followed by relative good health; and the gradual loss of abilities and eventual death. Effects on both the patient and his/her affected family and friends are considered, as are special cultural sensitivities, particularly in the Hispanic population. The mental health professional's emotions in dealing with a client with HIV positivity or AIDS are also discussed.

Reviewers' Comments: This video covers a broad range of issues, perhaps too many. The summary at the end of the film, however, is excellent. The recommendations for handling issues related to mental health professionals and AIDS/HIV are very good.

▲ For Ordering Information, see p. 216

PUBLIC SAFETY AND SUPPORT WORKERS

BROCHURES

◯ **AIDS Information For New York State Correctional Services Department Employees**

New York State Department of Health

❶ **Facts On AIDS - A Law Enforcement Guide**

New Jersey Department of Health AIDS Education Unit
4 panels; 1987; English/Spanish.

▲ For Ordering Information, see p. 224

PAMPHLETS

❷ **AIDS And Emergency Responders**

Channing L. Bete Co., Inc.
15 pages; illustrations; 1988; special rates / discounts; English.

This pamphlet, addressed to emergency responders, notes that while the risk of infection HIV small, it's not possible to know whether patients or accident victims have the virus by looking at them. Emergency responders are advised to treat the body fluids of all persons as if they are infected. It suggests on-the-job preventive measures including use of protective gloves and other devices, hand washing, and caution when using needles. Personal protection methods are listed as well, including limiting sexual partners, using condoms, and not shooting drugs. The HIV antibody test and what to do if the test is positive are explained.

Reviewers' Comments: The cartoons and illustrations make this book easy to understand and appealing for people who don't like to read a lot of information. The content is accurate and includes some general information on HIV transmission.

▲ For Ordering Information, see p. 217

VIDEOS / FILMS

❷ **AIDS: The Challenge For Corrections**

National Sheriffs' Association
18:02 min.; VHS; 1987; rental fee: $25.00/10 days; special rates / discounts; English.

This video focuses on the responsibilities and concerns of corrections professionals. Spokespersons include a Fairfax County, Virginia, sheriff; a corrections officer; a physician from the National Institute of Health; and a roundtable of other concerned professionals. Discussions include: a definition of HIV; high risk behaviors and populations; modes of transmission; how to perform arrests, and cell and body searches; CPR; housing; liability; and mandatory testing.

Reviewers' Comments: The video contains good demonstrations on how to reduce risk. There is an appropriate emphasis on training and the need for written policies. It should be accompanied by other training in order to help management understand the inmate's perspective.

▲ For Ordering Information, see p. 224

◯ **AIDS: The Silent Killer**

Syndistar, Inc.

❷ **AIDS: Con To Con**

Georgia Department of Corrections
30 min.; VHS; 1987; $100.00; English.

This video features inmates with AIDS/HIV who discuss the disease, its causes, transmission, and prevention. Inmates describe the impact of HIV infection on their lives and urge other inmates to protect themselves by implementing risk reduction measures.

Reviewers' Comments: This video gives an excellent presentation of its issues. It may be somewhat long. However, it could be useful for a wide range of audiences, especially drug users, street youth, and corrections workers. It contains good diversity in ethnicity and gender.

▲ For Ordering Information, see p. 220

❶ 1ST EDITION RECOMMENDED   ❷ 2ND EDITION RECOMMENDED   ◯ NOT RECOMMENDED

◯ **Nobody's Immune (Military)**

Walter Reed Army Institute of Research

❶ **On Guard - Infection Control For Safety And Health Care Professionals**

Focal Point Productions
23 min.; VHS; 1988; $295.00; English.

This video uses case studies to illustrate the U.S. Centers for Disease Control's "Universal Precautions" designed to minimize the risks of contracting a contagious disease from body fluids. Hospital and field scenarios alternate with scenes of drug dealer activity, police officers, ambulance drivers, and emergency room personnel. The video identifies specific ways public safety personnel can avoid contracting AIDS/HIV or hepatitis.

Reviewers' Comments: This dramatic, comprehensive presentation of infection control procedures will have wide appeal to police officers, rescue workers, and other public safety personnel. It advocates antibody testing for personnel who suffer needle-stick exposure to blood or body fluids.

▲ For Ordering Information, see p. 219

SEXUALLY ACTIVE ADULTS

BOOKS / MANUALS

❶ The Complete Guide To Safe Sex

The Exodus Trust
217 pages; 1987; $6.00; English.

This book strives to "turn people on to safe sex." Chapters cover AIDS/HIV, its transmission, the relative risk levels of certain sexual practices, methods of prevention, "safe-sex lifestyles," and ways to talk with partners. It includes an extensive glossary of academic and slang sex terms.

Reviewers' Comments: This manual offers helpful, straightforward suggestions for creating an enjoyable safer sex lifestyle. Although it is intended for sexually active adults in the general population, the manual uses technical and sophisticated language that may elude that reading audience.

▲ For Ordering Information, see p. 229

BROCHURES

❶ AIDS: A Virus That Doesn't Discriminate

North Central Florida AIDS Network
2 panels; illustrations; free, limited copies; Sep 1987; English.

▲ For Ordering Information, see p. 225

❶ AIDS: Am I At Risk? A Checklist For Modern Lovers

ETR Associates/Network Publications
3 panels; illustrations; $.22; special rates / discounts; 1988; English.

▲ For Ordering Information, see p. 219

◯ AIDS: Am I At Risk? A Self-Assessment Guide

Maine Department of Human Services Office on AIDS

◯ AIDS And Pregnancy / SIDA Y El Embarazo

Maternity Center Association

❶ AIDS And Safer Sex / AIDS/SIDA Y El Sexo Seguro

AIDS Foundation Houston, Inc.
1 panel; free, limited copies; Aug 1987; English/Spanish.

▲ For Ordering Information, see p. 213

❶ AIDS Does Not Discriminate / El SIDA No Descrimina

New York State Department of Health
1 panel; illustrations & photographs; free, limited copies; Mar 1987; English/Spanish.

▲ For Ordering Information, see p. 225

◯ AIDS Facts And Myths

San Mateo County AIDS Project

❶ AIDS-Guidelines For Risk Reduction

New Mexico AIDS Services, Inc.
4 panels; illustrations; English.

▲ For Ordering Information, see p. 225

❶ AIDS Hotline

Gay Men's Health Crisis, Inc.
5 panels; photographs; $.30; special rates / discounts; English/Spanish.

▲ For Ordering Information, see p. 219

❶ 1ST EDITION RECOMMENDED   ❷ 2ND EDITION RECOMMENDED   ◯ NOT RECOMMENDED

❶ AIDS Info: Facts You Should Know / Información Sobre El SIDA: Verdades Que Ud. Debes Saber

Cook County Hospital AIDS Service
2 panels; free, limited copies; 1987; English/Spanish.

▲ For Ordering Information, see p. 218

❷ AIDS Risk Questionnaire

Merced County Health Department
1 page; free; 1988; English.

This leaflet contains simple yes/no questions to determine a client's risk of HIV infection. It was developed for use with young people and others who practice high risk behaviours. It also offers suggestions on how to reduce risk and obtain assistance or information in Merced or Los Banos, CA.

▲ For Ordering Information, see p. 223

❷ AIDS Risk Reduction: Sex And AIDS

NO/AIDS Task Force
3 panels; $.10; special rates / discounts; 1988; English.

This brochure advises that risk of HIV infection is determined not by ethnic or sexual group to which one belongs but by behaviors in which one engages. It outlines safest, possibly safe, and unsafe sex behaviors. It provides specific information on how to use condoms and suggests that condoms should be a normal part of sex life. Ideas for negotiating safer sex, including examples, are offered. The NO/AIDS TASK Force offers resources, and provides phone numbers for information and AIDS awareness seminars.

▲ For Ordering Information, see p. 225

❶ AIDS - Safer Sex

Denver Disease Control Service
3 panels; illustrations; free, limited copies; Sep 1987; English.

▲ For Ordering Information, see p. 218

❶ AIDS - The Sexually Active Heterosexual

Denver Disease Control Service
3 panels; illustrations; May 1987; English.

▲ For Ordering Information, see p. 218

❶ AIDS: The Straight Facts / El SIDA Información Para Heterosexuales

New York City Department of Health AIDS Education Training Unit
4 panels; illustrations; free; May 1987; English/Spanish.

▲ For Ordering Information, see p. 225

❶ AIDS - Think About It / SIDA O AIDS - Pienselo

ETR Associates/Network Publications
3 panels; illustrations; free; 1987; English/Spanish.

▲ For Ordering Information, see p. 219

◯ ANYONE Can Get AIDS - At Best Abstain - At Least Protect Yourself - Use A Condom

Center One Anyone In Distress

❶ Breaking The STD Chain

Stanford University Cowell Student Health Center
4 panels; illustrations; $.50; 1987; English.

▲ For Ordering Information, see p. 228

❶ Close Encounters Of The Safer Kind

Marin AIDS Support Network
3 panels; $.25; Mar 1987; English.

▲ For Ordering Information, see p. 222

◯ The Condom

ETR Associates/Network Publications

❷ Condom Cards

**AIDS Research and Education Project,
Psychology Department California State
University at Long Beach**
Card; illustrations; $1.00; special rates / discounts;
1988; English.

Attached inside each of these black and white greeting
cards is a latex condom wrapped to look like a gold coin.
Each of the six cards offers a different, humorous message
and drawing. On the back of the cards is text advising the
reader to learn more about AIDS/HIV and to prevent its
transmission by using condoms.

▲ For Ordering Information, see p. 213

❶ Condom Cards / Tarjetas Sobre Condones

AIDS Action Committee of Massachusetts, Inc.
2 panels; illustrations; $.35; 1987; English/Spanish.

▲ For Ordering Information, see p. 213

◯ Condom Information

**Maine Department of Human Services
Office on AIDS**

❶ Condom Sense

St. Louis Efforts for AIDS
3 panels; $.15; special rates / discounts; 1986; English.

▲ For Ordering Information, see p. 228

◯ Condoms And STD

ETR Associates/Network Publications

❶ Condoms For Couples

San Francisco AIDS Foundation
3 panels; illustrations; Feb 1988; English.

▲ For Ordering Information, see p. 227

❶ Condoms, Safer Sex And AIDS

**New York City Department of Health AIDS
Education Training Unit**
4 panels; illustrations; free, limited copies; May 1987;
English/Spanish.

▲ For Ordering Information, see p. 225

❶ Face It: Safer Sex Is A Decision You Can Live With

St. Louis Efforts for AIDS
3 panels; $.15; special rates / discounts; 1986; English.

▲ For Ordering Information, see p. 228

❷ Fact Sheet No. 1 - Safer Sex

Gay Community AIDS Project
3 panels; $.10; 1988; English.

The brochure stresses the need to make changes in sexual
practices to reduce the risk for contracting AIDS/HIV.
Frank descriptions of how HIV may be transmitted through
anal intercourse and other sexual practices are given. It outlines safe, possibly safe, and unsafe sexual practices. A list
of other GCAP fact sheets, publications, and how to obtain
them is provided.

▲ For Ordering Information, see p. 219

❷ Fact Sheet No. 14 - Safer Sex Negotiations

Gay Community AIDS Project
3 panels; $.10; 1988; English.

This brochure stresses the importance of discussing safer
sex practices with a would-be partner. Several situations
are reviewed, including discomfort with certain types of
sexual behavior or issues, and the importance of frank communication is encouraged.

▲ For Ordering Information, see p. 219

◯ Fact Sheet No. 16 - User's Guide To Condoms

Gay Community AIDS Project

◯ The Facts About AIDS And Other Sexually Transmitted Diseases

Positive Promotion

◯ Family Planning Facts About AIDS

Massachusetts Department of Public Health

❶ 1ST EDITION RECOMMENDED ❷ 2ND EDITION RECOMMENDED ◯ NOT RECOMMENDED

● **For Health Care Professionals And AIDS Virus (HIV) Counselors - Safe Sex**

Montana Department of Health & Environmental Sciences Montana AIDS Program

○ **Getting Married - Facts About AIDS**

Massachusetts Department of Public Health

○ **Getting Married? Get The Facts About AIDS**

Massachusetts Department of Public Health

❷ **How To Use A Condom**

North Carolina AIDS Control Program
4 panels; illustrations; free; 1988; English.

This wallet-size brochure offers a drawing of an erect penis and demonstrates putting on a condom in three steps. Other instructions for correct condom use are also listed.

▲ For Ordering Information, see p. 225

❶ **How To Use A Condom (Rubber) / Como Usar un Condon**

Health Education Resource Organization (HERO)
4 panels; illustrations; $.15, limited copies; special rates / discounts; 1987; English/Spanish.

▲ For Ordering Information, see p. 220

❶ **I Can't Cope With My Fear Of AIDS**

Gay Men's Health Crisis, Inc.
4 panels; illustrations; $.30; special rates / discounts; 1986; English.

▲ For Ordering Information, see p. 219

❷ **I Don't Need To Wear One Of Those**

People of Color Against AIDS Network
3 panels; photographs; free, limited copies; 1988; English.

The words, "I don't need to wear one of those," stand out in white on the black background of the brochure, followed by the phrase, "Famous last words." Inside, a photograph

of a condom appears with the headline "Keep your love alive." Encouragement to use condoms and instructions for use are given in straightforward language. The hotline number for People of Color Against AIDS Network is listed.

▲ For Ordering Information, see p. 226

❶ **If You're Pregnant, Your Baby Might Be Born With AIDS / Cree Estar Embarazada?...Su Bebe Puede Nacer Con SIDA (AIDS)**

New York State Department of Health
3 panels; free, limited copies; Jul 1987; English/Spanish.

▲ For Ordering Information, see p. 225

○ **If You've Ever Had VD, Learn About AIDS**

New York State Department of Health

❷ **Important Information On AIDS...As You Marry**

Georgia Department of Human Resources
4 panels; illustrations; free, limited copies; 1988; English.

This brochure is designed as a guide for couples seeking information about the AIDS virus before marriage. It provides facts about HIV and its transmission and suggests safer sex practices and precautions for IV drug users. It discusses the risks of passing the virus on to unborn babies, briefly describes the HIV antibody test, and lists toll-free Georgia phone numbers for more information.

▲ For Ordering Information, see p. 220

○ **Información Sobre El SIDA: Verdades Que Ud. Debes Saber / AIDS Info: Facts You Should Know**

Cook County Hospital AIDS Service

❶ **Information About AIDS For Marriage License Applicants**

West Virginia Department of Health AIDS Prevention Program
3 panels; illustrations; free; Nov 1987; English.

▲ For Ordering Information, see p. 231

◯ **La Mujer Debe Informarse Sobre El SIDA / Women Need To Know About AIDS**

Gay Men's Health Crisis, Inc.

❶ **Lesbians And AIDS: What's The Connection?**

San Francisco AIDS Foundation
3 panels; charts; free, limited copies; Oct 1987; English.

▲ For Ordering Information, see p. 227

◯ **Lesbians: Low Risk For AIDS, High Risk For Discrimination**

Southern California Women for Understanding

◯ **Making Choices About Sex**

San Diego Department of Health Services

❶ **Making Sex Safer**

American College Health Association
4 panels; $.50; special rates / discounts; 1987; English.

▲ For Ordering Information, see p. 214

❷ **Men, Sex, And AIDS**

American Red Cross National Headquarters
8 panels; free; 1989; English.

This brochure targets heterosexual men. It covers basic information about HIV infection, outlines "the safest protection" against transmission, and discusses risky sex, condom use, safer sex negotiation, drug use and AIDS/HIV, and HIV antibody testing.

▲ For Ordering Information, see p. 215

❶ **An Ounce Of Prevention - AIDS Risk Reduction Guidelines For Healthier Sex**

Seattle-King County Department of Public Health
4 panels; illustrations; $.15; Apr 1987; English.

▲ For Ordering Information, see p. 228

❶ **Pregnancy And AIDS**

San Francisco AIDS Foundation
2 panels; illustrations; $.30, limited copies; Feb 1988; English/Spanish.

▲ For Ordering Information, see p. 227

❶ **STD Facts - Sexually Transmitted Disease / ETS - Las Enfermedadas De Transmisión Sexual**

ETR Associates/Network Publications
8 panels; 1986; English/Spanish.

▲ For Ordering Information, see p. 219

❶ **Safe Sex - Risk Reduction Guidelines / Para Prevenir El SIDA (AIDS)**

San Mateo County AIDS Project
Card; 25@ .75; 1987; English/Spanish.

▲ For Ordering Information, see p. 227

◯ **Safe Sex Cards**

San Francisco AIDS Foundation

❶ **Safe Sex For Men And Women Concerned About AIDS**

Health Education Resource Organization (HERO)
3 panels; illustrations; 100 @ .30; 1987; English.

▲ For Ordering Information, see p. 220

◯ **Safe Sex Lowers Your Risk For AIDS**

Minnesota AIDS Project

---

❶ 1ST EDITION RECOMMENDED   ❷ 2ND EDITION RECOMMENDED   ◯ NOT RECOMMENDED

❷ Safer Sex

AIDS Prevention Project Dallas County Health Department
3 panels; free; 1988; English/Spanish.

This brochure provides graphic descriptions of safe and un-safe sexual practices for men and women. The Spanish language version is recommended for gay Latinos. Both the English and Spanish versions meet the minimum acceptance criteria.

▲ For Ordering Information, see p. 213

❷ Safer Sex

American College Health Association
4 panels; photographs; $.50; special rates / discounts; 1986; English.

With frank descriptions of sexual behaviors, this brochure features special sections on condoms, lubricants, drugs, and alcohol. It categorizes safe, less risky, risky, and dangerous behaviors.

▲ For Ordering Information, see p. 214

❷ Safer Sex

Krames Communications
3 panels; illustrations; $.50; special rates / discounts; 1988; English.

This brochure for sexually active adults and adolescents uses color illustrations and text to explain how AIDS/HIV and other STDs are spread, safer sex practices including the use of condoms, and planning for talking to a partner about safer sex practices. Also included is information on sexual behaviors and their relative risk.

▲ For Ordering Information, see p. 222

◯ Safer Sex

Wisconsin Division of Health, AIDS/HIV Program

❶ The Safer Sex Condom Guide For Men And Women

Gay Men's Health Crisis, Inc.
6 panels; illustrations; special rates / discounts; 1987; English.

▲ For Ordering Information, see p. 219

❶ Safer Sex, Condoms, And AIDS

Ohio Department of Health - AIDS Unit
3 panels; free, limited copies; Jul 1987; English.

▲ For Ordering Information, see p. 225

❶ Safer Sex: A Guide For Everyone Concerned About AIDS

Gay and Lesbian Community Services Center
4 panels; illustrations; free, limited copies; 1987; English/Spanish.

▲ For Ordering Information, see p. 219

❶ Safer Sex: Guidelines For The Prevention Of Transmission Of The AIDS Virus

Children's Hospital National Medical Center
3 panels; 1987; English.

▲ For Ordering Information, see p. 217

❶ Safer Sex - Your Responsibility - Your Choice

Good Samaritan Project
3 panels; illustrations; free, limited copies; Mar 1987; English.

▲ For Ordering Information, see p. 220

❶ Sex And AIDS

Rhode Island Department of Health AIDS Program
2 panels; illustrations; free, limited copies; Apr 1987; English.

▲ For Ordering Information, see p. 227

❶ Some Things You Should Know About AIDS

Planned Parenthood of Central Oklahoma Education Department
1 panel; 1-99 @ .25, limited copies; Jun 1987; English/Spanish.

▲ For Ordering Information, see p. 226

❶ **Straight Talk About Sex And AIDS /**
Información A Las Parejas Sobre
AIDS/SIDA

San Francisco AIDS Foundation
3 panels; illustrations; Mar 1986; English/Spanish.

▲ For Ordering Information, see p. 227

❶ **Talking With Your Partner About**
Safer Sex

ETR Associates/Network Publications
3 panels; illustrations; 50 @ $11.00; 1987; English.

▲ For Ordering Information, see p. 219

❶ **Using Condoms Shows You Care About**
Yourself And Your Partner

AIDS Task Force of Central New York
1 panel; free; 1987; English.

▲ For Ordering Information, see p. 213

❶ **Using A Condom**

Oregon Health Division, HIV Program
3 panels; illustrations; $.10; special rates / discounts;
1988; English/Spanish.

▲ For Ordering Information, see p. 226

❶ **What Is Safer Sex?**

ETR Associates/Network Publications
3 panels; illustrations; 50 @ $11.00; 1987; English.

▲ For Ordering Information, see p. 219

◯ **¿Que Tan Hombre Es Usted? /**
Are You Man Enough?

Community Outreach Risk Reduction Education
Program (CORE)

PAMPHLETS

❷ **Are You Safe In Bed?**

Minnesota AIDS Project
8 pages; illustrations; 1987; $.20; English.

This pamphlet, aimed at sexually active young people, discusses how safer sexual activities can reduce their risk of HIV infection. Illustrations of unmade beds and strewn clothes accompany each section of information. The pamphlet ends: "You know, if we have safe sex tonight, we'll love ourselves in the morning." Minnesota hotlines are listed.

Reviewers' Comments: This pamphlet is appropriate for all sexually active adults since it conveys a basic message on safer sex. However, neither the graphics nor the text explains the "how-to's" of safer sex, and the medical information contains some gaps.

▲ For Ordering Information, see p. 223

◯ **Condom Sense**

Eroticus Publications

❷ **STDs - How To Recognize, Treat, Prevent**
Them

Krames Communications
18 pages; illustrations & graphs; 1986; $1.25; special
rates / discounts; English.

Colorful graphics and charts are used in this pamphlet to illustrate sexually transmitted diseases, how to recognize their symptoms, how to get treatment, and preventive measures. Chlamydia, AIDS/HIV, Herpes, Veneral Warts, Vaginitis, Gonorrhea and Syphilis are listed with symptoms and brief descriptions of treatment and prevention.

This pamphlet is useful, but not comprehensive. The idea of risk "groups" should be changed to risk "behaviors." Also, vaginal fluid and other secretions should be mentioned as fluids which contain HIV; only blood and semen are named.

▲ For Ordering Information, see p. 222

❶ 1ST EDITION RECOMMENDED   ❷ 2ND EDITION RECOMMENDED   ◯ NOT RECOMMENDED

❷ Understanding Safer Sex

Krames Communications

8 pages; illustrations; 1988; $1.10; special rates / discounts; English.

Medical illustrations, diagrams, and text are used in this pamphlet to describe safer sex practices. Included are explanations of AIDS/HIV, other sexually transmitted diseases, and specific steps to take to avoid high risk behavior. Suggested dialogues are included to help develop skills in negotiating safer sex with sex partners.

This pamphlet is comprehensive. It contains excellent information, particularly regarding skills in negotiating safer sex.

▲ For Ordering Information, see p. 222

❷ VD! STD! Or WHAT?

Hawaii State Department of Health STD/AIDS Prevention Program

16 pages; 1988; free; English/English.

General protective measures against STDs are encouraged in this booklet. The following diseases and their symptoms are described: gonorrhea, syphilis, chlamydia, vaginitis, genital herpes, AIDS, and veneral warts. The section on AIDS lists symptoms and identifies high-risk "groups". Where to go for a checkup, treatment advice, and hotline numbers are included.

Reviewers' Comments: This pamphlet is most appropriate for sexually active teenagers and young adults. It properly places AIDS/HIV in the context of sexually transmitted diseases. However, it emphasizes high risk "groups" rather than high risk "behaviors." Resource information is specific to Hawaii. Translations in Chinese, Ilocano, Visayan, and Tagalog meet minimum screening criteria. Japanese, Thai, Korean, and Cambodian translations do not meet these criteria. Language reviewers were unable to assess translations in Vietnamese, Laotion, Samoan, Tongan, and Hawaiian.

▲ For Ordering Information, see p. 220

POSTERS

❶ AIDS Can Be Prevented - Learn And Live / SIDA (AIDS) - Se Puede Prevenir - Aprenda Y Viva

Massachusetts Department of Public Health

17 x 22; color; Aug 1987; free, limited copies; English/Spanish.

Printed on a field of broad pastel bands, this poster succinctly summarizes the ways one can and cannot contract AIDS/HIV. It also lists risk reduction measures and provides English and Spanish hotline numbers for Massachusetts. Both the English and Spanish versions meet the minimum screening criteria.

Reviewers' Comments: Although accurate and informative, the poster's overall visual impact is somewhat muted.

▲ For Ordering Information, see p. 222

❶ Bang, You're Dead

New York City Department of Health AIDS Education Training Unit

14 x 20; photographs; color; free, limited copies; English.

This black and white poster features a large photograph of a couple embracing in bed. Under the caption, the text emphasizes the seriousness of AIDS/HIV and the need both to know your sexual partners and to use condoms. It concludes, "AIDS: If you think you can't get it, you're dead wrong."

Reviewers' Comments: Although the bedroom scene catches the eye of the viewer, the poster uses fear excessively.

▲ For Ordering Information, see p. 225

❶ Condoms--You Have A Right to Insist

San Mateo County AIDS Project

16 x 20; photographs; color; 1987; $1.00; English.

This poster shows seven women of different ages, races, and occupations holding up packets of condoms. The caption is in large red block letters.

Reviewers' Comments: This poster presents a good, clear message and is a good referral device.

▲ For Ordering Information, see p. 227

❷ Don't Be A Casualty Of Casual Sex

Wisconsin Division of Health, AIDS/HIV Program
14 x 22; color; 1988; free; English.

The poster, aimed at the sexually active population, emphasizes the need for protection against HIV infection during casual sex. This all-print poster warns readers not to be a "casualty of casual sex." It lists telephone numbers for national and Milwaukee area AIDS/HIV information.

Reviewers' Comments: The emphasis on "casual" sex rather than unprotected sex may be misleading for some; however, the poster may be used to encourage sexually active adults to get more information.

▲ For Ordering Information, see p. 231

❷ Don't Die Of Embarrassment / No Se Muera De La Pena

New York State Department of Health
8 1/2 x 11; photographs; black & white; 1987; special rates / discounts; English/Spanish.

This mini-poster series includes five posters with photos of celebrities appealing to viewers among the sexually active population. The celebrities are: Cher, Esai Morales, Whoopi Goldberg, Richard Belzer, and for the poster in Spanish, Keith Hernandez. The message reads: "Don't die of embarrassment." In smaller print, readers are urged not to be embarrasssed to talk about using condoms, and to insist on using them with anyone whose health and drug history is unknown. The New York State AIDS hotline number is given.

Reviewers' Comments: The posters make good use of celebrities to get across an appropriate message. There is a appropriate focus on negotiation skills.

▲ For Ordering Information, see p. 225

❶ Don't Go Out Without Your Rubbers

New York City Department of Health AIDS Education Training Unit
14 x 20; photographs; 1987; free, limited copies; English.

The black-and-white photograph features two condoms among the spilled contents of a women's evening purse. The caption along the bottom reinforces the visual message with, "AIDS - if you think you can't get it, you're dead wrong." This poster encourages women to carry condoms and to insist on their use.

Reviewers' Comments: Not everyone will understand the double meaning of "rubbers." For those who do, this is a clever, eye-catching poster.

▲ For Ordering Information, see p. 225

❶ Dress For The Occasion

San Francisco AIDS Foundation
15 x 20; photographs; 1988; English.

This poster features a black-and-white photograph of a white man seated, hands on knees, legs slightly apart. Shown from the mouth to the shins, he is nude except for the condom he wears on his erect penis. The message promotes safer sex through condom use, emphasizing that its use does not necessarily detract from the sexual experience.

Reviewers' Comments: Though probably not suited for indiscriminate display, this graphic but articulate picture is probably worth the proverbial "1000 words."

▲ For Ordering Information, see p. 227

❶ During Sex, Use A Latex Condom And A Lubricant With Nonoxynol-9

AIDS Administration for the State of Maryland Maryland C.A.R.E.S.
17 x 22; color; 1987; free; English.

In this poster, a comic character named "Condom King" poses with a box of lubricated condoms and a tube of contraceptive jelly, both labeled as containing nonoxynol-9. It stresses the need for sexual partners to inform themselves about these items and encourages their use.

Reviewers' Comments: This poster adequately conveys its message, but is specific to Maryland.

▲ For Ordering Information, see p. 213

❷ He Loves Me. He Loves Me Not. He Loves Me.

AIDS Administration for the State of Maryland Maryland C.A.R.E.S.
11 x 14; photographs; color; 1988; free; English.

At the top of this poster, in large black and white letters read the words: "He Loves Me. He Loves Me Not." Beneath is a photo of a pastel green condom in its package, followed, also in large black letters, by the words, "He Loves Me." In smaller letters it says, "To love someone is to protect them. Condoms do. They help keep love alive. And lovers too." Further encouragement to use condoms is followed by the Maryland AIDS hotline number and the Baltimore hotline number.

Reviewers' Comments: The small print size may make this poster difficult to read from a distance. The message is clear and simple.

▲ For Ordering Information, see p. 213

❶ 1ST EDITION RECOMMENDED   ❷ 2ND EDITION RECOMMENDED   ○ NOT RECOMMENDED

❶ If You're Not Practicing Safe Sex, You Might Get Burned - Don't Play With Fire

AIDS Council of Northeastern New York
13 x 21; illustrations; color; free; English.

Using vivid, contrasting colors and frank language, the poster warns against contracting AIDS/HIV by practicing unsafe sex. The poster ranks sexual practices from no risk to high risk. A tagline across the bottom emphasizes the dangers of AIDS/HIV.

Reviewers' Comments: This poster is visually complex and it fails to mention a number of risk behaviors. Its message is somewhat negative and it uses fear to convey that message.

▲ For Ordering Information, see p. 213

❶ In A Community As Diverse As Ours, No Matter What You're Into...Get Into This First. Be Well Equipped.

Northwest AIDS Foundation
14 x 24; photographs; free, limited copies; English.

This black-and-white poster juxtaposes photographs of three men and one woman, each holding a packaged condom. The poster urges all sexually active, at-risk members of the community to practice safer sex by using condoms. Above each of the four photographs appears a double entendre quote from the photo-subject concerning the use of condoms. For example, the black lawyer comments, "Right after I file my briefs on a risky case, I slip into this."

Reviewers' Comments: This poster can be used in a variety of adult settings. However, it is somewhat contrived, and the double entendre quotes may be misunderstood.

▲ For Ordering Information, see p. 225

❷ In 1984 We Discovered The AIDS Virus. In 1850 We Discovered A Way To Stop It.

AIDS Administration for the State of Maryland Maryland C.A.R.E.S.
11 x 14; photographs; color; 1988; free; English.

Aimed at encouraging condom use in the general population, this poster reads in large black and white letters: "In 1984, We Discovered The AIDS Virus. In 1850, We Discovered a Way To Stop It." Beneath is a photo of five condoms in pastel colors. The poster notes that while AIDS/HIV is new, condoms have been stopping diseases for years and encourages condom use. The Maryland and Baltimore AIDS hotline numbers are at the bottom.

Reviewers' Comments: The message is clear and simple, and it is visually effective.

▲ For Ordering Information, see p. 213

❷ Invest In Life Insurance

Howard Brown Memorial Clinic
11 x 14; photographs; black & white; 1988; $3.50, limited copies; special rates / discounts; English.

This poster uses a black and white photograph of a condom vending machine to present a witty, yet serious message that urges the use of condoms as one of the best defenses against AIDS/HIV. It suggests making it a "policy" to wear one, that it's an "investment that's good for life." The State of Illinois AIDS hotline number is provided.

Reviewers' Comments: The poster is engaging and the writing is excellent. It will have broad appeal to all sexually active adults regardless of sexual preference.

▲ For Ordering Information, see p. 221

❷ Let Me Help You

CDC National AIDS Information and Education Program
16 x 22; black & white; Oct 1988; free; English.

This poster shows a black square with white lettering reading, "Let me help you." The copy below reads, "If you want him to use a condom, this is all you have to say." The National AIDS Hotline number is provided for more information.

Reviewers' Comments: While for many people, "let me help you" may not be enough to say to a partner, this poster presents a positive approach to partner negotiation and suggests making condom use part of the fun.

▲ For Ordering Information, see p. 216

❷ Lifesaver

Indiana State Board of Health
14 x 38; illustrations; black & white; Dec 1988; special rates / discounts; English.

This poster describes condoms in a novel and realistic way. The words "A Pack of Life Savers" appear at the top. Below is a square of foil adhering to the poster, pressed to look like a condom package, complete with a raised ring and the words "LIFE, one rolled latex condom." The Indiana State AIDS hotline number appears below the condom package.

Reviewers' Comments: This poster is simple, direct, creative, and attractive. It makes its point well and effectively engages the viewer.

▲ For Ordering Information, see p. 221

❷ Love Is The Only Thing Your Partner Should Give You

Howard Brown Memorial Clinic
11 x 14; photographs; black & white; 1988; $3.50, limited copies; special rates / discounts; English.

This poster presents a black and white photograph of a condom in an opened condom package. The message urges partners to share love, not AIDS/HIV, and advocates the practice of safer sex and the use of condoms. The State of Illinois AIDS Hotline number is provided.

Reviewers' Comments: This is a provocative and appropriate statement. The information should include the necessity of using a latex condom and spermicide.

▲ For Ordering Information, see p. 221

❷ Only A Fool Fools Around

Connecticut State Department of Health
15 x 21; photographs; black & white; 1988; special rates / discounts; English.

This poster has a dark background with very large white letters reading, "Only Fools Fool Around. Below is a photo of condoms and the words, "Say no to sex. Or yes to condoms. AIDS. You never know who's got it." The State of Connecticut Department of Health Services is credited.

Reviewers' Comments: This poster imparts a clear message with good design elements.

▲ For Ordering Information, see p. 218

❶ The Other Night Charlie Brought Home A Quart Of Milk...And A Case Of AIDS

New York City Department of Health AIDS Education Training Unit
14 x 20; photographs; free, limited copies; English.

This poster emphasizes that bisexual men run the risk of spreading HIV to their lovers, wives, and unborn children. The poster pictures a young man carrying home a bag of groceries. It implies that he is a carrier of AIDS/HIV.

Reviewers' Comments: This poster is particularly useful because it addresses the often overlooked bisexual male. Its very realistic image has an immediate impact.

▲ For Ordering Information, see p. 225

❷ People Who Play Safe

Columbus AIDS Task Force
19 x 25; black & white; 1988; free; English.

This poster announces that "People who play safe. . . are still here." For viewers who know about AIDS/HIV and safer sex, it is a reminder to continue protecting their lives. It also functions as a teaser for those viewers who might be unaware of safer sex practices and their importance. The Columbus AIDS Task Force and local hotline numbers are included.

Reviewers' Comments: This is a clear and direct message with a positive approach to safer sex.

▲ For Ordering Information, see p. 217

◯ Prevent Life And Death All In One Shot

Health Education Resource Organization (HERO)

❷ Putting On A Condom Is Just As Simple

CDC National AIDS Information and Education Program
16 x 22; photographs; black & white; Oct 1988; free; English.

This poster shows a photograph of a man putting on a sock and reads, "Putting On A Condom Is Just As Simple." Copy below the photograph emphasizes the ease with which one can protect oneself by using condoms. The National AIDS Hotline number is given. A 30 second TV public service announcement with a longer script is also available. Both print and TV versions can be changed to include local hotlines or contacts.

Reviewers' Comments: This wonderful, wry comment counters a common misconception about the difficulty of condom use. The photography is attractive and the message is excellent.

▲ For Ordering Information, see p. 216

❷ Roll On Protection

Howard Brown Memorial Clinic
11 x 14; photographs; black & white; 1988; $3.50, limited copies; special rates / discounts; English.

This poster uses a black and white photograph of a condom to communicate its simple, light-hearted message about protection against AIDS/HIV. It urges the use of a condom during intercourse and suggests that you'll "get protection and pleasure rolled into one." The State of Illinois AIDS Hotline number is provided.

❶ 1ST EDITION RECOMMENDED ❷ 2ND EDITION RECOMMENDED ◯ NOT RECOMMENDED

Reviewers' Comments: This is a provocative, well-written poster; however, it omits "latex" and "spermicides." It is an interesting take-off on a well recognized TV commercial.

▲ For Ordering Information, see p. 221

❷ These Days You Could Get Your Name In The Paper Just By Having Sex

Howard Brown Memorial Clinic
11 x 14; photographs; black & white; 1988; $3.50, limited copies; special rates / discounts; English.

This poster uses a black and white photograph of the obituaries to make the point that sex without a condom can kill you. It urges the use of a condom in order to be safe and not to become a statistic. The State of Illinois AIDS Hotline number is provided.

Reviewers' Comments: This poster is thought-provoking and good graphically; however, it omits the need to use latex condoms and relays its message by fear.

▲ For Ordering Information, see p. 221

❷ What Have You Got Against A Condom? / ¿Que Tienes En Contra De Un Condon?

CDC National AIDS Information and Education Program
16 x 22; photographs; black & white; Oct 1988; free; English/Spanish.

This poster comes in eight versions with photographs of one man or woman from white, black, and Hispanic backgrounds. The headline reads, "What Have You Got Against A Condom?" and copy at the bottom stresses the importance of using condoms during each sexual encounter. Hotline numbers are also provided for further information. Two versions are in Spanish, six in English. The Spanish language versions list hotlines for Spanish-speaking people.

Reviewers' Comments: The "challenge" of this message is good. The abruptness and simplicity of the presentation will get the viewer's attention. Some photographs play more successfully off the headline than others. The Spanish translations meet the minimum screening criteria.

▲ For Ordering Information, see p. 216

❶ Women Can Get AIDS, Too / Las Mujeres Tambien Pueden Contraer El AIDS (SIDA)

New York City Department of Health AIDS Education Training Unit
11 x 17; illustrations; color; free, limited copies; English/Spanish.

This poster, in English and Spanish editions, warns that women can get AIDS/HIV too. It gives very brief summaries of modes of transmission and protection guidelines, and gives English and Spanish hotline numbers. This poster targets women of color. Both language versions meet selection standards.

Reviewers' Comments: The poster's message is brief, accurate, and appropriate for the target audience.

▲ For Ordering Information, see p. 225

❶ You Can't Live On Hope / No Se Puede Vivir De Esperanzas

New York City Department of Health AIDS Education Training Unit
14 x 20; illustrations; free, limited copies; English/Spanish.

This poster depicts, in comic strip-like drawings, a man and woman embracing in bed. Their thoughts appear in comic strip balloons: hers, " I hope he doesn't have AIDS;" his, "I hope she doesn't have AIDS." The message advises using condoms or just saying no. Both English and Spanish versions meet the selection standards.

Reviewers' Comments: The comic book motif and clever text forcefully convey the poster's message. The Spanish version will reach Spanish-speaking groups effectively.

▲ For Ordering Information, see p. 225

PUBLIC SERVICE ADS (TV, RADIO, PRINT)

❷ AIDS Radio Public Service Campaign - "Adults"

Connecticut State Department of Health
60 sec.; 1988; special rates / discounts; English.

Two women office workers discuss what did and did not happen when one of them went on a date the night before. Her friend is amazed that she asked "Mr. Right" to wear a condom, saying he doesn't look sick to her. The message is: "Don't flirt with AIDS; say no to sex or yes to condoms."

Reviewers' Comments: This is a very good PSA with strong role models for women.

▲ For Ordering Information, see p. 218

❷ AIDS Television Public Service Campaign - "Adults"

Connecticut State Department of Health
30 sec.; 1988; free; English/Spanish.

This TV ad shows an open window, curtains blowing in a breeze, and the outline of two figures in a bed with rumpled sheets while voices of a man and woman are overheard. When the woman suggests that the man "put this on," he asks if she is afraid of becoming pregnant, and she replies that she is concerned about AIDS and that they should both protect themselves. Without explicitly mentioning condoms, their use is recommended.

Reviewers' Comments: This PSA is strong and cleverly written. In a non-threatening way it emphasizes the need for women to take responsibility for their behavior.

▲ For Ordering Information, see p. 218

❷ AIDS Television Public Service Campaign - "Brother"

Connecticut State Department of Health
30 sec.; 1988; special rates / discounts; English.

This TV ad opens on a street scene. A young man crosses the street and hands something to his younger sister, telling her to use it to prevent pregnancy or infection with HIV. When she asks if he is giving his approval for her to "fool around," he replies that he is not; that "Only a fool fools around." It promotes the use of condoms without mentioning them and without condoning premarital sex. Also available in a radio version.

Reviewers' Comments: This is a very strong, well-produced PSA. The word "condom" is not used and is not shown, but the message is clear. The actors are Black but the message has a universal appeal.

▲ For Ordering Information, see p. 218

❷ Do You Talk About AIDS On The First Date?

CDC National AIDS Information and Education Program
Multimedia; black & white; Oct 1988; free; English.

This America Responds To AIDS print ad presents a photograph of a man in his early thirties. The title of the ad is the first line of a dialogue between the man in the photo and another, unseen person. The conversation encourages the reader to talk about AIDS/HIV, and especially to bring up the subject with prospective sexual partners. The ad provides the number for the National AIDS hotline and is available in a variety of sizes; a radio public service announcement version is also available. Government agencies and AIDS organizations are free to localize it to meet their needs.

Reviewers' Comments: This ad has an eye-catching headline.

▲ For Ordering Information, see p. 216

❷ Have You Talked With Your Wife About AIDS?

CDC National AIDS Information and Education Program
Multimedia; Oct 1988; free; English.

In this America Responds To AIDS print ad a photograph of a construction worker is accompanied by a conversation between him and an unseen person. Although he worries about AIDS/HIV a lot, "Bob" is resistant to the idea of talking to his wife about it. He realizes during the conversation that she probably worries about it, too, and he seems to acknowledge the importance of communication. The ad provides the number of the National AIDS Hotline and is available in a variety of sizes. Government agencies and AIDS organizations are free to localize it to meet their needs.

Reviewers' Comments: A noteworthy aspect of this print ad is that the implication of infidelity emphasizes the importance in all marriages of discussing AIDS/HIV. Worrying about it is not enough. Versions with more ethnically diverse images would be helpful.

▲ For Ordering Information, see p. 216

❶ 1ST EDITION RECOMMENDED　　❷ 2ND EDITION RECOMMENDED　　○ NOT RECOMMENDED

❷ I Love Sex /
Me Encanta Hacer El Amor

CDC National AIDS Information and Education Program
Multimedia; Oct 1988; free; English/Spanish.

This *America Responds To AIDS* print ad presents a photo of a male hand with a wedding band caressing a woman's bare abdomen. The man explains in the text that he's not afraid of getting AIDS/HIV because he's never shot drugs and he and his wife are mutually faithful. The ad in English provides the number for the National AIDS Hotline and in Spanish provides the National SIDA Hotline phone number. It is available in a variety of sizes, and government agencies and AIDS organizations are free to localize it to meet their needs.

Reviewers' Comments: The headline piques the reader's interest immediately and the message about monogamy is clear. However, it is very moralistic and the emphasis on fidelity can lead to misconceptions about risk. Socially sanctioned relationships do not prevent infection. The Spanish translation is good and meets the minimum acceptance criteria.

▲ For Ordering Information, see p. 216

❷ It Can Happen To You

Indiana State Board of Health
60 sec.; TV; 1987; $15.00; English.

This PSA encourages people to go to anonymous test sites for tests and counseling. Several people state various reasons why they thought they would not contract AIDS/HIV. Local phone numbers of each test site appear on individual tapes.

Reviewers' Comments: The vignettes in this PSA are compelling and reality-based, but they use stereotypes--the gay male is white, the prostitute is black. The piece also inaccurately implies that the "test" is for AIDS although it is actually for HIV antibodies.

▲ For Ordering Information, see p. 221

❷ Mathematical Equation

Indiana State Board of Health
30 sec.; TV; Sep 1988; special rates / discounts; English.

Targeted to young, sexually active adults, this PSA warns viewers that the more one has sex with different partners, the greater the chances are of contracting AIDS/HIV. The narrator states, "this is the woman who made love to the man who made love to the woman who made love to the man...who gave her AIDS."

Reviewers' Comments: The theme of this PSA is fair, but the visual is boring. The audio mix levels are very close to the voice-over, making it difficult to hear the message clearly.

▲ For Ordering Information, see p. 221

❶ Nightcap

Health Education Resource Organization (HERO)
30 sec.; TV; color; 1987; $75.00; English.

This public service announcement, featuring a young couple in an intimate setting, encourages condom use. Local agencies can easily customize this spot to promote regional resources.

Reviewers' Comments: This excellent, well-designed video targets sexually active, heterosexual, young adults.

▲ For Ordering Information, see p. 220

❷ Sexually Active Young Adults

Pima County Health Department
60 sec.; radio; 1988; free; English.

These three radio ads present the story of a man and a woman, each of whom overcomes timidity to discuss AIDS/HIV with the other. In the first, the woman and a friend discuss the need to broach the subject of AIDS/HIV with the new boyfriend. The second offers the man's version as he talks to a friend about his anxieties and reluctance to discuss AIDS/HIV. In the third ad, the man and woman overcome their apprehension and converse about AIDS/HIV.

Reviewers' Comments: This is a "good starter" piece for discussions on AIDS/HIV. It needs follow-up information on safer sex practices. The message that "straight people get AIDS too," is good and needed.

▲ For Ordering Information, see p. 226

❷ **Three Good Reasons For Not Being Out With The Boys /**
Tres Razones Para No Andar En La Calle Con Los Muchachos

CDC National AIDS Information and Education Program
Multimedia; Oct 1988; free; English/Spanish.

This America Responds To AIDS print ad presents a photograph of a man and his family. His message illustrates how he used to "score with others" to have a good time, but because of the risk of AIDS/HIV he has changed his behavior so he doesn't bring AIDS/HIV home. The English version provides the number for the National AIDS Hotline, and the Spanish version provides the National SIDA Hotline number. The print ad is available in a variety of sizes; a TV public service spot version (English and Spanish) is also available. Government agencies and AIDS organizations are free to localize these ads to meet their needs.

Reviewers' Comments: This ad is visually appealing and piques the reader's interest. However, it doesn't provide information about transmission and prevention. The message is also misleading: if this person became infected with HIV, discontinuing the risk of exposure won't protect his current sexual partner from infection. The Spanish language text is good and meets minimum acceptance criteria.

▲ For Ordering Information, see p. 216

VIDEOS / FILMS

❶ **AIDS: Changing The Rules**

AIDSFILMS
30 min.; VHS; 1987; $30.00; English.

Hosted by Ron Reagan, former president Reagan's son; model Beverly Johnson; and Salsa star Ruben Blades; this documentary discusses some of the basic facts about AIDS/HIV: its transmission, symptoms, current statistics, and rules for safer sex. The film features a segment on people with AIDS/HIV describing how they became sick and the effect of the disease on their lives. One scene shows three women discussing feelings and attitudes about condoms and sexual behavior. In another, Blades uses a banana to demonstrate the proper way to put on a condom. A discussion guide includes a film outline, suggestions for group discussion, a personal inventory on attitudes about AIDS/HIV, and fact sheets. A version with Spanish subtitles is available. This film is also available in a 60-minute version with a panel discussion produced by WETA/TV and moderated by Judy Woodruff.

Reviewers' Comments: This video is superb. The highly professional production contains touching scenes of people with AIDS/HIV, excellent information on AIDS/HIV prevention, and attractive, articulate narrators of different races.

▲ For Ordering Information, see p. 214

○ **AIDS In Your Life**

Medical Video Productions

○ **Condoms: A Responsible Option**

Focus International

❷ **Eddie's Story: How To Protect Yourself From STD's And AIDS**

New York State Department of Health
12 min.; VHS; 1988; $20.00, limited copies; special rates / discounts; English.

This video, a fictional story designed to reach teens and young adults, opens as Eddie and his three friends finish a pick-up game of basketball and head for a bar. Dave boasts of his many girlfriends and another tells them that he and his girlfriend had the AIDS/HIV test, tested negative, and have decided to be safe by being faithful to each other. He encourages the others to use condoms and to limit who they sleep with, and notes that if you have open sores from some other form of sexually transmitted disease, it's easier to get AIDS/HIV.

Reviewers' Comments: This is very well done with realistic situations, medically and scientifically accurate information and a positive portrayal of minorities. The portrayal of women is somewhat sexist. One of the scenes shows a condom being opened and put on a salt shaker.

▲ For Ordering Information, see p. 225

❶ 1ST EDITION RECOMMENDED   ❷ 2ND EDITION RECOMMENDED   ○ NOT RECOMMENDED

SPECIAL AUDIENCES

BROCHURES

❶ AIDS And Risk Reduction For Women & Men In Prostitution

Genesis House
Card; illustrations; special rates / discounts; Mar 1987; English.

▲ For Ordering Information, see p. 219

❷ AIDS And The Navajo

Shiprock Community Health Center
3 panels; illustrations; special rates / discounts; 1988; English.

This brochure uses color drawings of Indians to illustrate ways in which AIDS/HIV is and is not spread. Statistics dated March, 1988 and projections to the end of 1991 show the number of cases in the USA, Arizona, the Navajo Nation, and New Mexico. Prevention of infection through safer sex is urged. The importance of education and sharing information is also stressed. A long list of New Mexico resources for AIDS/HIV information and services is provided.

▲ For Ordering Information, see p. 228

❷ AIDS: Can Indian Kids Get It?

People of Color Against AIDS Network
3 panels; illustrations; free, limited copies; 1988; English.

This brochure pictures American Indians and uses Indian symbols throughout. It intends to dispel the myth that Indians don't get AIDS/HIV, gives statistics, and describes high-risk behavior. AIDS/HIV prevention advice is included along with Seattle area information numbers.

▲ For Ordering Information, see p. 226

❶ AIDS Information For Inmates

New York City Department of Health AIDS Education Training Unit
4 panels; illustrations; free, limited copies; Jul 1987; English/Spanish.

▲ For Ordering Information, see p. 225

❷ AIDS Is Also An Indian Problem

California Rural Indian Health Board, Inc.
8 panels; illustrations; special rates / discounts; 1988; English.

This brochure provides basic facts about AIDS/HIV, answering questions about the disease, how it is transmitted, how it can be prevented, and whether Indians are at risk for infection. Toll free numbers for more information are provided for Northern and Southern California.

▲ For Ordering Information, see p. 216

◯ AIDS: Know The Facts

Native American Women's Health Education Resource Center

❷ Are Indians At Risk For AIDS?

People of Color Against AIDS Network
3 panels; illustrations; free, limited copies; 1988; English.

This brochure addresses the myth that isolation protects Indians from AIDS/HIV by pointing out how many travel off the reservation. It notes that since some Indians shoot drugs and some have sex with people engaged in high risk behavior, they can contract the virus. High risk behavior and preventive measures are described. Seattle area information and hotline numbers are listed.

▲ For Ordering Information, see p. 226

❶ Asian Americans And AIDS

Multicultural Prevention Resource Center (MPRC)
3 panels; $.25, limited copies; English/Japanese/Korean/Chinese/Vietnamese/Tagalog.

▲ For Ordering Information, see p. 223

◯ If You Get Money For Having Sex

Hartford Health Department AIDS Prevention Program

❶ Information For People Of Color - Asians - Blacks - Latinos - Native Americans

San Francisco AIDS Foundation
3 panels; illustrations; free, limited copies; Dec 1985; English.

▲ For Ordering Information, see p. 227

○ Preservons Notre Futur: Evitons SIDA

Haitian & Caribbean Foundation for Education and Development

○ Prostitutes And AIDS

Genesis House

❷ You And AIDS - Be Safe

Planned Parenthood of South Palm Beach and Broward Counties
3 panels; illustrations; 1988; English.

Using graphic designs, this brochure indicates major ways AIDS/HIV can and cannot be contracted, and offers advice on how to prevent the spread of the disease. It is directed toward audiences that have a low literacy level.

▲ For Ordering Information, see p. 226

INSTRUCTIONAL PROGRAMS

○ AIDS Education Project For Sheltered & Incarcerated Youth

Sequoia YMCA Youth Development Department

❷ AIDS High Risk Adolescent Prevention

- **Training Curriculum Trainer's Manual**
- **Training Curriculum Participant's Manual**

Westover Consultants, Inc.

Designed for a wide range of youth services professionals who work with adolescents at high risk for AIDS/HIV infection, the three-day course instructs participants on how to acquire skills and information for initiating for enhancing AIDS prevention work with teens. The training is funded by the National Institute on Drug Abuse and will be held in numerous cities throughout the U.S. in 1989 and 1990.

The curriculum's nine units discuss practical skills, techniques, and approaches to adolescent-focused AIDS/HIV intervention, including modules on adolescent sexuality, substance abuse, AIDS/HIV risk assessment and risk reduction, HIV antibody testing issues, basic AIDS/HIV facts, and overcoming personal and agency barriers to AIDS/HIV prevention programming. The trainer's manual includes, at the beginning of each unit, additional guidelines, objectives, and suggestions for presentation of the material.

Reviewers' Comments: This curriculum is comprehensive in scope with valuable details and background informration. Goals, objectives and intended outcomes are spelled out for the user. While the facilitator/presenter role is complete, more focus should be given to participants, role playing, and small group activities. The curriculum is overwhelming in size and may present difficulty since participants will not have enough time to become familiar with the material prior to the session.

▲ For Ordering Information, see p. 231

○ AIDS High Risk Adolescent Prevention

Westover Consultants, Inc.

○ Training Of Peer Educators For AIDS: An Outline Of Technique

Dixwell Preventive Health Program

MULTICOMPONENT PROGRAMS

❷ AIDS Prevention On Navajoland

Shiprock Community Health Center
1988; special rates / discounts; English.

This multi-component program includes slides, a script, and an audiocassette and is an introduction to AIDS/HIV for the Navajo community. With facts about AIDS/HIV in the Native American Community and transmission and prevention, this package places an emphasis on education and caring for members of the community who have AIDS and who are at risk for AIDS/HIV. The script notes that Native Americans are not immune to AIDS/HIV, that the increased mobility of members of the community can place them in high risk situations. Community members are encouraged to become knowledgeable about modes of transmission and to educate their children about AIDS/HIV. The package is available in English and Navajo.

❶ 1ST EDITION RECOMMENDED   ❷ 2ND EDITION RECOMMENDED   ○ NOT RECOMMENDED

Reviewers' Comments: The IV needle sharing scenes are phoney - the settings are more like hospitals than "shooting galleries" and the needles are the wrong type. This package was well received, however, by non-Navajo tribes and is better than the non-Indian material available.

▲ For Ordering Information, see p. 228

PAMPHLETS

❷ AIDS And Prisons: The Facts For Inmates And Officers

ACLU National Prison Project
14 pages; 1988; special rates / discounts; English.

This pamphlet is directed at prisoners, corrections staff, and AIDS/HIV service providers. It addresses commonly asked questions concerning AIDS/HIV, the available medical treatments, and legal rights and responsibilities of inmates and officers regarding treatment of HIV positive individuals.

Reviewers' Comments: While the content of this pamphlet is accurate and complete, the reading level is high for the target audience.

▲ For Ordering Information, see p. 213

❷ AIDS Kills Women, Men, And Babies

AIDS Prevention Project Dallas County Health Department
2 panels; illustrations; 1988; free; English.

Through use of simple cartoons and brief sentences, this pamphlet is designed to reach the learning disabled population with prevention messages. The messages are: don't have sex or have sex with one person--not many; use rubbers; do not use drugs; and before you get pregnant, call a doctor. Cartoons of "Safe Things" are also depicted, such as swimming pools, sneezing, and toilet seats. Dallas, Texas area AIDS information phone numbers are listed.

Reviewers' Comments: This is one of the few items available for the learning disabled. It is good pictorially, but some of the written material may be confusing, for example, "Don't have sex/Have sex with one person." It should include information on condom use and the pamphlet should be used in combination with other resources.

▲ For Ordering Information, see p. 213

❷ Mom And Son Series

Native American Women's Health Education Resource Center
10 pages; illustrations; 1988; special rates / discounts; English.

This cartoon includes information for parents and other adults seeking to educate Native American children, grades K-5, about AIDS/HIV. It presents a cartoon as a starting point for conversation. In the cartoon, a son asks his mother whether Hulk Hogan, He-Man, or Rambo is tougher than the AIDS monster. His mother explains that none of them is stronger because the AIDS virus is too small to see, and once it gets in the blood stream it can't be gotten out. The son also asks if he can still be friends with John, a boy at school who has AIDS, and his mother reassures him that one can't get AIDS/HIV through casual contact. Information on what AIDS/HIV is, and how the virus is and is not transmitted is included.

Reviewers' Comments: The illustrations in this book are weak and take away from the messages, although the tone is suitable for young children. In order to be truely useful for adults and children, more backgound information on AIDS/HIV should be available.

▲ For Ordering Information, see p. 224

❷ SIDA / AIDS

Haitian Women's Program/AFSC
16 pages; 1988; $.45; special rates / discounts; Haitian/Crole/Eng..

This pamphlet is designed for Haitian or Creole speaking persons who are learning English as a second language. It provides basic information about AIDS transmission, disease process, and prevention and care. It is an instructional tool for the student and the teacher, for vocabulary, spelling, and grammar. The English translation is included on a per page basis.

Reviewers' Comments: The pamphlet not only gives an accurate presentation of AIDS information; it also takes into consideration a primary need of the Haitian population--English language development. The language is clear and to the point, and it addresses many important AIDS-related topics.

▲ For Ordering Information, see p. 220

POSTERS

❷ AIDS Is Not A Quick Kill

American Indian Health Care Association
17 x 22; photographs; color; 1989; $5.00; English.

A close-up of the full moon rests on a black background. Below the moon is a night owl with spread wings, glowing red eyes, and outstretched talons. The text indicates the significance of the situation faced by persons with AIDS/HIV, urging viewers to make the decision to avoid HIV infection.

Reviewers' Comments: The owl is an excellent symbol for most tribes; it normally connotes a messenger or death. The poster will have a good impact on traditional people.

▲ For Ordering Information, see p. 215

◯ AIDS...It Kills Indians Too!

California Rural Indian Health Board, Inc.

❷ No Glove No Love

American Indian Health Care Association
17 x 22; illustrations; color; 1989; $5.00; English.

A painting of a young heterosexual couple is the focus of this poster. He is looking at her. She holds a condom packet and looks knowingly at the viewer. The caption, "No Glove No Love," indicates her attitude. The poster encourages women to demand the use of condoms during sex to prevent HIV transmission.

Reviewers' Comments: The term "glove" used to mean condom is not familiar to many Native Americans; however, the message is a good one and the poster is well done and engaging. It gives a positive message of empowerment to hetrosexual females.

▲ For Ordering Information, see p. 215

❷ Practice Safer Sex

Native American Women's Health Education Resource Center
16 x 22; illustrations; color; 1988; free, limited copies; special rates / discounts; English.

This large yellow poster, directed at a sexually active Native American population, reads in large black letters at the top: "Prevent AIDS and other sexually transmitted diseases. PRACTICE SAFER SEX." A cartoon shows a "condom" running after a man and woman who are arm in

arm. The condom says, "Wait, don't forget me!" Further information about where to get condoms and lubricants follows the cartoon, and the address and phone of NACB Women's Resource Center are included.

Reviewers' Comments: The humor is typical of Sioux humor and will make most Indians feel that the piece is "Indian." The message is clear and important, and reaches those who cannot read as well as to those who can.

▲ For Ordering Information, see p. 224

❷ SIDA/ AIDS

Haitian & Caribbean Foundation For Education and Development
1989; free; Creole/French.

This poster is intended for an audience of Haitian descent with an ability to speak and read Creole and French. It seeks to convey a message about HIV transmission prevention. It describes the types of support and human interaction needed by a person who has AIDS. It provides the address and phone number of the Haitian & Caribbean Foundation for Education and Development.

Reviewers' Comments: Some corrections are necessary in language and grammar in order for this poster to best convey its message.

▲ For Ordering Information, see p. 220

❷ Stop AIDS In Indian Country

California Rural Indian Health Board, Inc.
18 x 24; illustrations; color; 1988; special rates / discounts; English.

The white poster shows a red international symbol for prohibition with the word "AIDS" in the center and beaded feathers hanging from it. It says, "STOP AIDS IN INDIAN COUNTRY." Toll free phone numbers for more information are provided for Northern and Southern California.

Reviewers' Comments: The use of the medicine wheel and the international "stop" symbol is a good blend for Native Americans. The message focuses on encouraging people to get more information; the graphics are good for this population.

▲ For Ordering Information, see p. 216

❶ 1ST EDITION RECOMMENDED   ❷ 2ND EDITION RECOMMENDED   ◯ NOT RECOMMENDED

VIDEOS / FILMS

❷ David's Song

Center for Indian Youth Program Development
12:54 min; 1988; $30.00; English.

This video targets American Indian adolescents. David, an Osage Indian with AIDS, talks with Indian teens about his concerns. Six New Mexico Indian teens ask David questions that were collected from their friends and classmates. The video encourages the audience to discuss issues such as: increased risk of IV drug use and risky sexual activities; increased risk of AIDS/HIV coming into an Indian community through transient events such as pow-wows, rodeos, concerts, jewelry buying and selling, and conferences. A study guide is included. Person(s) using the video are encouraged to use the accompanying study guide and to become familiar with the issues of AIDS/HIV and the local community's values. The study guide includes definitions of terms used in the video, statistics on AIDS/HIV, guidelines for schools, and listings of other resources.

Reviewers' Comments: There are many inaccuracies in this video, and the information is vague. Many terms are not explained, such as monogamy. Although the video features young people, the questions they ask are answered at too high and inappropriate a level. It is recommended as an exception to the usual acceptance criteria because it targets young Native Americans, for whom there is little group-specific educational material. It should be used with the study guide and an AIDS/HIV knowledgeable person.

▲ For Ordering Information, see p. 216

❷ Her Giveaway

Minnesota American Indian AIDS Task Force c/o The Minneapolis Indian Health Board
20 min.; VHS; May 1988; $100.00; English.

This video is an uplifting biography of one Objibwe Indian woman, Carole Lafavor, which details her experience as a person with AIDS/HIV. Ms. Lafavor talks about how she contracted AIDS, living with the virus, and her changed relationships with family and friends. Besides presenting insight into the life of this woman, the video addresses mythologies about Indians and sexuality, Indians and IV drug use, and Indians and their level of risk for contracting AIDS/HIV. Traditional images and music augment the educational narrative and underscore the spiritual perspective with which Ms. Lafavor views AIDS/HIV and her own illness, and with which the film is produced.

Reviewers' Comments: This well-made video is valuable to Native American audiences. Viewers in this community will appreciate its holistic view and emphasis on traditional spiritual healing. They will easily be able to identify with Ms. Lafavor's life experiences--alcohol and other drug abuse, but above all her spiritual path. The film captures the viewers attention on an emotional level while providing accurate information, and although the perspective is Native American, the film is applicable to a wide range of audiences.

▲ For Ordering Information, see p. 223

❷ Teaching People With Disabilities To Better Protect Themselves

Young Adult Institute
30 min.; VHS; 1987; $145.00; special rates / discounts; English/Spanish.

This video and 21-page trainer's manual offer step-by-step instructions on how to teach people with disabilities about the hazards of AIDS/HIV and precautions which they should take to protect themselves. The emphasis is that the disease is deadly and incurable and that anyone can become infected. The video graphically depicts the correct use of a condom on life-size replicas of male and female genitals. People enact scenes in which the use of condoms becomes a cause of dispute between sexual partners. The manual proposes objectives for training and offers instructions on how the course should be conducted including questions teachers may ask.

Reviewers' Comments: This video is recommended only as part of a total program. The presentation is somewhat condescending and the role-playing is stilted. It does allow time for discussion on each major point raised. The depiction of sexual intercourse is true to life and is used to illustrate safer sex practices.

▲ For Ordering Information, see p. 232

❷ Preventing AIDS: It's A Matter Of Life Or Death / La Prevención Del AIDS (SIDA): Es Cuestión De Vida O Muerte

National Sheriffs' Association
1987; rental fee: $25.00/10 Days; special rates / discounts; English/Spanish.

The concerns of incarcerated people, their friends and families are addressed in this video, which opens with several inmates offering a mix of opinion, rumor, and facts about HIV transmission. The issues they mention-- modes of transmission, prevention, and who can get the AIDS virus--are all addressed. The fact that anyone can get HIV is emphasized, as is the fact that many who carry and can transmit the virus show no sign of illness. Reassurance that HIV can't be transmitted simply by sharing a cell, food, or cigarettes is given, along with the admonition not to share razors, toothbrushes, and needles. The English version of this video is 14:58 minutes, and the Spanish version is 17:48 minutes.

Reviewers' Comments: The video gives a bland presentation of facts about the AIDS virus using the format of an expert giving a lecture. Inmates may lose interest.

▲ For Ordering Information, see p. 224

❷ Se Met Ko - An Educational Film On AIDS

Haitian Women's Program/AFSC

1989; $160.00; rental fee: $35.00/2 Weeks; special rates / discounts; Haitian Creole/English.

This film is an exposé of the AIDS problem in a crosscultural context, that of the Haitian family in the United States. It is designed to explicate the process from ignorance and denial to consideration of safer sexual behaviors. It is in Creole with English subtitles. Its story unfolds in the midst of a family and addresses AIDS as a family problem.

Reviewers' Comments: This video is sharp, to the point, and medically accurate. It is consistent with community values and easily understood by a range of audiences. The music is excellent. Through this film the producers successfully convey important messages about AIDS in the Haitian context.

▲ For Ordering Information, see p. 220

❶ 1ST EDITION RECOMMENDED ❷ 2ND EDITION RECOMMENDED ○ NOT RECOMMENDED

WOMEN

BOOKS / MANUALS

② **Advice For Life: A Woman's Guide To AIDS Risks And Prevention**

National Women's Health Network
179 pages; softcover; 1987; $6.95; special rates / discounts; English.

This book is an examination of personal AIDS/HIV prevention and policy issues for women. Chapters focus on personal prevention, including talking to men, the specifics of transmission, and the risks from both sex and drug abuse. The book examines the need for focused education on prevention, and for public policy initiatives, including the appropriate use of testing and partner notification. A personal AIDS risk-assessment for women questionnaire is included.

Reviewers' Comments: This very readable book provides a good discussion on the impact of testing and general information on AIDS/HIV for heterosexual women. Some of the information on hemophilia is incorrect or unclear.

▲ For Ordering Information, see p. 224

BROCHURES

❶ **AIDS And Pregnancy: How To Protect Your Unborn Child**

San Mateo County AIDS Project
4 panels; illustrations; $.10; 1987; English.

▲ For Ordering Information, see p. 227

❶ **AIDS And Women / El AIDS (SIDA) Y Las Mujeres**

Texas Department of Health Bureau of AIDS and STD Control
3 panels; illustrations; free, limited copies; Mar 1987; English/Spanish.

▲ For Ordering Information, see p. 229

❶ **AIDS Kills Women And Babies / AIDS (SIDA) Mata A Las Mujeres Y A Los Niños**

San Francisco AIDS Foundation
3 panels; illustrations; $.30; special rates / discounts; 1988; English/Spanish.

▲ For Ordering Information, see p. 227

❶ **AIDS - What A Woman Needs To Know**

AIDS Services of Austin
4 panels; illustrations; 1987; English.

▲ For Ordering Information, see p. 213

❶ **AIDS: What Every Woman Needs To Know**

National Women's Health Network
3 panels; $10.00; Sep 1987; English/Spanish.

▲ For Ordering Information, see p. 224

❶ **AIDS: Women Beware - AIDS Information For Women**

Dimension Communications Network (DCN)/RAMSCO Publishing Co.
2 panels; illustrations; $.20; special rates / discounts; 1986; English.

▲ For Ordering Information, see p. 218

② **All Women Need To Know About AIDS**

NO/AIDS Task Force
2 panels; $.10; special rates / discounts; 1988; English.

This brochure urges women to become informed about AIDS/HIV and how it affects their lives. It includes a definition of AIDS and a description of basic transmission modes and risk reduction. Mother-fetus transmission is detailed and discussed, and some statistics are presented regarding the impact of AIDS/HIV on women as a group. The brochure emphasizes the importance of education, and local and statewide hotline numbers are provided.

▲ For Ordering Information, see p. 225

❷ Facing AIDS: Advice For Women

Hawaii State Department of Health STD/AIDS Prevention Program
3 panels; free; 1988; English.

This brochure describes what AIDS/HIV is, how it spreads, and why women and their unborn babies are at risk. Preventive measures and testing are explained. Hawaii hotline numbers are provided.

▲ For Ordering Information, see p. 220

◯ Fact Sheet No.9 - Women And AIDS

Gay Community AIDS Project

❷ Having A Baby?

New York State Department of Health
1 panel; special rates / discounts; 1988; English/Spanish.

This flyer for women who are or may become pregnant states "Hundreds of babies have been born with AIDS. Most die by age 5," It explains that babies get AIDS/HIV from their mothers during pregnancy and lists ways women contract the virus. It encourages women who are having a baby to take an HIV antibody test and lists the testing hotline number.

▲ For Ordering Information, see p. 225

❷ Having A Baby?: Have A Test For AIDS Virus First

New York State Department of Health
3 panels; special rates / discounts; 1988; English/Spanish.

This brochure tells women that babies can contract AIDS/HIV from their mothers during pregnancy. It also explains that women may become infected by sharing IV drug needles, having sex with a man who shares needles, is bisexual, or whose health and drug use history aren't known. Women are encouraged to be tested for HIV before they get pregnant and to avoid high-risk behaviors.

▲ For Ordering Information, see p. 225

◯ If You Are Pregnant...

Illinois Alcoholism and Drug Dependence Association

❷ Love As If Your Life Depended On It

Mayor's Task Force On AIDS, New Haven
4 panels; special rates / discounts; 1988; English.

This brochure alerts female residents of New Haven, CT, that it is usually women who get AIDS/HIV through hetorosexual sex, and nearly half of the reported AIDS cases in Connecticut are in New Haven. Photographs of the serious faces of women help make this point. Safer sex choices are outlined, as is a warning about drugs and alcohol. The correct use of condoms is explained. Information on AIDS/HIV and pregnancy, counseling, and testing is provided. The fact that AIDS is a killer, but preventable, is stressed. Connecticut phone numbers of AIDS information and drug treatment are listed.

▲ For Ordering Information, see p. 222

❷ OK, But Next Time You Have To Wear One

People of Color Against AIDS Network
3 panels; photographs; free, limited copies; 1988; English.

The message offered by this brochure is that women have the right to protect themselves. A condom is pictured and women are encouraged to keep condoms available, insist on their use, and use them according to instructions. The fact that a woman can transmit AIDS/HIV to her unborn baby is emphasized.

▲ For Ordering Information, see p. 226

◯ Safer Sex

**South Carolina Dept. of Health and Environmental Control
Bureau of Preventive Health Services**

❶ What Every Woman Should Know About AIDS

North Carolina AIDS Control Program
4 panels; free, limited copies; Sep 1987; English.

▲ For Ordering Information, see p. 225

❶ 1ST EDITION RECOMMENDED   ❷ 2ND EDITION RECOMMENDED   ◯ NOT RECOMMENDED

❷ What Women Ask...AIDS

Georgia Department of Human Resources
4 panels; free, limited copies; 1987; English.

This brochure discusses facts about AIDS, including the numbers of women and children infected by HIV, symptoms of the disease, and how they become infected with the virus. It suggests preventive measures and briefly discusses the transmission of HIV during pregnancy and breastfeeding. It lists phone numbers in Georgia for more information.

▲ For Ordering Information, see p. 220

◯ What Women Should Know About AIDS

ETR Associates/Network Publications

❷ What You Should Know About AIDS And Pregnancy

Planned Parenthood Alameda/San Francisco
3 panels; $.18; special rates / discounts; 1988; English.

This brochure begins with brief questions for women who are pregnant or considering pregnancy. Answering yes to any of these questions implies a risk of exposure to the virus. The second part of the brochure gives explanations of the AIDS virus, modes of transmission, and how the virus affects pregnant women and their unborn children. Information about the HIV antibody test and its results is also included. Women are urged to take part in a counseling program for testing and to get further information through Planned Parenthood.

▲ For Ordering Information, see p. 226

❷ Women And AIDS

American College Health Association
5 panels; illustrations; $.50; special rates / discounts; 1988; English.

This brochure features safer sex guidelines for women and information on the transmission of HIV, decision making, and suggestions for precautions that may be taken in a sexual relationship. Special sections address intravenous needle sharing, drugs and alcohol, sex without consent, pregnancy, lesbian and bisexual women, and the HIV antibody test. A panel on protection includes ten tips on condom use and information on spermicides and latex squares.

▲ For Ordering Information, see p. 214

❶ Women And AIDS

New York City Department of Health AIDS Education Training Unit
3 panels; illustrations; free, limited copies; English/Spanish.

▲ For Ordering Information, see p. 225

❷ Women And AIDS

Ohio Department of Health - AIDS Unit
4 panels; free, limited copies; Mar 1987; English.

This brochure emphasizes to women that they are vulnerable to AIDS/HIV, regardless of race, and that they can pass the virus on to their unborn children. Causes, symptoms, transmission, prevention, and condom use are discussed. AIDS/HIV testing, and Ohio and U.S. Public Health Service hotline numbers are given.

▲ For Ordering Information, see p. 225

❷ Women And AIDS

Rhode Island Department of Health AIDS Program
3 panels; free; 1987; English.

This brochure offers women a list of criteria for estimating their risk of exposure to AIDS/HIV, emphasizing the dangers of sharing IV needles. Risks to unborn children and babies are discussed. It lists some of the symptoms of AIDS and explains that persons with AIDS may have no symptoms. Actions for reducing the risk of contracting AIDS/HIV are outlined with specific suggestions for safer sex practices. A list of Rhode Island counseling and test sites is provided.

▲ For Ordering Information, see p. 227

❷ Women And AIDS

Seattle-King County Department of Public Health
3 panels; illustrations; $.20; 1988; English.

Using a question and answer format, this brochure provides information on AIDS/HIV for women. It discusses how to assess one's risk and one's partner's risk. It also addresses issues of concern for lesbians, prostitutes, IV drug users, and rape victims. Prevention information is included.

▲ For Ordering Information, see p. 228

○ Women And AIDS

South Carolina Dept. of Health and Environmental Control Bureau of Preventive Health Services

❶ Women And AIDS

St. Louis Efforts for AIDS
5 panels; 100 @ $15.00; 1987; English.

▲ For Ordering Information, see p. 228

❶ Women And AIDS

North Central Florida AIDS Network
4 panels; illustrations; free, limited copies; 1987; English.

▲ For Ordering Information, see p. 225

❶ Women And AIDS / Las Mujeres Y El SIDA

New York State Department of Health
3 panels; photographs; free, limited copies; Mar 1987; English/Spanish.

▲ For Ordering Information, see p. 225

❶ Women And AIDS - What You Know About It May Save Your Life

AID Atlanta, Inc.
4 panels; free, limited copies; May 1987; English.

▲ For Ordering Information, see p. 213

❷ Women And Children Have Special Needs

Sacramento AIDS Foundation
2 panels; $.20; special rates / discounts; 1988; English.

This brochure informs women with HIV infection of local services available to them through the Sacramento AIDS Foundation. It offers a brief description of needs specific to HIV-infected women, and a list of relevant SAF services, as well as a guide to other local community agencies with applicable services.

▲ For Ordering Information, see p. 227

❷ Women Are Getting AIDS, Too

Fenway Community Health Center
3 panels; charts & illustrations; $.10; special rates / discounts; 1987; English.

This brochure for women presents basic information about AIDS/HIV, the need for communication among sex partners, suggestions for safer sex practices, and precautions for IV drug users. It also recommends "healthy habits" such as rest, exercise, nutrition, and regular pap smears to protect oneself from AIDS/HIV and other illnesses. It lists the numbers for a Boston area HIV antibody testing site and hotline assistance centers.

▲ For Ordering Information, see p. 219

○ Women, Babies, And AIDS

Massachusetts Department of Public Health

❶ Women, Infants And AIDS

Health Education Resource Organization (HERO)
1 page; 1987; English.

▲ For Ordering Information, see p. 220

❶ Women Need To Know About AIDS

Gay Men's Health Crisis, Inc.
4 panels; photographs; $.30; special rates / discounts; 1988; English/Spanish.

▲ For Ordering Information, see p. 219

❶ Women Need To Know About AIDS / La Mujer Debe Informarse Sobre El SIDA

Gay Men's Health Crisis, Inc.
4 panels; free, limited copies; 1986; English/Spanish.

▲ For Ordering Information, see p. 219

❷ Women, Sex, And AIDS

American Red Cross National Headquarters
8 panels; free; 1989; English.

This brochure discusses basic AIDS/HIV information and informs the reader about how many women have become infected. It also discusses sexual transmission, condom use, pregnancy-related issues, and testing.

▲ For Ordering Information, see p. 215

❶ 1ST EDITION RECOMMENDED ❷ 2ND EDITION RECOMMENDED ○ NOT RECOMMENDED

INSTRUCTIONAL PROGRAMS

❶ AIDS Education Activities Workshop

National Women's Health Network
 31 pages; stapled; illustrations; 1987; $20.00; English.

This packet contains guidelines and support materials for leaders and participants in workshops for young, sexually active women. The curriculum encourages non-threatening but open and frank discussions in college groups, women's centers, and self-help groups. Seven activities, some humorous, address such areas as risk behavior, transmission of HIV, current sexual habits, and negotiating with sexual partners. The packet includes information on the biological, chemical, and epidemiological aspects of HIV, an evaluation form, and safer sex guidelines.

Reviewers' Comments: Overall the curriculum is excellent, but the objectives could be more explicitly stated. It stresses sexual transmission and prevention, but does not cover IV drug use as a method of transmission. It uses creative ways to help women talk about sexual activity and is culturally sensitive.

▲ For Ordering Information, see p. 224

PAMPHLETS

❷ AIDS/Sexually Transmitted Diseases / Vaginal Infections

Planned Parenthood of New York City
 14 pages; 1988; $.60; special rates / discounts; English/Spanish.

This brochure presents information for women on sexually transmitted diseases, including AIDS/HIV. Also included are tips on prevention, general symptoms, and hygiene.

Reviewers' Comments: The pamphlet is accurate and detailed. It does not cover lesbianism. The Spanish language version meets the minimum screening criteria. Both language versions require a fairly high reading level.

▲ For Ordering Information, see p. 226

❷ Protection Against Infection For Women Using Alternative Insemination

The Feminist Institute Clearinghouse
 9 pages; 1988; $4.60; special rates / discounts; English.

This pamphlet answers questions about risks and precautions to safeguard health for women pursuing alternative insemination (AI), with an emphasis on protections against HIV infection. An appendix lists common sexually transmitted diseases, including HIV infection, and recom-mended lab tests for semen donors. A second appendix suggests protective methods if using frozen or fresh sperm for AI. The pamphlet is intended for women using AI and for clinics to distribute to potential AI clients.

Reviewers' Comments: The information in this pamphlet is detailed and requires a high literacy level, but is worthwhile for women considering alternative insemination. The question and answer format is useful. Good negotiating strategies for working with doctors, clinics, and sperm banks are offered.

▲ For Ordering Information, see p. 229

❶ What Women Should Know About HIV Infections, AIDS And Hemophilia

National Hemophilia Foundation
 10 pages; illustrations; 1988; free, limited copies; English.

This pamphlet provides information on HIV infection (causes, symptoms, and prevention) for women, especially those whose sexual partners may have been exposed to HIV, such as persons with hemophilia. It recommends safer sex practices, explains the HIV antibody test, and suggests that people who may have been in contact with the virus should be tested. It encourages women to continue relationships in spite of HIV infection possibility, to practice safer sex, and to communicate with their partners about concerns and recommended changes.

Reviewers' Comments: This pamphlet provides good basic information on HIV infection for women, but provides no resource list. The format is dense and requires a high reading level.

▲ For Ordering Information, see p. 224

❷ Women And AIDS

Channing L. Bete Co., Inc.
 16 pages; illustrations; 1988; special rates / discounts; English.

This pamphlet uses simple comicstrip illustrations to suggest reasons why women should to learn about AIDS/HIV, to explain how one can become infected with the virus, and how it can be passed on to one's baby. It illustrates protective measures such as not using IV drugs and making informed choices about sex. Tips on talking with partners are offered. It discusses common misunderstandings about safer sex activities and offers advice on taking the test for HIV.

Reviewers' Comments: This pamphlet is easy to read and understand and discusses issues of sexual intercourse in a way that should be acceptable to most populations. The section on testing is a little weak and should promote informed consent.

▲ For Ordering Information, see p. 217

POSTERS

② If He Doesn't Have A Condom... Tell Him To Go Get One / Si El No Tiene Un Condon, Pídele Que Busque Uno

CDC National AIDS Information and Education Program
16 x 22; photographs; black & white; Oct 1988; free; English/Spanish.

This poster comes in four versions, with photographs of a woman of white, black or Hispanic background looking directly at the viewer under a headline which reads, "If he doesn't have a condom, you just have to take a deep breath and tell him to go get one." Copy beneath the photograph acknowledges the difficulty/awkwardness of conversations with a sexual partner, but the importance of talking about condom use. Hotline numbers are provided. One version of this poster is in Spanish.

Reviewers' Comments: This poster conveys a very important message for women. It acknowledges the difficulty of talking with uncooperative partners and points to the need to weigh the risks and benefits of urging condom use. The Spanish translation is a little stilted but accurate. In general, the photographs are effective and match the copy.

▲ For Ordering Information, see p. 216

② Last Night This Woman Slept With Every One Of Her Boyfriend's Ex-Lovers.

AIDS Administration for the State of Maryland Maryland C.A.R.E.S.
11 x 14; photographs; color; 1988; free; English.

The main message of this poster is directed at young women. A softly backlit color photo of a young woman sitting in a white wicker chair looking thoughtful is accompanied by the lines: "Like it or not, when you sleep with someone, you also sleep with the risk of getting AIDS. From all the lovers your partner ever had. That alone should give you countless reasons to use condoms. Please do." Following this are Maryland and Baltimore AIDS hotline numbers.

Reviewers' Comments: The slogan is effective in attracting the viewer's attention, however, the photograph is difficult to see unless viewed from a short distance. It seems to be directed at middle-class white women.

▲ For Ordering Information, see p. 213

○ Whoopi Says: "Having A Baby? Have A Test For AIDS Virus First"

New York State Department of Health

② Women's AIDS Coalition 14 Poster Campaign

Mayor's Task Force On AIDS, New Haven
18 x 23; photographs; black & white; 1988; special rates / discounts; English/Spanish.

This campaign targets the need for women to protect themselves from sexual exposure to HIV. The posters available in the campaign contain photographs of individuals and groups of varying ages, sexes, and races. The captions, some of which have Spanish translations, relate to transmission prevention. They include, "I'm serious about love. I use condoms," "Insist on condoms," and "AIDS doesn't discriminate," among others.

Reviewers' Comments: This series makes good use of portrait photography of "everyday" folks to convey the message that AIDS is every woman's problem.

▲ For Ordering Information, see p. 222

PUBLIC SERVICE ADS (TV, RADIO, PRINT)

② He Wouldn't Give Up Shooting Up... So I Gave Him Up / El No Dejó De Inyectarse Drogas... Por Eso Lo Deje

CDC National AIDS Information and Education Program
Multimedia; Oct 1988; free; English/Spanish.

This America Responds To AIDS print ad is also available as a poster. It contains a photograph of a young woman whose message encourages women to take responsibility for protecting themselves from HIV infection. She explains that she had a sex partner who was shooting up and sharing needles. He wouldn't stop, despite the danger of HIV infection for both of them, so she left him. The English version provides the number of the National AIDS Hotline, and the Spanish version provides the SIDA Hotline number. The ad is available in a variety of sizes, and government agencies and AIDS organizations are free to localize it to meet their needs.

Reviewers' Comments: The message of this ad is clear and has emotional appeal. It encourages the reader to take immediate action to protect herself from HIV infection and not to put herself at risk under any circumstances. Both

❶ 1ST EDITION RECOMMENDED   ❷ 2ND EDITION RECOMMENDED   ○ NOT RECOMMENDED

the English and Spanish versions meet the minimum acceptance criteria.

▲ For Ordering Information, see p. 216

❷ How About Dinner, A Movie, And A Talk About AIDS?

CDC National AIDS Information and Education Program
Multimedia; Oct 1988; free; English.

In this America Responds To AIDS print ad, "Marie" explains that although dinner, a movie, and a talk about AIDS/HIV is not her ideal date, AIDS/HIV is something that needs to be discussed. The ad encourages the reader to start talking about AIDS/HIV by suggesting that doing so isn't so difficult. It provides the number for the National AIDS Hotline and is available in a variety of sizes; a radio version for PSA use is also available. Government agencies and AIDS organizations are free to localize it according to their needs.

Reviewers' Comments: The extended message of this print ad is better than the headline. However, the effectiveness of urging readers to "be careful" would be increased if the ad included information about safer sex.

▲ For Ordering Information, see p. 216

❷ I Didn't Know I Had AIDS... Not Until My Baby Was Born With It

CDC National AIDS Information and Education Program
Multimedia; Oct 1988; free; English.

This America Responds To AIDS print ad is also available as a poster and in TV and radio spot versions. It contains a photograph of a black woman seated next to a crib. She explains that she got AIDS because her husband/lover, an IV drug user who shared needles, gave her the virus through sex. Had she known anything about AIDS, she continues, she would have demanded using condoms during sex. The ad provides the number for the National AIDS Hotline and is available in a variety of sizes. Government agencies and AIDS organizations are free to localize it to meet their needs.

Reviewers' Comments: The message of this ad is important, and it clearly defines condom use as a means of preventing transmission. However, the text doesn't clarify the difference between HIV infected and having AIDS. Babies aren't born with AIDS, and an HIV infected mother does not necessarily have AIDS.

▲ For Ordering Information, see p. 216

❷ If Your Man Is Dabbling In Drugs... He Could Be Dabbling With Your Life.

CDC National AIDS Information and Education Program
Multimedia; Oct 1988; free; English.

This America Responds To AIDS print ad contains copy and a photograph of a black woman with a serious expression. Her message is that the reader risks HIV infection and AIDS if she has a sex partner who is using IV drugs. The ad suggests a variety of strategies for the situation: get the man into counseling; insist on condom use during sex every time; and if a partner refuses to practice safer sex, leave. The ad provides the number for the National AIDS Hotline and is available in a variety of sizes. Government agencies and AIDS organizations are free to localize it to meet their needs.

Reviewers' Comments: This poster's message is straightforward and encourages the reader to be alert, careful, and responsible. There is some doubt as to whether the word "dabbling" will have much meaning to the IVDU population.

▲ For Ordering Information, see p. 216

❷ A Message To The Third Man In My Life / Un Mensaje Al Tercer Hombre En Mi Vida

CDC National AIDS Information and Education Program
Multimedia; Oct 1988; free; English/Spanish.

This America Responds To AIDS print ad presents a photograph of a woman and her two sons. In the copy she explains to "the third man" in her life that if he shoots drugs or has a problem with wearing a condom he should stay away from her. She and her sons are too important to her for her to make any mistakes. The English version provides the number for the National AIDS Hotline, and the Spanish version provides the National SIDA Hotline number. The ad is available in a variety of sizes, and government agencies and AIDS organizations are free to localize it to meet their needs.

Reviewers' Comments: The message is strong and piques the reader's interest, and it encourages the reader to be responsible. The Spanish translation is good, but not excellent. It is innovative and is appealing to Latino family values.

▲ For Ordering Information, see p. 216

VIDEOS / FILMS

❶ AIDS, Women And Sexuality

The Exodus Trust
17 min.; VHS; 1986; $150.00; English.

In this short videotape, seven sexually active women discuss their concerns about AIDS/HIV. They explore issues related to sexual identity, their own sexual relationships, changing roles of women, sexual decision-making, communicating with partners, and safer sex behavior. An accompanying six-page viewer's guide provides questions to stimulate group discussion.

Reviewers' Comments: The participants in this engaging video are candid, fluent, and believable. The discussion is conversational and reflects real life situations. There is good group interaction and support. While there is no explicit information about what constitutes safer sex, the discussion guide does provide additional information on this topic.

▲ For Ordering Information, see p. 229

❷ Beverly's Story: Pregnancy And The Test For AIDS Virus

New York State Department of Health
12:30 min.; VHS; 1988; $20.00, limited copies; special rates / discounts; English.

This video, targeted to pregnant women and those who are considering pregnancy, suggests that they should consider being tested for AIDS/HIV. It begins by showing several babies who are hospitalized with AIDS and continues with a fictional story of Beverly who conveys news of her pregnancy to her friend Linda. Linda is concerned because Beverly's husband uses drugs. She convinces Beverly to go with her to the free clinic for a confidential HIV antibody test. Beverly is very fearful at the clinic, but she follows through and later comes back to get the news. There, she sees an acquaintance coming out of the clinic who has received a positive HIV test. However, Beverly herself tests negative. She does insist that her husband get a test, since she could still get the virus from him while pregnant and pass it on to the baby.

Reviewers' Comments: The film reinforces the message that women are motivated only by fear of transmitting HIV to their babies, not by the need to take care of themselves. Also, the focus is on avoidance of anal sex only. The list of "do's" and "don't's" includes knowing your partner's sexual history as a preventive measure.

▲ For Ordering Information, see p. 225

❷ Joan's Story: How Women Can Protect Themselves From AIDS

New York State Department of Health
8 min.; VHS; 1988; $20.00, limited copies; special rates / discounts; English.

This fictional story is designed to show women that they are at risk for AIDS/HIV and that they can and must protect themselves. A friend tells Joan that her boyfriend, Jack, may be involved with drugs and that even though he isn't sick, Joan could still get the AIDS virus from him. The friend tells Joan that buying condoms is no more embarrassing than buying sanitary napkins for the first time and goes with her to the drugstore to get some. Joan then gives the condoms to Jack and tells him that they both need to protect themselves. At first Jack resists, but he eventually agrees.

Reviewers' Comments: The positive approach of showing women empowering themselves and each other is lessened by some inaccuracies or misleading information. The major fallacy is that women can choose partners carefully and limit the number of partners to avoid AIDS/HIV.

▲ For Ordering Information, see p. 225

❷ Women And AIDS

Gay Men's Health Crisis, Inc.
28 min.; VHS; 1987; $79.95; special rates / discounts; English.

This video explores the underlying issues of how AIDS/HIV highlights problems such as racism, sexism, childcare, and lack of adequate health care for women. These issues are personalized by using diverse interviews with women. AIDS/HIV prevention information is integrated throughout.

Reviewers' Comments: This video is directed at AIDS/HIV service providers/health care workers, and stands as a good justification for developing programs for women. It is also a good piece on sensitizing audiences to the social needs of women and the social problems they face. It is one of the few videos that stress that lesbians are potentially at risk.

▲ For Ordering Information, see p. 219

❶ 1ST EDITION RECOMMENDED   ❷ 2ND EDITION RECOMMENDED   ○ NOT RECOMMENDED

WORKPLACE

BOOKS / MANUALS

❶ The AIDS Book - Information For Workers, 3rd Edition

Service Employees International, AFL-CIO, CLC
64 pages; Apr 1988; $3.00; special rates / discounts; English.

This book provides general information on AIDS/HIV and a comprehensive guide for a safe working environment. Twenty questions and answers address work related AIDS/HIV topics. One section describes the union's role regarding AIDS/HIV, while another outlines worker protection guidelines; appendicies provide pertinent federal and other guidelines.

Reviewers' Comments: Well written and comprehensive, this pamphlet's question and answer section covers many concerns of health care workers. This publication offers information only, even though one of its stated objectives is instructional strategies for union management. It calls for excellent reading and comprehension skills.

▲ For Ordering Information, see p. 228

❷ Understanding AIDS: A Personal Handbook For Employees And Managers

Employee Benefits Review
54 pages; paperback; 1988; $4.50; special rates / discounts; English.

This book addresses AIDS/HIV in the workplace, providing medical facts about AIDS/HIV such as how HIV attacks the body, the physiology of transmission, methods of prevention, and antibody testing. It examines health standards for workers in general as well as for specific occupations such as food handling, personal service, medical care, and emergency care. A chapter provides information on resources and training guidelines. Corporate and federal government guidelines regarding AIDS/HIV-infected employees and guidelines for a management/employee dialogue are also provided. It lists public health regional administrators, state AIDS/HIV-prevention project directors, and federal coordination committees.

Reviewers' Comments: This book covers topics in a detailed fashion, but should be used only as supplemental reading since it offers little gudiance for companies trying to develop their own policies for managers and employees.

▲ For Ordering Information, see p. 219

BROCHURES

❷ AIDS And The Workplace

San Diego Department of Health Services
2 panels; illustrations; free, limited copies; 1988; English.

Designed for employees in office settings, this leaflet includes ways AIDS/HIV is transmitted and suggests preventive measures that may be taken both in and out of the workplace.

▲ For Ordering Information, see p. 227

❶ AIDS And The Workplace

Texas Department of Health Bureau of AIDS and STD Control
2 panels; illustrations; free, limited copies; Sep 1987; English.

▲ For Ordering Information, see p. 229

❷ AIDS And The Workplace: What You Need To Know

Howard Brown Memorial Clinic
4 panels; special rates / discounts; 1988; English.

This brochure explains that AIDS/HIV is not spread through casual, everyday contacts that occur at work. It advises that people with the AIDS virus should continue to work as long as they are able and that they may have a special need for compassion. Four ways that the AIDS virus is transmitted are outlined, and some of the symptoms are listed. Measures to protect oneself and others are explained.

▲ For Ordering Information, see p. 221

◯ AIDS Awareness Game

American Red Cross Columbus Area Chapter

◯ AIDS In The Workplace

North Central Florida AIDS Network

❷ AIDS In The Workplace

NO/AIDS Task Force

3 panels; $.10; special rates / discounts; 1988; English.

This brochure speaks to adults concerned about casual contact transmission. It describes AIDS and the transmission of HIV, and briefly discusses the evidence against the possibility of casual contact transmission. It clarifies that special precautions against transmission are not necessary in the workplace setting and raises the reader's awareness of the issue of mandatory testing of employees. Local and statewide hotline phone numbers are included.

▲ For Ordering Information, see p. 225

❶ AIDS - What Workers Should Know

National Safety Council

5 panels; $.57; Oct 1987; English.

▲ For Ordering Information, see p. 224

❷ Your Job And AIDS: Are There Risks?

American Red Cross National Headquarters

6 panels; free; 1989; English.

This brochure discusses workplace-related topics such as working with someone who is HIV infected, HIV transmission, testing, and what employees and employers should know about AIDS including the needs of HIV infected workers and the importance of having AIDS-related policies.

▲ For Ordering Information, see p. 215

INSTRUCTIONAL PROGRAMS

❷ AIDS Training Manual

Georgia Department of Human Resources

167 pages; looseleaf; charts; 1988; free, limited copies; English.

Developed by the Georgia Department of Human Resources, this manual is part of a "train the trainer" program to educate all members of the department about AIDS. The objective is to prepare employees to handle questions on AIDS/HIV and to enable supervisors to address employee concerns about AIDS. The following topics are discussed: the clinical spectrum of HIV infections, the mechanism of transmission, recommendations for prevention of transmission, and the psychosocial aspects of the disease.

The role of the trainer in planning workshops, assessing the needs of the audience, and answering questions is discussed. A model for an AIDS/HIV training program is presented that includes AIDS knowledge assessment and AIDS values exercises and course evaluation forms. Detailed contents of the program, a script of an AIDS/HIV slide presentation, and commonly asked AIDS/HIV questions and answers are provided. A reference section contains a glossary of AIDS terms, Georgia and national resources, the Surgeon General's report on AIDS, precautions to prevent transmission of AIDS/HIV in health care settings, Georgia State regulations on AIDS/HIV, and pretest and post-test counseling brochures.

Reviewers' Comments: This is a well-organized manual with clear objectives. It does not, however, provide an opportunity for participants to examine their own psychosocial responses to AIDS or to PWA/HIVs. Some of the medical information may be dated; therefore, users may want to check for updates.

▲ For Ordering Information, see p. 220

❷ Managing AIDS In Your Workplace - A Workbook For Nonprofit Organizations

Minnesota AIDS Project

66 pages; spiral; charts; 1988; $35.00; English

The workbook is for use by managers developing a pro-active plan for AIDS/HIV in the workplace. It is a collection of worksheets with introductory explanations to be disassembled and used at the discretion of each organization. Components include: forming a task force; assessing the readiness of the organization; approval strategies; and preparing a policy, management procedures, a communication plan, and a training plan. Included as resource materials in the workbook are: an employee survey; awareness case study exercises; a detailed description of appropriate organization policies and procedures, and their use, and legal guidelines. It is sold only in conjunction with a workshop.

This manual is well organized and easy to use, with excellent worksheets and a comprehensive step-by-step approach. It does, however, assume that team leaders and employees have access to acceptable information on HIV and AIDS. This manual should be used in conjunction with an AIDS "101" piece and with training.

---

❶ 1ST EDITION RECCOMENDED   ❷ 2ND EDITION RECCOMENDED   ○ NOT RECCOMENDED

MULTICOMPONENT PROGRAMS

❶ AIDS In The Workplace

- **AIDS Antibody Testing AT Alternative Test Sites**
  4 panels; $.45; English.

- **AIDS Lifeline**
  3 panels; $.45; English.

- **An Educational Guide For Managers**
  68 pages; looseleaf; $65.00; English.

- **An Epidemic Of Fear**
  23 min; 1987; $275.00; English.

- **A Guide For Employees**
  4 panels; English.

- **When A Friend Has AIDS**
  3 panels; $.45; English.

- **Strategy Manual And Appendix**
  53 pages; $60.00; English.

San Francisco AIDS Foundation

This multi-media educational program addresses the specific needs of small and large businesses and was developed cooperatively by the San Francisco AIDS Foundation and senior executives and health officers of seven major corporations. It includes a videotape, a manager's guide, a strategy and resource manual, and a series of multilingual brochures.

The video, "An Epidemic of Fear: AIDS in the Workplace," educates managers and employees with real-life work situations and includes interviews with medical experts, corporate managers, employees with AIDS/HIV, and their co-workers.

The "Educational Guide for Managers" is a how-to guide that tells decision makers what they need to know about AIDS/HIV, providing a model for educating employees and a list of resources arranged in a notebook format.

The "Strategy Manual and Appendix" provides hands-on suggestions for the development of workplace policies and guidelines from companies who have dealt successfully with these issues. A comprehensive collection of resource materials, samples of corporate policies and guidelines, newsletter articles, educational evaluation forms, and other information dealing with medical, legal and ethical issues are included.

"AIDS in the Workplace: A Guide for Employees," is a brochure that addresses employee concerns about AIDS/HIV in the work environment and lists state and local hotlines throughout the U.S. "AIDS LIfeline," is availabe in English and Braille, Spanish and Chinese. It provides answers to common questions about HIV. "AIDS Antibody Testing at Alternative Test Sites" describes free antibody testing programs in the San Francisco area, discusses the meaning of test results, and the pros and cons of testing.

This package also includes the brochure, "When a Friend Has AIDS," which gives several humane and concrete suggestions for friends and co-workers, along with a list of support services and hotlines in the San Francisco area.

Reviewers' Comments: This package is well designed in content, instructional design, and technical production. The video portrays good human interest, but does not cover specific treatment or prevention measures. It should be augmented by discussion and information provided by the brochures. The program components are best used in an integrated fashion rather than as stand-alone products.

▲ For Ordering Information, see p. 227

❶ AIDS in the Workplace - An Employee Education Program

Dartnell Corporation
Oct 1987; $565.00; English.

This integrated employee education program consists of a videotape entitled "One of Our Own" and seven printed products. A 27-page "Guide for Management" discusses the strategic planning required in developing a workforce educational program; provides basic facts on the disease; and reviews legal issues dealing with discrimination, testing, and confidentiality. The guide presents sample workplace policies and procedures and lists AIDS (800) number hotlines and service organizations by state.

The 30-minute video, "One of our Own," is a dramatization of the issues and effects of having an employee with AIDS/HIV. It conveys basic information on AIDS/HIV, portrays management's concern with employee rights, presents both management and employee perspectives on dealing with AIDS/HIV in the workplace, sensitizes viewers to ethical and human implciations, and stresses the importance of a strong corporate strategy and information program.

A companion 36-page "Meeting Leader's Guide" includes the complete script of the video and detailed suggestions for post-viewing discussion and follow-up workshops. Other printed materials include a 24-page pamphlet, "What a Manager Should Know About AIDS in the Workplace;" and three brochures entitled: "Questions and Answers about AIDS," "When a Co-worker has AIDS," "10 Myths about AIDS," and a poster.

Reviewers' Comments: This high quality package is an effective training tool for managers and white collar workers. Written materials compliment the video and are necessary for a complete program. They provide a good overview of the issues involved and what management should do when confronted with an employee with AIDS/HIV. They also are very supportive when addressing how to handle employees and initiate policy making. The poster is particularly eye-catching and good for office settings.

▲ For Ordering Information, see p. 218

❶ Managing AIDS In The Workplace

- **All About AIDS**
  VHS; 1989; special rates / discounts; English.
- **An Executive Briefing And Training Manual**
  120 pages; 3 ring binder; special rates / discounts; English.
- **Caring About AIDS**
  23 pages; stapled; English.
- **AIDS Training Tools For Employees -**
  Slides or video; English.

Workplace Health Communications Corporation

This multi-component training package with the overall theme, "Managing AIDS in the Workplace," includes a manager's training manual, a video and guidebook, a general information pamphlet for employees and managers, and a bi-monthly newsletter.

The video version of a slideshow is accompanied by a guidebook including a complete script of the show, suggestions on how the material should be presented, quizzes, and exercises. The presentation is divided into five units, each approximately 15 minutes in length contained in three cassettes. Topics covered include: medical facts about AIDS/HIV, employee rights, laws concerning the disease, working with people with AIDS/HIV, and preventing its transmission.

The manual is designed to provide managers with the information needed to manage AIDS/HIV issues effectively in the workplace. Sections cover: demystifying AIDS/HIV, economic issues, corporate education, testing and confidentiality, employee relations, public relations, and a summary of guidelines. Appendices are provided on: case law, training exercises, evaluation instruments, CDC guidelines, AIDS/HIV referral sources, and reading and videos.

The pamphlet for employees, managers, families and their friends, uses a question and answer format to cover facts about AIDS/HIV, reducing fear of AIDS/HIV, working with people with AIDS/HIV, and employee legal rights. Hotline numbers are listed for each state.

These materials may be augmented by a bi-monthly, two-page newsletter.

Reviewers' Comments: The "Executive Briefing and Training Manual" provides executives and managers with a comprehensive and objective approach to managing AIDS/HIV in the workplace. The manual's production and presentation are excellent. Its analysis of CDC/Workplace Guidelines is particularly noteworthy, but its resource lists are incomplete, and in some cases, inaccurate. It's overall level of sophistication and recommended policies and operational guidelines make it more suitable for larger organizations.

The "Slides and Guidebook" kit is excellent in content and organization, and is well suited for the training of both managers and employees. The slides can be tailored to specific presentations. The pamphlet, "Caring About AIDS," helps employees explore fears, feelings, and emo-

tions as well as understand the facts about AIDS/HIV. The design makes the information readily accessible.

▲ For Ordering Information, see p. 232

❶ Working Beyond Fear

- **Working Beyond Fear**
  33 min.; VHS 3/4; 1987.
- **Administrative And Marketing Guide**
  50 pages; paperback; 1987.
- **Facilitator's Manual**
  89 pages; paperback; 1987.

American Red Cross National Headquarters

The American Red Cross AIDS Prevention Program for the Workplace, whose overall theme is "Working Beyond Fear," includes a videotape, a facilitator's manual, and an administrative marketing guide. The 33-minute videotape, presented in documentary style, discusses the AIDS virus, transmission, symptoms of AIDS and ARC, research, testing, and safety of the blood supply. It briefly identifies high risk behavior and discusses transmission and prevention. It shows people with AIDS, IV drug users injecting drugs, and HIV antibody positive prostitutes discussing their concerns. It demonstrates how some cities are meeting the need of people with AIDS and the public, and discusses education programs. Three 3-minute workplace scenarios deal with the issues of first aid response to people with AIDS, protection of one's sexual partner, personal choices, confidentiality, gossip, misinformation, and personal ethics. The 89-page facilitator's manual describes the purpose and objective of the Program and provides practical information on the development of employee/employer training programs. It discusses facilitator preparation and program presentation outlines. It covers discussion guidelines, preparation checklists, and program presentation options, including use of the companion videotape, Working Beyond Fear. Appendices include references, a booklist, journal list, general information about AIDS, questions and answers on AIDS, community resources, evaluation instruments, company policies, and procedures related to AIDS, and U.S. Federal Centers for Disease Control guidelines on AIDS in the workplace and healthcare settings. It also includes a guide to services and information on AIDS from the Personnel Journal. The 50-page marketing guide for Red Cross administrators reviews methods for customizing a workplace program, Red Cross Chapter and facilitator preparation for the workplace program, and facilitator selection and training.

Reviewers' Comments: This video provides a good historical perspective and basic understanding of AIDS, and is particularly effective in discussing blood supply issues and concerns such as blood donations, transmission of the disease via transfusions, and blood testing. It is somewhat out of date (e.g. it refers to HTLV-III) and does not adequately deal with treatment, high risk behaviors, or safe sex practices. It needs to be supplemented with facilitated discussions and additional materials, as provided in the accompanying facilitator's manual and administrative guide.

▲ For Ordering Information, see p. 215

❶ 1ST EDITION RECCOMENDED   ❷ 2ND EDITION RECCOMENDED   ○ NOT RECCOMENDED

PAMPHLETS

○ **AIDS In The Workplace**

Channing L. Bete Co., Inc.

❶ **AIDS - Risk Prevention Understanding**

National Leadership Coalition on AIDS
8 pages; Oct 1987; English.

This pamphlet, for use in the workplace, provides information on AIDS/HIV, how it is spread, and what precautions can be taken to prevent infection. It also offers suggestions for employees and supervisors on how to treat co-workers with AIDS. It lists AIDS information resources and the National AIDS Hotline telephone number.

Reviewers' Comments: This pamphlet is designed to educate employees with high reading levels who are AIDS/HIV aware and knowledgeable about the basics of transmission and prevention. It is not a rudimentary education tool. The language can sometimes be unclear, but this is a good tool for sensitizing readers to people with AIDS. It addresses issues of homophobia.

▲ For Ordering Information, see p. 224

○ **What All Businesses Need To Know About AIDS**

United Way of America

VIDEOS / FILMS

❷ **AIDS In The Workplace: One Company's Response**

Equitable Life Assurance Society of U.S.
15 min.; VHS; 1989; rental fee: $5.00/2 Weeks; English.

This video describes Equitable's efforts to educate employees about the causes and prevention of AIDS/HIV. It also discusses the policies they have established for dealing with AIDS/HIV in the work environment.

Reviewers' Comments: This video gives sound business arguments for why management should implement an AIDS/HIV program and may be persuasive for managers and company policy makers who are undecided about committing to AIDS/HIV education. Both the length and production quality are good.

▲ For Ordering Information, see p. 219

○ **At Work - At Risk**

Hennepin County Administration

○ **A Corporate Response to AIDS**

National Association of Manufacturers

❷ **Living And Working With AIDS**

New England Corporate Consortium For AIDS Education
22:15 min.; VHS; 1989; $190.00; special rates / discounts; English.

This video is designed to familiarize employees in diverse work environments with the concerns and needs of people who have AIDS/HIV, and to emphasize that AIDS/HIV is not transmitted by casual contact in the workplace. In interviews, people with AIDS/HIV relate their apprehensions and considerations when informing employers and co-workers of being diagnosed as having the disease. Company policies and the rights of people with AIDS/HIV are discussed. The video offers information about HIV transmission and briefly explains how the virus attacks the immune system. It also identifies high-risk behaviors and suggests precautions.

Reviewers' Comments: This is a high quality video that covers the basic issues with a postive human interest approach. The production of the video is excellent.

▲ For Ordering Information, see p. 224

❶ **Not Ready To Die Of AIDS**

Films for the Humanities & Sciences, Inc.
52 min.; VHS; 1987; $149.00; English.

This documentary chronicles the experiences of Paul Cronan, a New England Telephone Company employee, as he faces the implications of his AIDS diagnosis. He endures conflict and finally reconciliation with family members, goes to court to win the right to return to work, and struggles with the loneliness of a restricted social life. Viewers see him go through many of the stages of grief associated with terminal illness - anger, denial, resignation, and determination to lead a worthwhile life with the time remaining.

Reviewers' Comments: As a profile of one man's struggle with discriminatory action and the litigation process, this is a good video.

▲ For Ordering Information, see p. 219

○ **Talk About AIDS**

San Francisco AIDS Foundation

○ **Universal Precautions**

Indiana State Board of Health

❶ **When Facts Are Not Enough - Managing AIDS In The Workplace**

American Hospital Association
20 min.; VHS; 1986; rental fee: 300.00; English.

This video addresses hospital management's response to their employees' fears of AIDS/HIV. Al Mitchell of the American Hospital Association asks questions about managment issues related to AIDS/HIV and two experts on employee relations respond. The discussion assumes a basic knowledge of AIDS/HIV. Questions and answers cover strategies for dealing with employees who refuse to work with patients or co-workers infected with HIV, employee education, and legal issues.

The advice presented includes having written policies and maintaining confidentiality for employees with AIDS/HIV. The package includes a program guide with suggested discussion points, facts about HIV transmission, recommendations for care of patients with HIV infection, personnel management issues, and communication strategies. Appendicies contain a sample AIDS/HIV position statement, a model policy, an AIDS/infectious disease audit, a list of resources, and a bibliography.

Reviewers' Comments: This is an effective training tool for hospital management in the development of AIDS/HIV policies for employees. Some terminology, e.g., HTLV--III/LAV, needs to be updated.

▲ For Ordering Information, see p. 214

❶ 1ST EDITION RECCOMENDED   ❷ 2ND EDITION RECCOMENDED   ○ NOT RECCOMENDED

References and Resources 2

REFERENCES

The first section of this chapter lists AID/HIV-related materials that provide reference or supplementary information for educational programs or activities. These materials are alphabetically listed under the following categories: Books, Directories, Films, Guidelines/Policy Statements, Monographs, Periodicals, and Reports. The following information is provided for each item: title, producer, target audience, publication date, and a reference to ordering information. Below is a sample item.

● AIDS And The Law: A Guide For The Public

Yale University Press
General Community; $7.95; 1987.
▲ For Ordering Information, see p. 221

RESOURCES

The final section of this chapter contains: 1) names, address, and telephone numbers of state and federal agencies involved in AIDS education /prevention; 2) titles of AIDS/HIV educational materials available from the World Health Organization along with ordering information.

● Guidelines For Nursing Management Of People Infected With HIV

World Health Organization, Global Programme on AIDS
Health Care Professionals; $7.20; special rates / discounts; 1988.
▲ For Ordering Information, see p. 221

REFERENCES AND RESOURCES

AUDIO TAPES

● **AIDS Medicine And Miracles**

Exploring AIDS
General Community; cost not specified; 1988.
▲ For Ordering Information, see p. 219

● **Audiocassettes Of Various Radio Programs On AIDS**

Pacifica Program Service and Radio Archive
General Community; cost not specified; 1986.
▲ For Ordering Information, see p. 226

● **Conversations On AIDS**

Illinois State Medical Society
Health Care Professionals; free; 1987.
▲ For Ordering Information, see p. 221

● **Relaxation And Visualization**

UCSF AIDS Health Project
General Community; $5.00; 1985.
▲ For Ordering Information, see p. 231

● **Sally Fisher - Visualizations For Discovery And Release**

Northern Lights Alternatives, Inc.
General Community; $10.00; 1988.
▲ For Ordering Information, see p. 225

BOOKS / MANUALS

● **Acquired Immune Deficiency Syndrome**

Florida Department of Health and Rehabilitative Services
Health Care Professionals; free, limited copies; 1988.
▲ For Ordering Information, see p. 219

● **Acquired Immune Deficiency Syndrome: II International Conference On AIDS (June 1986)**

Elsevier Science Publishing Company, Inc.
Health Care Professionals; $45.00; 1986.
▲ For Ordering Information, see p. 218

● **AIDS: A Guide For Survival**

Harris County Medical Society Houston Academy of Medicine
General Community; special rates / discounts; 1987.
▲ For Ordering Information, see p. 220

● **AIDS: Administrative Reference Manual**

Massachusetts Hospital Association
Health Care Professionals; cost not specified; 1987.
▲ For Ordering Information, see p. 222

● **AIDS And Patient Management**

National Health Publishing
Health Care Professionals; $38.00; 1986.
▲ For Ordering Information, see p. 224

● **AIDS And The Dental Team**

Year Book Medical Publishers
Health Care Professionals; $21.50;
special rates / discounts; 1988.
▲ For Ordering Information, see p. 232

● **AIDS And The Law: A Guide For The Public**

Yale University Press
General Community; $7.95; 1987.
▲ For Ordering Information, see p. 232

● **AIDS And The Nursing Home**

American Health Care Association
Health Care Professionals; $10.95; 1988.
▲ For Ordering Information, see p. 214

● **The AIDS Challenge: Prevention Education For Young People**

ETR Associates/Network Publications
Parents, Educators, And Administrators; $24.95; special rates / discounts; 1988.
▲ For Ordering Information, see p. 219

● **The AIDS Crisis**

SIRS - Social Issues Resources Series, Inc.
General Community; $80.00; 1988.
▲ For Ordering Information, see p. 228

● **AIDS Education Instructor's Manual**

American Red Cross Hawkeye Chapter
General Community; $7.00; Sep 1988.
▲ For Ordering Information, see p.

● **AIDS Facts And Issues**

Rutgers University Press
General Community; $10.95, limited copies; 1987.
▲ For Ordering Information, see p. 227

● **AIDS: Facts For Life**

Illinois Department of Public Health
 AIDS Facts for Life
Parents, Educators, And Administrators; free; 1987.
▲ For Ordering Information, see p. 221

● **AIDS: Facts For Life - HIV In The Health Care Setting**

Illinois Department of Public Health
 AIDS Facts for Life
Health Care Professionals; free; 1987.
▲ For Ordering Information, see p. 221

● **The AIDS Fighter**

Keats Publishing, Inc.
General Community; special rates / discounts; 1988.
▲ For Ordering Information, see p. 221

● **AIDS/HIV Infection: A Reference Guide For Nursing Professionals**

W.B. Saunders
Health Care Professionals; $19.95; 1988.
▲ For Ordering Information, see p. 231

● **AIDS/HIV Reference Guide For Medical Professionals, 3rd Ed.**

CIRID at UCLA
Health Care Professionals; $21.00; special rates / discounts; 1988.
▲ For Ordering Information, see p. 217

● **AIDS Hotline Training Manual**

San Francisco AIDS Foundation
Psychologists And Social Workers; $25.00; 1987.
▲ For Ordering Information, see p. 227

● **AIDS: Impact On The Schools**

Capitol Publications
Parents, Educators, And Administrators; $45.00; 1986.
▲ For Ordering Information, see p. 216

● **AIDS: Improving The Response Of The Correctional System**

National Sheriffs' Association
Policy Makers And Lawyers; $10.00; special rates / discounts; 1986.
▲ For Ordering Information, see p. 224

● **AIDS In Children, Adolescents, And Heterosexual Adults: An Interdisciplinary Approach To Prevention**

Elsevier Science Publishing Company, Inc.
Health Care Professionals; $34.95; Feb 1987.
▲ For Ordering Information, see p. 218

● **AIDS Legal Guide**

Lambda Legal Defense and Education Fund, Inc.
Policy Makers And Lawyers; $50.00; special rates / discounts; Dec 1987.
▲ For Ordering Information, see p. 222

● **The AIDS Manual**

National Health Publishing
Health Care Professionals; $149.00; 1988.
▲ For Ordering Information, see p. 224

● **AIDS On The College Campus - ACHA Special Report**

American College Health Association
College And University Students; cost not specified; 1986.
▲ For Ordering Information, see p. 214

● **AIDS Papers From SCIENCE, 1982-1985**

American Association for the Advancement of Science
General Community; $19.95; Mar 1986.
▲ For Ordering Information, see p. 214

● **AIDS Practice Manual: A Legal And Educational Guide**

National Gay Rights Advocates
Policy Makers And Lawyers; $35.00; special rates / discounts; 1987.
▲ For Ordering Information, see p. 224

● **AIDS Practice Manual: A Legal And Educational Guide**

National Lawyers Guild AIDS Network
Policy Makers And Lawyers; $35.00; special rates / discounts; 1987.
▲ For Ordering Information, see p. 224

● **AIDS Public Policy Dimensions**

United Hospital Fund
General Community; cost not specified; 1986.
▲ For Ordering Information, see p. 230

● **AIDS Reference And Research Collections: 1980-1988**

University Publishing Group
General Community; $315.00; 1988.
▲ For Ordering Information, see p. 231

● **AIDS Service Providers**

New York State Department of Social Services, Office of Human Resource Development
Health Care Professionals; cost not specified; Jan 1987.
▲ For Ordering Information, see p. 225

● **AIDS, Sexual Behavior, And IV Drug Use**

National Academy Press
General Community; $24.95; special rates / discounts; 1989.
▲ For Ordering Information, see p. 223

● **AIDS: The Caregiver's Handbook**

St. Martin's Press
People Who Care; $10.95; special rates / discounts; Dec 1988.
▲ For Ordering Information, see p. 228

● **AIDS: The Legal Issues**

American Bar Association
Policy Makers And Lawyers; $15.00; special rates / discounts; 1988.
▲ For Ordering Information, see p. 214

● **AIDSLaw**

AIDS Legal Referral Panel
Policy Makers And Lawyers; $81.00; special rates / discounts; 1988.
▲ For Ordering Information, see p. 213

● **And The Band Played On**

St. Martin's Press
General Community; $12.95; Oct 1988.
▲ For Ordering Information, see p. 228

● **Beyond AIDS: A Journey Into Healing**

Brotherhood Press
HIV Positive Individuals; $10.00; special rates / discounts; 1988.
▲ For Ordering Information, see p. 216

● **A Clinician's Guide To AIDS And HIV Infection**

Georgia Department of Human Resources
Health Care Professionals; $10.00; Nov 1988.
▲ For Ordering Information, see p. 220

● **Color Atlas Of AIDS And HIV Disease**

Year Book Medical Publishers
Health Care Professionals; $35.00; special rates / discounts; 1988.
▲ For Ordering Information, see p. 232

● **The Color Of Light: Daily Meditations For All Of Us Living With AIDS**

Hazelden Educational Materials
HIV Positive Individuals; $6.95; special rates / discounts; 1988.
▲ For Ordering Information, see p. 220

● **Confronting AIDS: Directions For Public Health, Health Care, And Research**

Institute of Medicine, National Academy of Sciences
General Community; $24.95; 1986.
▲ For Ordering Information, see p. 221

● **Confronting AIDS: Update 1988**

National Academy Press
General Community; $15.95; special rates / discounts; 1988.
▲ For Ordering Information, see p. 223

● **Developing AIDS Residential Settings**

Visiting Nurses and Hospice of San Francisco
Special Audiences; $95.00; special rates / discounts; 1988.
▲ For Ordering Information, see p. 231

- **Disease Prevention / Health Promotion: The Facts**

  U.S. Government,
    Department of Health and Human Services
    Office of Disease Prevention and Health
    Promotion
  Health Care Professionals; $22.95; 1988.
  ▲ For Ordering Information, see p. 230

- **Emergency Workers And The AIDS Epidemic: A Guidebook For Law Enforcement, Fire Service, And Ambulance Service Personnel**

  California Firefighter Foundation
  Public Safety And Support Workers; $2.00; 1987.
  ▲ For Ordering Information, see p. 216

- **Enhanced Health Promotion And AIDS Disease Program- Training In Interpersonal Problem-Solving (TIPS)**

  Center for Excellence in Addiction
    Treatment Research
  General Community; cost not specified; 1988.
  ▲ For Ordering Information, see p. 216

- **The Essential AIDS Fact Book: What You Need To Know To Protect Yourself, Your Family, And All Your Loved Ones**

  Pocket Books
  General Community; $3.95; 1987.
  ▲ For Ordering Information, see p. 226

- **Extended Health Care At Home: A Complete And Practical Guide**

  Celestial Arts Publishing
  People Who Care; $9.95; special rates / discounts; 1988.
  ▲ For Ordering Information, see p. 216

- **Financing Care For Persons With AIDS**

  University Publishing Group
  Health Care Professionals; $45.00; special rates / discounts; 1989.
  ▲ For Ordering Information, see p. 231

- **GMHC Volunteer Training Manual**

  Gay Men's Health Crisis, Inc.
  People Who Care; $25.00; Nov 1986.
  ▲ For Ordering Information, see p. 219

- **The Heterosexual Transmission Of AIDS In Africa**

  ABT Books, Inc.
  Health Care Professionals; $29.00; special rates / discounts; 1988.
  ▲ For Ordering Information, see p. 213

- **How To Persuade Your Lover To Use A Condom . . . And Why You Should**

  Prima Publishing
  Sexually Active Adults; $4.95; 1987.
  ▲ For Ordering Information, see p. 227

- **Human Sexuality: A Bibliography For Everyone**

  Sex Information and Education Council
    of The United States
  General Community; cost not specified.
  ▲ For Ordering Information, see p. 228

- **Laboratory Methods For The Diagnosis of Sexually Transmitted Diseases**

  American Public Health Association
  Health Care Professionals; $25.00;
  special rates / discounts; 1987.
  ▲ For Ordering Information, see p. 215

- **The Living Will And Other Advance Directives**

  Concern for Dying
  Policy Makers And Lawyers; $3.00.
  ▲ For Ordering Information, see p. 217

- **Managing AIDS In The Workplace**

  Addison-Wesley Publishing Company, Inc.
  Workplace; $19.95; special rates / discounts; 1988.
  ▲ For Ordering Information, see p. 213

- **Mortal Fear: Meditations On Death And AIDS**

  Cowley Publications
  General Community; $6.95.
  ▲ For Ordering Information, see p. 218

- **Plain Words About AIDS**

  Whitehall Press-Budget Publications
  General Community; $17.50.
  ▲ For Ordering Information, see p. 231

● **The Real Truth About Women And AIDS: How To Eliminate The Risks Without Giving Up Love And Sex**

Simon & Schuster, Inc.
Sexually Active Adults; $4.95; 1987.
▲ For Ordering Information, see p. 228

● **Reducing HIV Transmission - Lessons From The Recent Past**

AIDSCOM/Academy for Educational Development
General Community; cost not specified.
▲ For Ordering Information, see p. 214

● **Religious Publications On Sex Education And Sexuality**

Sex Information and Education Council of the United States
General Community; cost not specified.
▲ For Ordering Information, see p. 228

● **Report Of The CWLA Task Force On Children And HIV Infection: Initial Guidelines**

Child Welfare League of America
Children And Adolescents; $22.95; 1988.
▲ For Ordering Information, see p. 217

● **Responding To AIDS: Psychosocial Initiatives**

National Association of Social Workers
Psychologists And Social Workers; $12.95; 1986.
▲ For Ordering Information, see p. 223

● **Safe Sex In A Dangerous World**

Random House, Inc., Vintage Books
General Community; $3.95.
▲ For Ordering Information, see p. 227

● **Sex, Drugs & AIDS**

Bantam Books, Inc.
Children And Adolescents; $4.95; Jun 1987.
▲ For Ordering Information, see p. 215

● **The Social Impact Of AIDS In The U.S.**

ABT Books, Inc.
Health Care Professionals; $19.95; special rates / discounts; 1988.
▲ For Ordering Information, see p. 213

● **Social Security Self-Help Manual**

AIDS Legal Referral Panel
General Community; $25.00; 1988.
▲ For Ordering Information, see p. 213

● **The Sourcebook Of Lesbian/Gay Health Care**

National Lesbian and Gay Health Foundation
Health Care Professionals; $20.00; 1988.
▲ For Ordering Information, see p. 224

● **Strategies For Survival**

St. Martin's Press
Gay And Bisexual Men; $10.95; special rates / discounts; Dec 1987.
▲ For Ordering Information, see p. 228

● **Subject Index To Abstracts, III International Conference On AIDS**

Whitehall Press-Budget Publications
Health Care Professionals; $10.00.
▲ For Ordering Information, see p. 231

● **Surviving And Thriving With AIDS: Collected Wisdom, Volume 2**

PWA (People With AIDS) Coalition, Inc.
HIV Positive Individuals; $20.00; special rates / discounts; 1988.
▲ For Ordering Information, see p. 227

● **Surviving And Thriving With AIDS: Hints For The Newly Diagnosed, Volume 1**

PWA (People With AIDS) Coalition, Inc.
HIV Positive Individuals; $10.00; special rates / discounts; 1987.
▲ For Ordering Information, see p. 227

● **They Conquered AIDS: True Life Adventures**

Tree of Life Publications
General Community; $24.95; special rates / discounts; Jan 1989.
▲ For Ordering Information, see p. 230

● **2176 Medicaid Waivers TA Packet**

National AIDS Network (NAN)
Health Care Professionals; $15.00; special rates / discounts; 1988.
▲ For Ordering Information, see p. 223

- **Understanding AIDS, Volume 1**

  Century House Publications, Inc.
  General Community; $6.95; 1987.
  ▲ For Ordering Information, see p. 217

- **Understanding And Preventing AIDS: A Book For Everyone**

  Health Alert Press
  General Community; $24.95; special rates / discounts; 1988.
  ▲ For Ordering Information, see p. 220

- **Women And AIDS Clinical Resource Guide**

  San Francisco AIDS Foundation
  Women; $45.00; 1987.
  ▲ For Ordering Information, see p. 227

- **You Can Do Something About AIDS**

  The Stop AIDS Project
  General Community; $2.00; special rates / discounts; 1988.
  ▲ For Ordering Information, see p. 229

BROCHURES

- **Advance Directives (Living Wills)**

  Society for the Right to Die
  General Community; free, limited copies; 1988.
  ▲ For Ordering Information, see p. 228

- **AIDS: An Update For You And Your Family**

  Caremark Homecare
  General Community; free; Feb 1988.
  ▲ For Ordering Information, see p. 216

- **AIDS And Civil Liberties: ACLU Briefing Paper**

  American Civil Liberties Union Foundation
  Health Care Professionals; free, limited copies; Jun 1987.
  ▲ For Ordering Information, see p. 214

- **AIDS: Facts For Physicians**

  Illinois State Medical Society
  Health Care Professionals; free; 1987.
  ▲ For Ordering Information, see p. 221

- **AIDS: How And Where To Find Facts And Do Research**

  R & E Research, Inc.
  General Community; cost not specified; 1986.
  ▲ For Ordering Information, see p. 227

- **AIDS Projects**

  Macro Systems, Inc.
  Health Care Professionals; free; 1988.
  ▲ For Ordering Information, see p. 222

- **AIDSRISK: Risk Assessment Questionnaires For Men And Women**

  Polaris Research and Development
  General Community; $.65; special rates / discounts; 1988.
  ▲ For Ordering Information, see p. 226

- **AIDSTECH**

  Family Health International
  Workplace; cost not specified.
  ▲ For Ordering Information, see p. 219

- **Available Resources**

  NO/AIDS Task Force
  HIV Positive Individuals; $.10; special rates / discounts; 1988.
  ▲ For Ordering Information, see p. 225

- **Experimental Drug Treatment Information**

  Project Inform
  HIV Positive Individuals; free; 1988.
  ▲ For Ordering Information, see p. 227

- **Glossary Of AIDS Terms**

  Riverside County Department of Health AIDS Activities Program
  General Community; free, limited copies; May 1988.
  ▲ For Ordering Information, see p. 227

- **HIV Testing - AIDS**

  Richmond City Health Department
  General Community; cost not specified; 1985.
  ▲ For Ordering Information, see p. 227

- **Information Packet: Dartmouth College Comprehensive AIDS Education Program**

  Dartmouth College
  Department of Health Education
  College And University Students; special rates / discounts; 1988.
  ▲ For Ordering Information, see p. 218

- **Issues In Home Intravenous Antibiotic Therapy**

  Caremark Homecare
  Health Care Professionals; free; 1987.
  ▲ For Ordering Information, see p. 216

- **A Living Will**

  Concern for Dying
  General Community; free, limited copies; Jan 1984.
  ▲ For Ordering Information, see p. 217

- **Living Will Declaration**

  Society for the Right to Die
  General Community; free.
  ▲ For Ordering Information, see p. 228

- **The Predicted Disease Impact Of AIDS In Minnesota**

  Minnesota Department of Health (MDH)
  AIDS Program Unit
  Health Care Professionals; free; Apr 1987.
  ▲ For Ordering Information, see p. 223

- **Questions And Answers About The Living Will**

  Concern for Dying
  General Community; free, limited copies; 1987.
  ▲ For Ordering Information, see p. 217

- **Student Health Survey**

  Rhode Island Hospital
  Children And Adolescents; cost not specified.
  ▲ For Ordering Information, see p. 227

- **What Every Podiatric Physician Should Know About AIDS**

  American Podiatric Medical Association
  Health Care Professionals; special rates / discounts; 1986.
  ▲ For Ordering Information, see p. 215

- **What You Should Know About Durable Power Of Attorney**

  Society for the Right to Die
  General Community; cost not specified; Nov 1987.
  ▲ For Ordering Information, see p. 228

- **You And Your Living Will**

  Society for the Right to Die
  General Community; free.
  ▲ For Ordering Information, see p. 228

CATALOGS / BIBLIOGRAPHIES

- **The A.I.D.S. Catalog**

  R & E Research, Inc.
  General Community; $1.00; Feb 1988.
  ▲ For Ordering Information, see p. 227

- **AAAS Symposia Papers On AIDS, 1988**

  American Association for the Advancement of Science
  General Community; special rates / discounts; Oct 1988.
  ▲ For Ordering Information, see p. 214

- **Acquired Immune Deficiency Syndrome: An Annotated Bibliography**

  Sex Information and Education Council of the United States
  General Community; cost not specified; 1986.
  ▲ For Ordering Information, see p. 228

- **AIDS 1987**

  The Oryx Press
  Health Care Professionals; $29.50; Nov 1987.
  ▲ For Ordering Information, see p. 226

- **AIDS And Safer Sex Education: An Annotated Bibliography**

  Sex Information and Education Council of the United States
  General Community; cost not specified.
  ▲ For Ordering Information, see p. 228

- **AIDS Audiovisual Resources For Health Care Professionals**

  Health Information Network
  Health Care Professionals; $2.50; 1988.
  ▲ For Ordering Information, see p. 220

- **AIDS Audiovisual Resources For PWAs, PWARCs, HIV+s, High Risk Persons, Their Friends And Families, And On Safer Sex**

  Health Information Network
  Sexually Active Adults; $2.50; 1988.
  ▲ For Ordering Information, see p. 220

- **AIDS Audiovisual Resources For The General Public**

  Health Information Network
  General Community; $2.50; 1988.
  ▲ For Ordering Information, see p. 220

- **AIDS Audiovisual Resources For The Workplace**

  Health Information Network
  Workplace; $2.50; 1988.
  ▲ For Ordering Information, see p. 220

- **AIDS Audiovisual Resources For Young People And Schools**

  Health Information Network
  Parents, Educators, And Administrators; $2.50; 1988.
  ▲ For Ordering Information, see p. 220

- **AIDS Bibliography**

  National Library of Medicine
  Health Care Professionals; $12.00; 1988.
  ▲ For Ordering Information, see p. 224

- **AIDS Bibliography**

  University of California at San Francisco Institute for Health Policy Studies AIDS Resource Program
  General Community; cost not specified; Jun 1987.
  ▲ For Ordering Information, see p. 231

- **AIDS Bibliography: Selected Resources For Church Educators**

  Division of Education and Ministry National Council of Churches Task Force on AIDS
  Pastoral Counselors; $3.00; 1989.
  ▲ For Ordering Information, see p. 218

- **AIDS Computerized And Periodical Resources**

  Health Information Network
  Health Care Professionals; $2.50; 1988.
  ▲ For Ordering Information, see p. 220

- **AIDS In The Workplace Bibliography**

  Human Interaction Research Institute
  Workplace; $10.00; 1988.
  ▲ For Ordering Information, see p. 221

- **AIDS Information Resources For Health Care Professionals (Washington State List)**

  Health Information Network
  Health Care Professionals; $2.50; 1988.
  ▲ For Ordering Information, see p. 220

- **AIDS Information Resources For Health Care Professionals (National List)**

  Health Information Network
  Health Care Professionals; $2.50; 1988.
  ▲ For Ordering Information, see p. 220

- **AIDS Public Education Program**

  American Red Cross National Headquarters
  General Community; cost not specified; Dec 1985.
  ▲ For Ordering Information, see p. 215

- **AIDS/STD's Educational Resources Catalog**

  Kansas Department of Health and Environment Bureau of Epidemiology AIDS
  Parents, Educators, And Administrators; free; Dec 1987.
  ▲ For Ordering Information, see p. 221

- **AIDS: Law, Ethics And Public Policy**

  Georgetown University, Kennedy Institute of Ethics National Reference Center for Bioethics Literature
  Policy Makers And Lawyers; $3.00; 1988.
  ▲ For Ordering Information, see p. 220

- **AIDS: A Bibliography**

  R & E Research, Inc.
  General Community; $10.00; 1987.
  ▲ For Ordering Information, see p. 227

- **AIDS: A Guide To Research Resources**

  University of California, Berkeley: The Library
  College And University Students; $20.00; special rates / discounts; 1989.
  ▲ For Ordering Information, see p. 231

● **Bibliographic Search - Database**

**International Working Group on AIDS
and IV Drug Use
Narcotic and Drug Research, Inc.**
Special Audiences; free; 1988.
▲ For Ordering Information, see p. 221

● **Collected Papers On AIDS Research,
1986-1987**

BIOSIS
Special Audiences; $95.00; 1987.
▲ For Ordering Information, see p. 215

● **IV International Conference On AIDS,
Stockholm - June 12-16, 1988,
Abstracts, Two Volumes**

BioData Publishers
General Community; $90.00; special rates / discounts; 1988.
▲ For Ordering Information, see p. 215

● **Guide To AIDS Educational Materials**

Harris County Health Department
Parents, Educators, And Administrators; cost not specified;
Dec 1987.
▲ For Ordering Information, see p. 220

● **Immune System Support**

Alliance 7 Buyer's Club
HIV Positive Individuals; free; 1988.
▲ For Ordering Information, see p. 214

● **National Library Of Medicine Literature
Search: Acquired Immunodeficiency
Syndrome (AIDS) Series**

National Library of Medicine
General Community; free, limited copies.
▲ For Ordering Information, see p. 224

● **NOBCO AIDS Education Project:
Selected AIDS Bibliography**

**National Organization of Black County Officials,
Inc.**
Black Community; free; 1988.
▲ For Ordering Information, see p. 224

● **Resources For Educators - AIDS And
Adolescents**

Center for Population Options
Parents, Educators, And Administrators; $3.50;
special rates / discounts; 1988.
▲ For Ordering Information, see p. 217

● **School Curriculums On AIDS And STD**

Health Information Network
Parents, Educators, And Administrators; $2.50; 1988.
▲ For Ordering Information, see p. 220

● **Third International AIDS Conference
(June 1-5, 1987)**

InfoMedix
Health Care Professionals; cost not specified.
▲ For Ordering Information, see p. 221

● **III International Conference On AIDS,
Washington, DC - June 1-5, 1987,
Abstracts Volume, Reprint**

BioData Publishers
General Community; $30.00; special rates / discounts; 1987.
▲ For Ordering Information, see p. 215

COMPUTER INFORMATION SERVICES

● **AIDS Health Education Learning
Objectives Database**

**University of Louisville
Department of Psychiatry**
Health Care Professionals; free; 1988.
▲ For Ordering Information, see p. 231

● **AIDS History Files**

University Publishing Group
General Community; $860.00; 1989.
▲ For Ordering Information, see p. 231

● **AIDS In Focus**

BIOSIS
Health Care Professionals; cost not specified; 1988.
▲ For Ordering Information, see p. 215

● **AIDS Info On-Line**

**AIDS Research and Education Project,
Psychology Department
California State University at Long Beach**
College And University Students;
special rates / discounts; 1988.
▲ For Ordering Information, see p. 213

- **AIDS Information And Education Worldwide**

  CD Resources / Libraries-To-Go
  Health Care Professionals; special rates / discounts; Jul 1988.
  ▲ For Ordering Information, see p. 216

- **AIDS Stack**

  WIN Project Foundation
  General Community; special rates / discounts; 1988.
  ▲ For Ordering Information, see p. 231

- **AIDSLINE**

  National Library of Medicine
  Health Care Professionals; special rates / discounts; 1988.
  ▲ For Ordering Information, see p. 224

- **AIDSQUEST ONLINE**

  CDC AIDS Weekly
  General Community; free; special rates / discounts; 1988.
  ▲ For Ordering Information, see p. 216

- **CAIN - Computerized AIDS Information Network**

  Gay and Lesbian Community Services Center
  General Community; $49.95.
  ▲ For Ordering Information, see p. 219

- **CDC AIDS Weekly Computer Readable Diskette Edition**

  CDC AIDS Weekly
  Health Care Professionals; $676/year; special rates / discounts; 1988.
  ▲ For Ordering Information, see p. 216

- **CDC AIDS Weekly Electronic Edition**

  CDC AIDS Weekly
  General Community; special rates / discounts.
  ▲ For Ordering Information, see p. 216

- **CDC AIDS Weekly Infoline**

  CDC AIDS Weekly
  General Community; free; 1988.
  ▲ For Ordering Information, see p. 216

- **First Medic AIDS Computerized Medical History Reporting System**

  WIN Project Foundation
  Health Care Professionals; special rates / discounts; Jan 1989.
  ▲ For Ordering Information, see p. 231

- **Grateful Med**

  National Library of Medicine
  Health Care Professionals; $29.95; Feb 1988.
  ▲ For Ordering Information, see p. 224

- **Indian AIDS Network**

  National Native American AIDS Prevention Center
  Special Audiences; cost not specified; 1989.
  ▲ For Ordering Information, see p. 224

- **L.I.N.K.**

  Planned Parenthood Federation of America
  Health Care Professionals; cost not specified; 1987.
  ▲ For Ordering Information, see p. 226

- **Local AIDS Database**

  U.S. Conference of Mayors; U.S. Conference of Local Health Officers
  Policy Makers And Lawyers; cost not specified; 1988.
  ▲ For Ordering Information, see p. 230

- **NLA Online AIDS Bibliographic/Abstract Service**

  Northern Lights Alternatives, Inc.
  HIV Positive Individuals; cost not specified; 1988.
  ▲ For Ordering Information, see p. 225

- **WAIDS-AIDS In The Workplace Computer Bulletin Board**

  Human Interaction Research Institute
  Workplace; cost not specified; 1988.
  ▲ For Ordering Information, see p. 221

- **Where To Find AIDS Information Online**

  University of California at Irvine
  General Community; cost not specified.
  ▲ For Ordering Information, see p. 231

- **WIN AIDS Dataline**

  WIN Project Foundation
  General Community; special rates / discounts; Feb 1989.
  ▲ For Ordering Information, see p. 231

- **WIN AIDS Laser Disk Library**

  WIN Project Foundation
  General Community; special rates / discounts; 1988.
  ▲ For Ordering Information, see p. 231

DIRECTORIES

● **AIDS: A Public Health Challenge**

George Washington University
 Intergovernmental Health Policy Project
Policy Makers And Lawyers; $150.00; 1987.
▲ For Ordering Information, see p. 220

● **AIDS: A Resource Guide For Connecticut**

Connecticut Department of Health Services
 AIDS Program
General Community; free; 1987.
▲ For Ordering Information, see p. 218

● **AIDS: A Resource Guide For New York City**

New York City Department of Health
 AIDS Education Training Unit
General Community; free, limited copies; May 1987.
▲ For Ordering Information, see p. 225

● **AIDS Coalition Of Southern California Resources Guide**

Camden County Health Department AIDS Program
Health Care Professionals; free; Oct 1988.
▲ For Ordering Information, see p. 216

● **AIDS Community Resource Directory**

Texas Department of Health
 Bureau of AIDS and STD Control
General Community; cost not specified; Dec 1986.
▲ For Ordering Information, see p. 229

● **AIDS Database Directory**

Medical Data Exchange
General Community; cost not specified; 1988.
▲ For Ordering Information, see p. 222

● **AIDS Funding: A Guide To Giving By Foundations & Charitable Organizations**

The Foundation Center
Special Audiences; $35.00; special rates / discounts; 1988.
▲ For Ordering Information, see p. 229

● **The AIDS/HIV Record Directory Of Key Program Officials In Federal, State, County, And City Governments**

BioData Inc.
General Community; $47.95; special rates / discounts; 1988.
▲ For Ordering Information, see p. 215

● **AIDS Information And Education Resources**

Massachusetts Department of Public Health
General Community; free; Jul 1987.
▲ For Ordering Information, see p. 222

● **AIDS Information Sourcebook**

The Oryx Press
General Community; $24.50.
▲ For Ordering Information, see p. 226

● **AIDS Program Resource List**

Tennessee Department of Health and Environment
General Community; cost not specified.
▲ For Ordering Information, see p. 229

● **AIDS Related Resources For Referral In Minnesota**

Minnesota AIDS Project
Health Care Professionals; $7.50; 1987.
▲ For Ordering Information, see p. 223

● **AIDS Resource Manual For Wyoming**

State of Wyoming, Division of Health and Medical STD/AIDS
General Community; free.
▲ For Ordering Information, see p. 228

● **AIDS Resource Materials For Schools**

Monmouth Ocean AIDS Information Group, Inc.
Parents, Educators, And Administrators; free.
▲ For Ordering Information, see p. 223

● **AIDS Resources**

Louisville and Jefferson County Board of Health
General Community; free, limited copies; Dec 1988.
▲ For Ordering Information, see p. 222

- **AIDS Resources For Greater Houston**

  Harris County Health Department
  HIV Positive Individuals; free, limited copies; Nov 1987.
  ▲ For Ordering Information, see p. 220

- **AIDS Service Directory For Hispanics**

  National Coalition of Hispanic Health and Human Services Organizations (COSSMHO)
  Latino Community; $7.50; Apr 1987.
  ▲ For Ordering Information, see p. 224

- **AIDS Service Directory For The Chicago Area**

  Northwest University Medical School AIDS Mental Health Education and Evaluation Project
  Health Care Professionals; cost not specified.
  ▲ For Ordering Information, see p. 225

- **AIDS Speaker Bureau**

  Kansas Department of Health and Environment Bureau of Epidemiology AIDS
  General Community; free; Feb 1988.
  ▲ For Ordering Information, see p. 221

- **Bilingual Directory Of Health Services For Hispanics / Directorio Bilingüe De Servicios De Salud Para Hispanos**

  Oregon Council for Hispanic Advancement
  Latino Community; $1.00; 1988.
  ▲ For Ordering Information, see p. 225

- **Client Services Directory**

  Gay Men's Health Crisis, Inc.
  Health Care Professionals; free.
  ▲ For Ordering Information, see p. 219

- **A Community Resource Guide For Assisting People With AIDS**

  Massachusetts Department of Public Health
  HIV Positive Individuals; free; Apr 1987.
  ▲ For Ordering Information, see p. 222

- **Compendium Of International Focal Points, Programmes, And Policy Initiatives In Response To . . . (SIDA/AIDS)**

  Worthington Associates Worldwide
  Health Care Professionals; $10.00;
  special rates / discounts; 1989.
  ▲ For Ordering Information, see p. 232

- **Directory And Database Of AIDS-Specific Periodicals And Computer-Readable Databases**

  CDC AIDS Weekly
  General Community; special rates / discounts; 1989.
  ▲ For Ordering Information, see p. 216

- **Directory And Database Of Antiviral And Immunomodulatory Therapies For AIDS (DAITA)**

  CDC AIDS Weekly
  General Community; special rates / discounts; 1989.
  ▲ For Ordering Information, see p. 216

- **Directory Of Points Of Contact In International Organizations Working Globally To Combat AIDS/SIDA**

  UNICEF, The Non-Governmental Organizations Committee
  General Community; cost not specified; 1988.
  ▲ For Ordering Information, see p. 230

- **Express "Mini Pack" - AIDS**

  Florida Department of Education Florida Prevention Center
  Parents, Educators, And Administrators; cost not specified.
  ▲ For Ordering Information, see p. 219

- **Health Care Resources For People With HIV Infection**

  Health Information Network
  HIV Positive Individuals; $2.50; 1988.
  ▲ For Ordering Information, see p. 220

- **Legal Docket: AIDS And The Law; Sexuality**

  American Civil Liberties Union Foundation
  Policy Makers And Lawyers; $10.00; Jun 1987.
  ▲ For Ordering Information, see p. 214

- **Local AIDS Services**

  U.S. Conference of Mayors;
  U.S. Conference of Local Health Officers
  General Community; $12.00; special rates / discounts; 1988.
  ▲ For Ordering Information, see p. 230

- **NAN Directory Of AIDS-Related Periodicals**

  National AIDS Network (NAN)
  Health Care Professionals; $5.00; special rates / discounts; 1988.
  ▲ For Ordering Information, see p. 223

- **NAN Directory Of AIDS-Related Videos**

  National AIDS Network (NAN)
  Health Care Professionals; $5.00; special rates / discounts; 1988.
  ▲ For Ordering Information, see p. 223

- **NLA National Directory Of Alternative Approaches**

  Northern Lights Alternatives, Inc.
  HIV Positive Individuals; cost not specified; 1988.
  ▲ For Ordering Information, see p. 225

- **NOBCO AIDS Education Resource Guide**

  National Organization of Black County Officials, Inc.
  Black Community; free; 1988.
  ▲ For Ordering Information, see p. 224

- **Ohio AIDS Foundation - Resources Directory**

  Ohio AIDS Foundation
  General Community; cost not specified; 1988.
  ▲ For Ordering Information, see p. 225

- **Resource Directory: AIDS Related Services For Michigan**

  United Community Services of Metropolitan Detroit
  Health Care Professionals; $3.00; Feb 1988.
  ▲ For Ordering Information, see p. 230

- **Resource Guide For Persons With AIDS/ARC**

  Tampa AIDS Network
  HIV Positive Individuals; free, limited copies; Nov 1987.
  ▲ For Ordering Information, see p. 229

- **Resource List**

  Rhode Island Department of Health AIDS Program
  General Community; cost not specified; Feb 1988.
  ▲ For Ordering Information, see p. 227

- **Statewide AIDS/HIV Resource Guide**

  South Carolina Dept. of Health and Environmental Control Bureau of Preventive Health Services
  Health Care Professionals; free; 1988.
  ▲ For Ordering Information, see p. 228

- **Women's Centers And AIDS Project: A Guide To Educational Materials**

  Women's Action Alliance
  Women; $2.25; Nov 1988.
  ▲ For Ordering Information, see p. 232

- **Women's Centers And AIDS Project: New Jersey Service Guide**

  Women's Action Alliance
  Women; $2.25; Nov 1988.
  ▲ For Ordering Information, see p. 232

- **Women's Centers And AIDS Project: New York Service Guide**

  Women's Action Alliance
  Women; $2.25; Nov 1988.
  ▲ For Ordering Information, see p. 232

- **The Workplace And AIDS - A Guide To Services And Information**

  A. C. Croft, Inc.
  Workplace; cost not specified; 1988.
  ▲ For Ordering Information, see p. 213

INSTRUCTIONAL PROGRAMS

● **Acquired Immune Deficiency Syndrome (AIDS) Breaking The Chain Of Infection**

National Organization of Black County Officials, Inc.
Black Community; free; 1988.
▲ For Ordering Information, see p. 224

● **Acquired Immune Deficiency Syndrome: The Basics**

National Native American AIDS Prevention Center
Special Audiences; $5.00; 1988.
▲ For Ordering Information, see p. 224

● **AIDS: A Caring Response: A Program For Religious Leadership**

Roanoke AIDS Project
Pastoral Counselors; free; 1988.
▲ For Ordering Information, see p. 227

● **AIDS: Culturally Specific Education Instructional Manual**

African Americans Taking Action Against AIDS Council
c/o American Red Cross Hawkeye Chapter
Black Community; $3.00; Dec 1988.
▲ For Ordering Information, see p. 213

● **AIDS Education: A Training Program For School Board Members**

National School Boards Association
Parents, Educators, And Administrators; cost not specified; Sep 1988.
▲ For Ordering Information, see p. 224

● **AIDS Resource Manual For Educators**

Iowa Department of Education
Parents, Educators, And Administrators; cost not specified; Sep 1987.
▲ For Ordering Information, see p. 221

● **Cultural Aspects Of Counseling**

Statewide Minority Advocacy Group for Alcohol and Drug Prevention, Inc.
General Community; cost not specified.
▲ For Ordering Information, see p. 228

● **Educator's Guide To Sexually Transmitted Dieseases**

Texas Department of Health Bureau of AIDS and STD Control
Parents, Educators, And Administrators; free.
▲ For Ordering Information, see p. 229

● **Eroticizing Safer Sex Workshop Manual**

Gay Men's Health Crisis, Inc.
Gay And Bisexual Men; $8.00.
▲ For Ordering Information, see p. 219

● **Instructional Outcomes For AIDS Education**

Rhode Island Department of Health AIDS Program
Parents, Educators, And Administrators; free, limited copies; May 1987.
▲ For Ordering Information, see p. 227

● **Parrish-Based AIDS 101**

AIDS Ministries Program
General Community; cost not specified; May 1988.
▲ For Ordering Information, see p. 213

● **Resource Unit For Family Life Education**

Chicago Public Schools Bureau of Science
Children And Adolescents; cost not specified; 1984.
▲ For Ordering Information, see p. 217

● **STD/AIDS Professional Development**

Gay and Lesbian Community Services Center
Health Care Professionals; cost not specified.
▲ For Ordering Information, see p. 219

● **Stop AIDS Start-Up Manual**

Stop AIDS Resource Center (Stop AIDS Project)
Special Audiences; free; 1989.
▲ For Ordering Information, see p. 228

● **The Three Rivers PAL Project Training Manual**

Pittsburgh AIDS Task Force, Inc.
People Who Care; free, limited copies; 1985.
▲ For Ordering Information, see p. 226

- **University Curriculum**

  George Washington University School of Medicine and Health Sciences
  College And University Students; cost not specified; 1988.
  ▲ For Ordering Information, see p. 220

MICROFILMS / SLIDES

- **Quilt Of Sorrow/Quilt Of Hope: I Want To Know What Love Is**

  Health Matters, Inc.
  General Community; $79.95; 1989.
  ▲ For Ordering Information, see p. 220

MULTICOMPONENT PROGRAMS

- **AIDS: Corporate America Responds (Report)**

  Allstate Insurance Company Allstate Forum on Public Issues
  Workplace; free, limited copies; Jan 1988.
  ▲ For Ordering Information, see p. 214

- **AIDS: Corporate America Responds (Video)**

  Allstate Insurance Company Allstate Forum on Public Issues
  Workplace; $12.00; Jan 1988.
  ▲ For Ordering Information, see p. 214

- **AIDS Programs In Medical Education Audio Cassettes, Videos, Guides**

  Audio-Video Digest Foundation
  Health Care Professionals; cost not specified.
  ▲ For Ordering Information, see p. 215

- **Basic And Advanced AIDS Prevention And Knowledge Study Questionnaires, Guides, Tests**

  AIDS Virus Education and Research Institute (AVERI)
  Health Care Professionals; cost not specified; Jan 1988.
  ▲ For Ordering Information, see p. 214

- **Exploring The Heart Of Healing**

  The Access Group
  Health Care Professionals; cost not specified; 1988.
  ▲ For Ordering Information, see p. 229

- **Infection Control Package (Pamphlets, Articles, Brochure, Chart)**

  American Dental Association Division of Communications
  Health Care Professionals; $3.00; 1987.
  ▲ For Ordering Information, see p. 214

- **Listen, Look, And Learn - AIDS (Audio Cassette, Slide, Text)**

  Health and Education Resources
  Health Care Professionals; $245.00; $50.00/month; 1987.
  ▲ For Ordering Information, see p. 220

PAMPHLETS

- **Acquired Immune Deficiency Syndrome (AIDS) Or AIDS-Related Complex (ARC) Case Report**

  World Hemophilia AIDS Center
  Parents, Educators, And Administrators; special rates / discounts; 1988.
  ▲ For Ordering Information, see p. 232

- **AIDS And Your Legal Rights: What Everyone Needs To Know**

  National Gay Rights Advocates
  HIV Positive Individuals; $2.00; special rates / discounts; 1987.
  ▲ For Ordering Information, see p. 224

- **AIDS Kills**

  Ohio Department of Health - AIDS Unit
  IV Drug Users; free, limited copies; 1988.
  ▲ For Ordering Information, see p. 225

- **AIDS - Ten Articles For Teachers, Counselors, School Nurses And School Administratorsrators**

  Truckee Meadows Community College - AIDS Education Project
  Parents, Educators, And Administrators; free, limited copies; Jan 1989.
  ▲ For Ordering Information, see p. 230

- **Checklist And Guidelines For AIDS Policy**

  University of Pittsburgh
  Workplace; free, limited copies; 1987.
  ▲ For Ordering Information, see p. 231

- **Children And AIDS: The Challenge For Child Welfare**

  Child Welfare League of America
  Policy Makers And Lawyers; $6.95; 1988.
  ▲ For Ordering Information, see p. 217

- **Coping With AIDS: Psychological And Social Considerations In Helping People With HTLV-III Infection**

  U.S. Government,
  Department of Health and Human Services
  National Institute of Mental Health
  Psychologists And Social Workers; free; 1986.
  ▲ For Ordering Information, see p. 230

- **Diet Guidelines For Children With AIDS**

  Children's Hospital of New Jersey Children's Hospital AIDS Program (CHAP)
  Parents, Educators, And Administrators; free; 1986.
  ▲ For Ordering Information, see p. 217

- **Disability**

  Social Security Administratorsration
  Department of Health and Human Services
  General Community; free; Jan 1988.
  ▲ For Ordering Information, see p. 228

- **Financing Health Care For AIDS Patients Under HCFA Programs**

  U.S. Government,
  Department of Health and Human Services
  Health Care Financing Administratorsration
  General Community; cost not specified; Feb 1988.
  ▲ For Ordering Information, see p. 230

- **Guidelines For Handling Health Data On Individuals Tested Or Treated For HIV Infection**

  American Medical Record Association
  Health Care Professionals; $5.00; 1987.
  ▲ For Ordering Information, see p. 215

- **Knight Vision Battles The Hidden Enemy**

  Planned Parenthood of New York City
  Special Audiences; special rates / discounts; 1989.
  ▲ For Ordering Information, see p. 226

- **Pamphlets For Individuals And Self-Help Groups**

  New York City Parents and Friends of Lesbians and Gay Men, Inc.
  General Community; $.15.
  ▲ For Ordering Information, see p. 225

- **A Physicians Guide To HIV Counseling & Treating Of Women Of Childbearing Age**

  New York State Department of Health
  Health Care Professionals; special rates / discounts; 1988.
  ▲ For Ordering Information, see p. 225

- **Pros And Cons Of The HTLV-III Antibody Test**

  National Gay Rights Advocates
  HIV Test Recipients; $2.00; special rates / discounts; May 1986.
  ▲ For Ordering Information, see p. 224

- **Resources For Healing Services**

  AIDS Ministries Program
  Pastoral Counselors; free, limited copies; special rates / discounts; Sep 1987.
  ▲ For Ordering Information, see p. 213

- **The Role Of Biotechnology In AIDS Research: A Progress Report**

  Industrial Biotechnology Association
  General Community; free; Dec 1987.
  ▲ For Ordering Information, see p. 221

- **Skin Conditions Related To AIDS And HIV Infection**

  American Academy of Dermatology
  Health Care Professionals; free, limited copies; 1988.
  ▲ For Ordering Information, see p.

- **Social Security: How It Works For You**

  Social Security Administratorsration
  Department of Health and Human Services
  General Community; free; Jan 1988.
  ▲ For Ordering Information, see p. 228

● **Women And AIDS: The Silent Epidemic**

Women and AIDS Resource Network (WARN)
Women; free; 1988.
▲ For Ordering Information, see p. 232

● **A World Of Difference**

Caremark Homecare
Health Care Professionals; free; 1988.
▲ For Ordering Information, see p. 216

PERIODICALS

● **AIDS Alert**

American Health Consultants
Health Care Professionals; $109.00/year.
▲ For Ordering Information, see p. 214

● **AIDS And Public Policy Journal**

University Publishing Group
Policy Makers And Lawyers; $95.00.
▲ For Ordering Information, see p. 231

● **AIDS Bulletin**

U.S. Government,
   National Institute of Justice NCJRS
Policy Makers And Lawyers; free, limited copies.
▲ For Ordering Information, see p. 230

● **AIDS Cabisco News**

Carolina Biological Supply Company
General Community; free.
▲ For Ordering Information, see p. 216

● **The AIDS Educator**

American Red Cross St. Paul Area Chapter
Health Care Professionals; free.
▲ For Ordering Information, see p.

● **AIDS Facts Magazine: A Magazine For
   You And Your Family**

Classroom Connections, Inc.
Parents, Educators, And Administrators; cost not specified.
▲ For Ordering Information, see p. 217

● **AIDS Health Education Risk Reduction**

State of Wyoming, Division of Health and
   Medical STD/AIDS
General Community; free.
▲ For Ordering Information, see p. 228

● **The AIDS/HIV Record**

BioData Inc.
General Community; $275.00/year; special rates / discounts.
▲ For Ordering Information, see p. 215

● **AIDS In Indian Country**

National Native American AIDS Prevention Center
Special Audiences; free.
▲ For Ordering Information, see p. 224

● **AIDS Information Exchange**

U.S. Conference of Mayors;
   U.S. Conference of Local Health Officers
Policy Makers And Lawyers; $50.00; special rates / dis-
counts.
▲ For Ordering Information, see p. 230

● **AIDS Law And Litigation Reporter**

University Publishing Group
Public Safety And Support Workers; $95.00.
▲ For Ordering Information, see p. 231

● **The AIDS Law Reporter**

National Legal Research Group, Inc.
Policy Makers And Lawyers; $75.00.
▲ For Ordering Information, see p. 224

● **AIDS Literature And News Review**

University Publishing Group
General Community; $95.00.
▲ For Ordering Information, see p. 231

● **AIDS Medical Update**

UCLA AIDS Clinical Research Center
Health Care Professionals; $24.00.
▲ For Ordering Information, see p. 230

● **AIDS Nursing Update**

UCLA AIDS Clinical Research Center
Health Care Professionals; $10.00.
▲ For Ordering Information, see p. 230

● **AIDS Patient Care**

Mary Ann Liebert Inc., Publishers
Health Care Professionals; $69.00.
▲ For Ordering Information, see p. 222

● **AIDS Policy & Law**

Buraff Publications, Inc.
Policy Makers And Lawyers; $337.00/year.
▲ For Ordering Information, see p. 216

● **AIDS: Mental Health Interventions**

Florida Mental Health Institute,
Department of Community Mental Health
Special Audiences; cost not specified.
▲ For Ordering Information, see p. 219

● **The AIDS Project**

Premier Hospitals Alliance, Inc.
Health Care Professionals; $99.00; special rates / discounts.
▲ For Ordering Information, see p. 227

● **AIDS Protection**

National AIDS Prevention Institute
General Community; $78.00.
▲ For Ordering Information, see p. 223

● **AIDS Research And Human Retroviruses**

Mary Ann Liebert Inc., Publishers
Special Audiences; $145.00.
▲ For Ordering Information, see p. 222

● **AIDS Research Today**

BIOSIS
Special Audiences; $120.00.
▲ For Ordering Information, see p. 215

● **AIDS/STDateline**

Rhode Island Department of Health
AIDS Program
Parents, Educators, And Administrators; free.
▲ For Ordering Information, see p. 227

● **AIDS Treatment News**

AIDS Treatment News
Health Care Professionals; $50.00; special rates / discounts.
▲ For Ordering Information, see p. 214

● **AIDS Update**

Lambda Legal Defense and Education Fund, Inc.
Public Safety And Support Workers; $75.00; special rates / discounts.
▲ For Ordering Information, see p. 222

● **AIDS Update**

New York State Department of Social Services,
Office of Human Resource Development
Health Care Professionals; free, limited copies.
▲ For Ordering Information, see p. 225

● **AIDS Update**

Santa Barbara County Health Care Services
Health Care Professionals; free.
▲ For Ordering Information, see p. 228

● **AIDS Update, Hemophilia Information Exchanges**

National Hemophilia Foundation
Blood And Tissue Recipients; cost not specified.
▲ For Ordering Information, see p. 224

● **AIDS Update Monthly**

Ohio AIDS Foundation
General Community; cost not specified.
▲ For Ordering Information, see p. 225

● **AIDS Working Group Newsletter**

University of Texas Health Services Center,
AIDS Working Group
General Community; cost not specified..
▲ For Ordering Information, see p. 231

● **AIDS Workplace Update**

Panel Publishers, Inc.
Workplace; $135.00.
▲ For Ordering Information, see p. 226

● **AIDSFILE**

San Francisco General Hospital Medical Center
Medical Special Care Unit for Treatment of AIDS
Health Care Professionals; cost not specified.
▲ For Ordering Information, see p. 227

● **ALERT**

**Universal Fellowship of Metropolitan
Community Churches**
General Community; cost not specified.
▲ For Ordering Information, see p. 231

● **American Journal Of Public Health
Special Issue On AIDS**

American Public Health Association
General Community; $6.00; special rates / discounts.
▲ For Ordering Information, see p. 215

● **Being Alive Newsletter**

Being Alive
HIV Positive Individuals; free.
▲ For Ordering Information, see p. 215

● **BETA (Bulletin Of Experimental
Treatment For AIDS)**

San Francisco AIDS Foundation
HIV Positive Individuals; cost not specified.
▲ For Ordering Information, see p. 227

● **Body Positive Magazine**

Body Positive of New York
HIV Positive Individuals; $15.00;
special rates / discounts.
▲ For Ordering Information, see p. 216

● **Brown University STD Update**

Manisses Communications Group, Inc.
Health Care Professionals; $127.00.
▲ For Ordering Information, see p. 222

● **CAAA Reports**

California Association of AIDS Agencies
Health Care Professionals; $50.00/year.
▲ For Ordering Information, see p. 216

● **CDC AIDS Weekly Print Edition**

CDC AIDS Weekly
General Community; $676/year.
▲ For Ordering Information, see p. 216

● **Clinical Update Monthly**

Gay Men's Health Crisis, Inc.
Health Care Professionals; cost not specified.
▲ For Ordering Information, see p. 219

● **Correctional Information Bulletin (AIDS)**

American Correctional Health Services Association
Public Safety And Support Workers; cost not specified.
▲ For Ordering Information, see p. 214

● **Designing An Effective AIDS Risk
Reduction Program For San Francisco**

San Francisco AIDS Foundation
Health Care Professionals; $25.00.
▲ For Ordering Information, see p. 227

● **East Bay AIDS News**

AIDS Project of the East Bay
HIV Positive Individuals; cost not specified.
▲ For Ordering Information, see p. 213

● **The Exchange**

National Lawyers Guild AIDS Network
Policy Makers And Lawyers; $10.00.
▲ For Ordering Information, see p. 224

● **Executive Briefing**

Foundation for Public Communication
Workplace; $100.00; special rates / discounts.
▲ For Ordering Information, see p. 219

● **FDA Talk Paper: Update On
Experimental AIDS Therapies And
Vaccines**

**U.S. Government,
Food & Drug Administration**
General Community; free.
▲ For Ordering Information, see p. 230

● **FOCUS: A Guide To AIDS Research**

UCSF AIDS Health Project
Health Care Professionals; $36.00; special rates / discounts.
▲ For Ordering Information, see p. 231

● **Heads, Hearts, And Hands**

National AIDS Network (NAN)
Special Audiences; special rates / discounts.
▲ For Ordering Information, see p. 223

● **Hemophilia World**

World Hemophilia AIDS Center
Blood And Tissue Recipients; free.
▲ For Ordering Information, see p. 232

- **HIV Legal Issues: An Introduction For Developmental Services**

  National Association of Protection and Advocacy Systems
  Health Care Professionals; free.
  ▲ For Ordering Information, see p. 223

- **Infection Control Recommendations For Dental Practice**

  AIDS Prevention Project for Dental Health Professionals University of California Dental School
  Health Care Professionals; free.
  ▲ For Ordering Information, see p. 213

- **LIAAC Newsletter**

  Long Island Association for AIDS Care, Inc.
  People Who Care; free.
  ▲ For Ordering Information, see p. 222

- **Long-Term Care Management**

  McGraw-Hill Healthcare Information Center
  Health Care Professionals; cost not specified.
  ▲ For Ordering Information, see p. 222

- **Minnesota AIDS Project Newsletter**

  Minnesota AIDS Project
  General Community; $1.25.
  ▲ For Ordering Information, see p. 223

- **Morbidity And Mortality Weekly Report**

  U.S. Government, Department of Health and Human Services Centers for Disease Control
  Health Care Professionals; cost not specified.
  ▲ For Ordering Information, see p. 230

- **NAF Newsletter**

  Nevada AIDS Foundation
  General Community; free.
  ▲ For Ordering Information, see p. 224

- **The NAN Monitor**

  National AIDS Network (NAN)
  General Community; $25.00; special rates / discounts.
  ▲ For Ordering Information, see p. 223

- **NAN Multi-Cultural Notes On AIDS Education And Service**

  National AIDS Network (NAN)
  Health Care Professionals; $25.00; special rates / discounts.
  ▲ For Ordering Information, see p. 223

- **NAPWA News**

  National Association of PWA's (NAPWA)
  HIV Positive Individuals; cost not specified.
  ▲ For Ordering Information, see p. 223

- **Network News**

  National AIDS Network (NAN)
  General Community; $50.00; special rates / discounts.
  ▲ For Ordering Information, see p. 223

- **New Views In Healing And AIDS Update**

  Tree of Life Publications
  General Community; $48.00; special rates / discounts.
  ▲ For Ordering Information, see p. 230

- **Newsletter Of The International Working Group On AIDS And IV Drug Use**

  International Working Group on AIDS and IV Drug Use, Narcotic and Drug Research, Inc.
  Special Audiences; free.
  ▲ For Ordering Information, see p. 221

- **Newsline**

  PWA (People With AIDS) Coalition, Inc.
  General Community; $20.00; special rates / discounts.
  ▲ For Ordering Information, see p. 227

- **NGRA Newsletter**

  National Gay Rights Advocates
  Policy Makers And Lawyers; cost not specified.
  ▲ For Ordering Information, see p. 224

- **Oral Aspects Of HIV Disease For Dental Practice**

  AIDS Prevention Project for Dental Health Professionals University of California Dental School
  Health Care Professionals; free.
  ▲ For Ordering Information, see p. 213

● **P.I. Perspective**

Project Inform
HIV Positive Individuals; cost not specified.
▲ For Ordering Information, see p. 227

● **Prevention Notes - A Newsletter On State Preventive Health Services**

Association of State and Territorial Health Officials
Policy Makers And Lawyers; free, limited copies.
▲ For Ordering Information, see p. 215

● **Rhode Island AIDS Alert**

Rhode Island Department of Health AIDS Program
Health Care Professionals; free.
▲ For Ordering Information, see p. 227

● **SIECUS Reports**

Sex Information and Education Council of the United States
General Community; cost not specified.
▲ For Ordering Information, see p. 228

● **State AIDS Reports**

AIDS Policy Center IHPP, George Washington University
Special Audiences; $145.00.
▲ For Ordering Information, see p. 213

● **Street Pharmacologist**

Up Front Drug Information
Psychologists And Social Workers; $25.00.
▲ For Ordering Information, see p. 231

● **Support Newsletter**

Howard Brown Memorial Clinic
Special Audiences; free, limited copies.
▲ For Ordering Information, see p. 221

● **Treatment Issues**

Gay Men's Health Crisis, Inc.
Health Care Professionals; cost not specified.
▲ For Ordering Information, see p. 219

● **Update**

Pittsburgh AIDS Task Force, Inc.
People Who Care; cost not specified.
▲ For Ordering Information, see p. 226

● **Update: AIDS Products In Development**

Pharmaceutical Manufacturers Association
HIV Positive Individuals; cost not specified.
▲ For Ordering Information, see p. 226

● **The Volunteer**

Gay Men's Health Crisis, Inc.
People Who Care; cost not specified.
▲ For Ordering Information, see p. 219

POLICY STATEMENTS / GUIDELINES

● **AIDS: A Social Work Response**

National Association of Social Workersrs
Psychologists And Social Workers; free; Nov 1987.
▲ For Ordering Information, see p. 223

● **AIDS: Administrative Reference Manual**

Massachusetts Hospital Association
Health Care Professionals; $35.00; special rates / discounts; Oct 1987.
▲ For Ordering Information, see p. 222

● **AIDS: An Educational Reference Manual**

Massachusetts Hospital Association
Health Care Professionals; $35.00; special rates / discounts; Jun 1988.
▲ For Ordering Information, see p. 222

● **AIDS And Adolescents: The Time For Prevention Is Now**

Center for Population Options
Policy Makers And Lawyers; $10.00; special rates / discounts; 1988.
▲ For Ordering Information, see p. 217

● **AIDS And Handicapped Discrimination: A Survey Of The 50 States And The District Of Columbia**

National Gay Rights Advocates
Policy Makers And Lawyers; $10.00; special rates / discounts; 1986.
▲ For Ordering Information, see p. 224

- **AIDS And Schools: A Position Statement**

  National Association of Social Workers
  Parents, Educators, And Administrators; cost not specified; Aug 1987.
  ▲ For Ordering Information, see p. 223

- **AIDS And The Employer**

  The New York Business Group on Health
  Workplace; $15.00; Dec 1985.
  ▲ For Ordering Information, see p. 229

- **AIDS And The Public Schools: Leadership Reports, Volume 1**

  National School Boards Association
  Parents, Educators, And Administrators; $15.00; 1986.
  ▲ For Ordering Information, see p. 224

- **AIDS/ ARC Nursing Care Plan**

  Gay Men's Health Crisis, Inc.
  Health Care Professionals; cost not specified.
  ▲ For Ordering Information, see p. 219

- **AIDS Guidelines For The Hawaii Council Of Churches**

  Hawaii Council of Churches
  Pastoral Counselors; free, limited copies; Jul 1987.
  ▲ For Ordering Information, see p. 220

- **AIDS In The Workplace; Guidelines For AIDS Information And Education And For Personnel Management Issues**

  U.S. Government,
  Office of Personnel Management
  Policy Makers And Lawyers; free, limited copies; Mar 1988.
  ▲ For Ordering Information, see p. 230

- **AIDS Infection Policy: Insuring A Safe Hospital Environment**

  American Hospital Association
  Health Care Professionals; free, limited copies; Nov 1987.
  ▲ For Ordering Information, see p. 214

- **AIDS - Management Of HTLV-III/LAV Infection In The Hospital**

  American Hospital Association
  Health Care Professionals; $4.25; Jan 1986.
  ▲ For Ordering Information, see p. 214

- **AIDS - Overview; Policies; Strategic Options; 1987 Projects; Feasibility Study For AIDS Education**

  The National Foundation for Infectious Diseases
  Policy Makers And Lawyers; cost not specified; 1987.
  ▲ For Ordering Information, see p. 229

- **AIDS Policy Statements**

  Brookline Health Department;
  Brookline School Department
  Parents, Educators, And Administrators; free; 1985.
  ▲ For Ordering Information, see p. 216

- **AIDS Prevention Model**

  Kaiser Permanente Medical Care Program
  Health Care Professionals; free.
  ▲ For Ordering Information, see p. 221

- **AIDS Recommendations And Guidelines**

  CDC AIDS Program Technical Information Activity
  Health Care Professionals; $21.95; 1988.
  ▲ For Ordering Information, see p. 216

- **Acquired Immunodeficiency Syndrome (AIDS) Recommendations And Guidelines November 1982 - May 1987**

  U.S. Government,
  Department of Health and Human Services
  Centers for Disease Control
  General Community; cost not specified; 1987.
  ▲ For Ordering Information, see p. 230

- **Clinical Guidelines For Optometrists Regarding AIDS**

  American Academy of Optometry
  Health Care Professionals; cost not specified; Dec 1988.
  ▲ For Ordering Information, see p. 214

- **Confidentiality Of Medical Information Pertaining To AIDS**

  Kaiser Permanente Medical Care Program
  Health Care Professionals; free; 1988.
  ▲ For Ordering Information, see p. 221

- **Criteria For Evaluating An AIDS Curriculum**

  National Coalition of Advocates for Students
  Parents, Educators, And Administrators; $4.00; Jul 1987.
  ▲ For Ordering Information, see p. 223

● **Criterios Para Evaluar Un Curriculo Sobre El SIDA**

National Coalition of Advocates for Students
Latino Community; $2.00; 1988.
▲ For Ordering Information, see p. 223

● **Effective AIDS Education: A Policy Maker's Guide**

National Association of State Boards of Education
Policy Makers And Lawyers; $7.00; special rates / discounts; 1988.
▲ For Ordering Information, see p. 223

● **Facts About AIDS For The Dental Team**

American Dental Association Division of Communications
Health Care Professionals; free, limited copies; Feb 1988.
▲ For Ordering Information, see p. 214

● **Florida Department Of Education Guidelines For District AIDS Policies And Procedures**

Florida Department of Education Florida Prevention Center
Parents, Educators, And Administrators; cost not specified.
▲ For Ordering Information, see p. 219

● **General Statement On Institutional Response To AIDS**

American College Health Association
Health Care Professionals; free, limited copies; 1985.
▲ For Ordering Information, see p. 214

● **Governor's Task Force On AIDS**

Massachusetts Department of Public Health
General Community; free; Jun 1987.
▲ For Ordering Information, see p. 222

● **Guide To Public Health Practice: AIDS Confidentiality And Anti-Discrimination Principles**

Public Health Foundation
Health Care Professionals; $13.50; special rates / discounts; Mar 1988.
▲ For Ordering Information, see p. 227

● **Guide To Public Health Practice: HIV Partner Notification Strategies**

Public Health Foundation
Health Care Professionals; $8.50; special rates / discounts; Sep 1988.
▲ For Ordering Information, see p. 227

● **Guide To Public Health Practice: State Health Agency Programmatic Response To HTLV-III Infection**

Public Health Foundation
Health Care Professionals; $10.00; special rates / discounts; Mar 1986.
▲ For Ordering Information, see p. 227

● **Guidelines For Disclosing AIDS Antibody Test Results**

UCSF AIDS Health Project
Health Care Professionals; $10.00; special rates / discounts; Apr 1987.
▲ For Ordering Information, see p. 231

● **Guidelines For Effective School Health Education To Prevent The Spread Of AIDS**

U.S. Government, Department of Health and Human Services Centers for Disease Control
Parents, Educators, And Administrators; cost not specified; Jan 1988.
▲ For Ordering Information, see p. 230

● **Guidelines For Personal Management Issues**

Kaiser Permanente Medical Care Program
Health Care Professionals; free; 1988.
▲ For Ordering Information, see p. 221

● **Guidelines For Preventing AIDS Transmission In Day Care**

North Carolina AIDS Control Program
Workplace; free, limited copies; Jul 1986.
▲ For Ordering Information, see p. 225

● **Guidelines For Review**

Center for Population Options
Special Audiences; $1.00; special rates / discounts; 1988.
▲ For Ordering Information, see p. 217

- **Guidelines For Schools With Children Who Have Hepatitis B Virus Or HIV Infections**

  Oregon Department of Human Resources Oregon Health Division, AIDS Education Program
  Parents, Educators, And Administrators; $.10; Nov 1985.
  ▲ For Ordering Information, see p. 225

- **Guidelines For Social Service Agencies: Universal Precautions For Hepatitis B And The AIDS Virus**

  Dixwell Preventive Health Program
  Psychologists And Social Workers; $.20; 1988.
  ▲ For Ordering Information, see p. 218

- **The Hemophilia Patient / Family Model**

  National Hemophilia Foundation
  Blood And Tissue Recipients; cost not specified.
  ▲ For Ordering Information, see p. 224

- **HIV Counseling For Women Of Childbearing Age And TB Patients**

  North Carolina AIDS Control Program
  Health Care Professionals; free, limited copies; Mar 1987.
  ▲ For Ordering Information, see p. 225

- **Human Immumodeficiency Virus (HIV) Infection Codes. Official Authorized Addendum To The International Class Of Diseases**

  U.S. Government, Department of Health and Human Services Centers for Disease Control
  Health Care Professionals; cost not specified; Dec 1987.
  ▲ For Ordering Information, see p. 230

- **Infection Control For The Electroneurodiagnostic Laboratory**

  American Society of Electroneurodiagnostic Technologists
  Health Care Professionals; $5.00; special rates / discounts; 1989.
  ▲ For Ordering Information, see p. 215

- **Information And Procedural Guidelines For Providing Health And Social Services To Persons With AIDS**

  Florida Department of Health and Rehabilitative Services
  Health Care Professionals; free, limited copies; 1985.
  ▲ For Ordering Information, see p. 219

- **Insurance Coverage For People With Disabilities**

  Madison AIDS Support Network
  Policy Makers And Lawyers; free; 1988.
  ▲ For Ordering Information, see p. 222

- **Joint Advisory Notice - Protection Against Occupational Exposure To Hepatitis B Virus (HBV) And HIV**

  U.S. Department of Labor/OSHA
  Workplace; free; Nov 1987.
  ▲ For Ordering Information, see p. 230

- **Management Of Chronic Infectious Diseases in School Children**

  Illinois Department of Public Health AIDS Facts for Life
  Parents, Educators, And Administrators; free, limited copies; 1989.
  ▲ For Ordering Information, see p. 221

- **Model Communicable Disease Control Policy**

  Michigan Department of Education
  Parents, Educators, And Administrators; free, limited copies; 1988.
  ▲ For Ordering Information, see p. 223

- **NASW Education Commission Guidelines On School Policies Regarding AIDS**

  National Association of Social Workersrs
  Parents, Educators, And Administrators; cost not specified; Nov 1985.
  ▲ For Ordering Information, see p. 223

- **Nursing Care**

  Delaware Department of Health and Social Services Division of Public Health, AIDS Program Office
  Health Care Professionals; free, limited copies.
  ▲ For Ordering Information, see p. 218

- **Nursing Care Plan**

  Delaware Department Of Health and Social Services Division of Public Health, AIDS Program Office
  Health Care Professionals; free, limited copies.
  ▲ For Ordering Information, see p. 218

● **The Philadelphia Commission On AIDS Report To The Community**

Philadelphia Commission on AIDS at University of Pennsylvania
Policy Makers And Lawyers; $15.00; 1988.
▲ For Ordering Information, see p. 226

● **Position Paper On Testing For Antibody To The Human Immunodeficiency Virus**

Iowa AIDS Legislature Task Force
Policy Makers And Lawyers; $3.00; Dec 1987.
▲ For Ordering Information, see p. 221

● **Prevention Of HIV Transmission In Schools**

North Carolina AIDS Control Program
Parents, Educators, And Administrators; free, limited copies; Jan 1986.
▲ For Ordering Information, see p. 225

● **Prostitutes And AIDS: Scapegoating And The Law**

Coyote
Policy Makers And Lawyers; $11.25; 1988.
▲ For Ordering Information, see p. 218

● **Protection Of Laboratory Workers From Infectious Diseases Transmitted By Blood And Tissue**

National Committee for Clinical Laboratory Standards (NCCLS)
Health Care Professionals; $15.00; 1987.
▲ For Ordering Information, see p. 224

● **Protocol For A Pilot Program Of Partner Outreach Services**

Minnesota Department of Health (MDH) AIDS Program Unit
Health Care Professionals; free; Nov 1986.
▲ For Ordering Information, see p. 223

● **Protocol For Statewide Follow-Up Of Blood Donors Infected With HIV And Recipients Of Blood Or Blood Components Potentially Contaminated With HIV**

Minnesota Department of Health (MDH) AIDS Program Unit
Health Care Professionals; free; Nov 1987.
▲ For Ordering Information, see p. 223

● **Public Health Fact Sheets First Series**

Massachusetts Department of Public Health
General Community; free; Sep 1987.
▲ For Ordering Information, see p. 222

● **Recommendations For Prevention Of HIV Transmission In Health Care Settings**

U.S. Government, Department of Health and Human Services Centers for Disease Control
Health Care Professionals; cost not specified; Aug 1987.
▲ For Ordering Information, see p. 230

● **Recommendations On Issues Of Ethics, Care, And Financing**

American College of Physicians
Policy Makers And Lawyers; free, limited copies; special rates / discounts; Jan 1988.
▲ For Ordering Information, see p. 214

● **Recommendations Regarding AIDS-Infected Food Service Workers**

North Carolina AIDS Control Program
Workplace; free, limited copies; Jul 1986.
▲ For Ordering Information, see p. 225

● **Recommended Additional Guidelines For HIV Antibody Counsel And Testing In The Prevention Of HIV Infection And AIDS**

U.S. Government, Department of Health and Human Services Centers for Disease Control
Psychologists And Social Workers; cost not specified; Apr 1987.
▲ For Ordering Information, see p. 230

● **Relationship Of AIDS/HIV Education To Indiana Health Education Proficiencies**

Indiana Department of Education
Parents, Educators, And Administrators; free; Dec 1988.
▲ For Ordering Information, see p. 221

● **Responding To AIDS: Ten Principles For The Workplace**

Citizens Commission on AIDS for New York City and Northern New Jersey
Workplace; free; Feb 1988.
▲ For Ordering Information, see p. 217

● **Revised Objectives Of The Statewide HIV Risk Reduction And Disease Prevention Plan, December 1987**

Minnesota Department of Health (MDH) AIDS Program Unit
Health Care Professionals; free; Dec 1987.
▲ For Ordering Information, see p. 223

● **Revision Of The CDC Surveillance Case Definition For Acquired Immunodeficiency Syndrome**

U.S. Government, Department of Health and Human Services Centers for Disease Control
Health Care Professionals; cost not specified; Aug 1987.
▲ For Ordering Information, see p. 230

● **Screening Tool For Identification Of Risk For HIV/AIDS**

Kent County Health Department
Health Care Professionals; free; Feb 1988.
▲ For Ordering Information, see p. 221

● **State Board Of Education Regulation And Policies**

State of New Mexico AIDS Prevention Program Health & Environment Department
Parents, Educators, And Administrators; free; Jul 1988.
▲ For Ordering Information, see p. 228

● **State Board Of Education Regulations On AIDS**

New Mexico State Department of Education
Parents, Educators, And Administrators; cost not specified; 1987.
▲ For Ordering Information, see p. 225

● **State Of Georgia Five-Year Plan And Five-Year Plan Interim Report**

Georgia Department of Human Resources
Policy Makers And Lawyers; free, limited copies; 1988.
▲ For Ordering Information, see p. 220

● **TCADA Guidelines For AIDS Precautions In Substance Abuse**

Texas Commission on Alcohol and Drug Abuse
Health Care Professionals; cost not specified; 1987.
▲ For Ordering Information, see p. 229

● **UNHCR Policy And Guidelines Regarding Refugee Protection And Assistance And AIDS**

United Nations High Commissioner for Refugees
Policy Makers And Lawyers; free; 1988.
▲ For Ordering Information, see p. 230

● **Working with AIDS: A Resource Guide For Mental Health Professionals**

UCSF AIDS Health Project
Health Care Professionals; $30.00; special rates / discounts; Jun 1987.
▲ For Ordering Information, see p. 231

● **Workplace Guidelines For Employers With International Responsibilities And Operations**

UNICEF, The Non-Governmental Organizations Committee
Workplace; cost not specified; 1988.
▲ For Ordering Information, see p. 230

REPORTS / MONOGRAPHS

● **ACLU Policy Network**

American Civil Liberties Union Foundation
Policy Makers And Lawyers; free; Dec 1987.
▲ For Ordering Information, see p. 214

● **Acquired Immune Deficiency Syndrome And Chemical Dependency**

U.S. Department of Health and Human Services Public Health Service
Health Care Professionals; free; 1987.
▲ For Ordering Information, see p. 230

● **Adolescents And Youth: Some Educational And Epidemiological Aspects Of The AIDS Crisis**

Worthington Associates Worldwide
Parents, Educators, And Administrators; $2.50; special rates / discounts; 1986.
▲ For Ordering Information, see p. 232

- **An Agenda For AIDS Drug Development**

  Institute of Medicine,
  National Academy of Sciences
  Health Care Professionals; free; 1987.
  ▲ For Ordering Information, see p. 221

- **AIDS: A Report On Funding Sources**

  The Foundation Center
  General Community; $35.00; Aug 1988.
  ▲ For Ordering Information, see p. 229

- **AIDS: A Special Report For The People Of Syntex**

  Syntex Corporation
  Workplace; free, limited copies; Mar 1987.
  ▲ For Ordering Information, see p. 229

- **AIDS: A Status Report On Foundation Funding**

  The Foundation Center
  General Community; $20.00; Oct 1987.
  ▲ For Ordering Information, see p. 229

- **AIDS: Africa, USA, And Haiti, A Comparative Study**

  Latin Americans United
  General Community; free; 1988.
  ▲ For Ordering Information, see p. 222

- **AIDS And Drug Use: Breaking The Link**

  Citizens Commission on AIDS for New York City and Northern New Jersey
  Policy Makers And Lawyers; free; 1988.
  ▲ For Ordering Information, see p. 217

- **AIDS And Health Insurance: An OTA Survey**

  Office of Technology Assessment, U.S. Congress
  Policy Makers And Lawyers; $2.75; 1988.
  ▲ For Ordering Information, see p. 225

- **AIDS And Liberties Project**

  American Civil Liberties Union Foundation
  Policy Makers And Lawyers; cost not specified.
  ▲ For Ordering Information, see p. 214

- **AIDS And People Of Color: The Discrimination Impact**

  New York City Commission on Human Rights/AIDS Discrimination
  General Community; free; 1987.
  ▲ For Ordering Information, see p. 225

- **AIDS And The Law Enforcement Officer: Concerns & Policy Responses**

  U.S. Government,
  National Institute of Justice NCJRS
  Public Safety And Support Workers; free, limited copies; Jun 1987.
  ▲ For Ordering Information, see p. 230

- **AIDS And The Law: Responding To The Special Concerns Of Hospitals**

  American Hospital Association
  Policy Makers And Lawyers; $8.00; Nov 1987.
  ▲ For Ordering Information, see p. 214

- **AIDS And The Role Of The Health Care Financing Administration**

  U.S. Government,
  Department of Health and Human Services
  Health Care Financing Administration
  General Community; free; Dec 1987.
  ▲ For Ordering Information, see p. 230

- **AIDS: Basic Documents**

  American Civil Liberties Union Foundation
  Policy Makers And Lawyers; $5.00; Apr 1987.
  ▲ For Ordering Information, see p. 214

- **AIDS Children And Child Welfare**

  Macro Systems, Inc.
  Psychologists And Social Workers; free; 1987.
  ▲ For Ordering Information, see p. 222

- **AIDS, Civil Rights, And The Public Health: America's Leaders Speak Out**

  National Gay Rights Advocates
  Workplace; $10.00; special rates / discounts; 1987.
  ▲ For Ordering Information, see p. 224

- **AIDS Education Leadership Report**

  National School Boards Association
  Parents, Educators, And Administrators; cost not specified; Sep 1988.
  ▲ For Ordering Information, see p. 224

- **AIDS Education Materials**

  U.S. Conference of Mayors;
  U.S. Conference of Local Health Officers
  Policy Makers And Lawyers; free, limited copies; Oct 1987.
  ▲ For Ordering Information, see p. 230

- **AIDS '88 Summary: A Practical Synopsis Of The IV International Conference**

  Philadelphia Sciences Group
  Health Care Professionals; $295.00; special rates / discounts; 1988.
  ▲ For Ordering Information, see p. 226

- **AIDS In Correctional Facilities: Issues And Options**

  U.S. Government,
  National Institute of Justice NCJRS
  Public Safety And Support Workers; free, limited copies; May 1988.
  ▲ For Ordering Information, see p. 230

- **AIDS: Information / Education Plan To Prevent And Control AIDS In The United States**

  U.S. Government,
  Department of Health and Human Services
  Centers for Disease Control
  General Community; cost not specified; Mar 1987.
  ▲ For Ordering Information, see p. 230

- **AIDS Into The 90's: Strategies For An Integrated Response To The AIDS Epidemic**

  National AIDS Network (NAN)
  Policy Makers And Lawyers; $10.00; special rates / discounts; 1988.
  ▲ For Ordering Information, see p. 223

- **AIDS: Issues For Probation And Parole**

  U.S. Government, National Institute of Justice NCJRS
  Public Safety And Support Workers; free, limited copies; Jun 1988.
  ▲ For Ordering Information, see p. 230

- **AIDS Knowledge And Attitudes For October 1987: Provisional Data From The National Health Institute Survey**

  U.S. Government,
  Department of Health and Human Services
  Centers for Disease Control
  General Community; cost not specified; Mar 1988.
  ▲ For Ordering Information, see p. 230

- **AIDS Long Term Care Advisory Committee Report**

  AIDS Housing of Washington
  Health Care Professionals; free; May 1988.
  ▲ For Ordering Information, see p. 213

- **AIDS Prevention Activities - FY 1987**

  U.S. Government,
  Department of Health and Human Services
  Centers for Disease Control
  General Community; cost not specified; 1987.
  ▲ For Ordering Information, see p. 230

- **AIDS: The New Workplace Issues**

  American Management Association AMACOM
  Briefings And Surveys
  Workplace; free, limited copies; 1985.
  ▲ For Ordering Information, see p. 215

- **AIDS Weekly Surveillance Report: United States**

  U.S. Government, Department of Health and Human Services Centers for Disease Control
  General Community; cost not specified.
  ▲ For Ordering Information, see p. 230

- **American Corporate Policy: AIDS And Employment**

  National Gay Rights Advocates
  Workplace; $10.00; special rates / discounts; 1987.
  ▲ For Ordering Information, see p. 224

- **Americans Who Care**

  National AIDS Network (NAN)
  People Who Care; $25.00; special rates / discounts; 1987.
  ▲ For Ordering Information, see p. 223

- **An Assessment Of AIDS Knowledge**

  New Haven Health Department
  Health Care Professionals; free; 1988.
  ▲ For Ordering Information, see p. 224

- **Attention To AIDS: Responding To The Growing Number Of Children And Youth With AIDS**

  Child Welfare League of America
  General Community; $14.50; special rates / discounts; 1987.
  ▲ For Ordering Information, see p. 217

- **A Baseline Survey Of The AIDS-Related Knowledge, Attitudes, And Behaviors Of San Francisco's Black Population**

  Polaris Research And Development
  Health Care Professionals; $20.40; 1988.
  ▲ For Ordering Information, see p. 226

- **Business Response To AIDS**

  Fortune Magazine
  Workplace; cost not specified; 1988.
  ▲ For Ordering Information, see p. 219

- **Casual Contact And The Risk Of HIV Infection**

  American Public Health Association
  General Community; $3.00; special rates / discounts; Jul 1988.
  ▲ For Ordering Information, see p. 215

- **Comparative Review Of State-Only Expenditures For AIDS**

  George Washington University Intergovernmental Health Policy Project
  Policy Makers And Lawyers; $60.00; 1987.
  ▲ For Ordering Information, see p. 220

- **Comparative Review Of State-Only Expenditures For AIDS**

  AIDS Policy Center IHPP, George Washington University
  Special Audiences; special rates / discounts; Feb 1989.
  ▲ For Ordering Information, see p. 213

- **Contact Tracing And Partner Notification**

  American Public Health Association
  Policy Makers And Lawyers; $3.00; special rates / discounts; Nov 1988.
  ▲ For Ordering Information, see p. 215

- **The Costs Of AIDS And Other HIV Infections**

  Office of Technology Assessment, U.S. Congress
  Policy Makers And Lawyers; free; 1987.
  ▲ For Ordering Information, see p. 225

- **Current Protection And Advocacy AIDS-Related Services**

  National Association of Protection and Advocacy Systems
  Policy Makers And Lawyers; free; 1989.
  ▲ For Ordering Information, see p. 223

- **DC Teenagers And AIDS: Knowledge, Attitudes And Behavior**

  Center for Population Options
  Parents, Educators, And Administrators; special rates / discounts; 1988.
  ▲ For Ordering Information, see p. 217

- **Designing An Effective AIDS Risk Reduction Program For San Francisco: Results From Probability Samples**

  San Francisco AIDS Foundation
  Health Care Professionals; $25.00; 1984.
  ▲ For Ordering Information, see p. 227

- **Dignity For Latinos With AIDS: Final Report Of Minority AIDS Needs Assessment**

  Instituto Familiar De La Raza - Latino AIDS Project
  Latino Community; $12.00; special rates / discounts; 1988.
  ▲ For Ordering Information, see p. 221

- **Do Insects Transmit AIDS?**

  Office of Technology Assessment, U.S. Congress
  Policy Makers And Lawyers; cost not specified; 1987.
  ▲ For Ordering Information, see p. 225

- **The Elements Of A Comprehensive AIDS Prevention Campaign**

  Communication Technologies
  Health Care Professionals; $13.00; special rates / discounts; 1988.
  ▲ For Ordering Information, see p. 217

- **Evaluation Of AIDS Educational And Media Materials For English- And Spanish-Speaking Populations**

  San Francisco AIDS Foundation
  Health Care Professionals; cost not specified; 1987.
  ▲ For Ordering Information, see p. 227

- **Exploring Alternatives To Hospitalization Step-Down Care For People With AIDS**

  AIDS Housing of Washington
  Health Care Professionals; free; 1988.
  ▲ For Ordering Information, see p. 213

- **The Facts About AIDS: A Special Guide For NEA Members**

  National Education Association (NEA) Health Information Network
  Special Audiences; cost not specified.
  ▲ For Ordering Information, see p. 224

- **Health And Wholeness In The Midst Of Panic: A Pronouncement**

  United Church Board for Homeland Ministries AIDS Program
  Pastoral Counselors; $.35; 1987.
  ▲ For Ordering Information, see p. 230

- **Health Education For AIDS Risk Reduction In The Gay/Bisexual Male Community**

  San Francisco AIDS Foundation
  Health Care Professionals; $4.00; 1985.
  ▲ For Ordering Information, see p. 227

- **How Effective Is AIDS Education?**

  Office of Technology Assessment, U.S. Congress
  Special Audiences; $6.00; 1988.
  ▲ For Ordering Information, see p. 225

- **Human Immuno Deficiency Virus Infection In The United States A Review Of Current Knowledge**

  U.S. Government,
  Department of Health and Human Services
  Centers for Disease Control
  General Community; cost not specified; Nov 1987.
  ▲ For Ordering Information, see p. 230

- **Humanity Under Seige: AIDS, International Relations And Development**

  Worthington Associates Worldwide
  Policy Makers And Lawyers; $3.00; special rates / discounts; Jun 1987.
  ▲ For Ordering Information, see p. 232

- **The Impact Of AIDS In The Native American Community**

  Native American Women's Health Education Resource Center
  Special Audiences; $5.00; 1988.
  ▲ For Ordering Information, see p. 224

- **The Impact Of AIDS On The Kaiser Permanente Medical Care Program**

  Office of Technology Assessment, U.S. Congress
  Special Audiences; $2.25; 1988.
  ▲ For Ordering Information, see p. 225

- **Information And Recommendations For Child Care And Pediatric AIDS, HIV Infection And Related Conditions**

  Wisconsin Division of Health, AIDS/HIV Program
  Health Care Professionals; $3.00; 1988.
  ▲ For Ordering Information, see p. 231

- **Information And Recommendations For Social, Psychological, And Neuro-Psychiatric Aspects Of HIV Infections**

  Wisconsin Division of Health, AIDS/HIV Program
  Health Care Professionals; $2.50; 1988.
  ▲ For Ordering Information, see p. 231

- **Information And Recommendations For The Chronically Ill: Services For People With AIDS In Wisconsin**

  Wisconsin Division of Health, AIDS/HIV Program
  Health Care Professionals; $2.50; 1988.
  ▲ For Ordering Information, see p. 231

- **Information Brochure**

  Stop AIDS Resource Center (Stop AIDS Project)
  Special Audiences; free; 1988.
  ▲ For Ordering Information, see p. 228

- **Interim Report Of The Presidential Commission On The Human Immunodeficiency Virus Epidemic**

  U.S. Government,
  Executive Office of the President
  General Community; free; Mar 1988.
  ▲ For Ordering Information, see p. 230

- **Local Policies In Response To Acquired Immunodeficiency Syndrome (AIDS) And HIV Infection**

  U.S. Conference of Mayors;
  U.S. Conference of Local Health Officers
  Policy Makers And Lawyers; free, limited copies; Jul 1986.
  ▲ For Ordering Information, see p. 230

- **Medical Evaluation Of Persons At Risk**

  San Francisco AIDS Foundation
  Health Care Professionals; cost not specified; 1987.
  ▲ For Ordering Information, see p. 227

- **Meeting The Challenge: Foundation Responses To AIDS**

  The Foundation Center
  General Community; $6.50; Oct 1987.
  ▲ For Ordering Information, see p. 229

- **Missionworks: AIDS And The Church**

  United Church Board for Homeland Ministries
  AIDS Program
  General Community; $.60; 1987.
  ▲ For Ordering Information, see p. 230

- **Moving Beyond Counseling And Knowledge Enhancing Interventions**

  Stop AIDS Resource Center (Stop AIDS Project)
  Special Audiences; free; 1988.
  ▲ For Ordering Information, see p. 228

- **Overview Of Psycho-Social Issues Concerning AIDS**

  Gay Men's Health Crisis, Inc.
  Psychologists And Social Workers; cost not specified.
  ▲ For Ordering Information, see p. 219

- **Perspectives On Oral Manifestations Of AIDS**

  Office Sterilization and Asepsis Procedures
  Research Foundation
  University of Texas Health Science Center
  Dental School at San Antonio
  Health Care Professionals; $10.00; special rates / discounts; 1988.
  ▲ For Ordering Information, see p. 225

- **Position Statements**

  American Association of Physicians for Human Rights (AAPHR)
  General Community; free; 1987.
  ▲ For Ordering Information, see p. 214

- **Preventing The Transmission Of HIV In Dental Practice**

  Wisconsin Division of Health, AIDS/HIV Program
  Health Care Professionals; $1.75; 1988.
  ▲ For Ordering Information, see p. 231

- **Preventing The Transmission Of HIV In The Home Setting**

  Wisconsin Division of Health, AIDS/HIV Program
  Health Care Professionals; $2.50; 1988.
  ▲ For Ordering Information, see p. 231

- **Preventing The Transmission Of HIV Through Serologic Screening**

  Wisconsin Division of Health, AIDS/HIV Program
  Health Care Professionals; $2.00; 1988.
  ▲ For Ordering Information, see p. 231

- **Preventing The Transmission Of HTLV-III During Post-Mortem Examination, Autopsy, And Funeral Preparation**

  Wisconsin Division of Health, AIDS/HIV Program
  Health Care Professionals; $3.25; 1988.
  ▲ For Ordering Information, see p. 231

- **Preventing The Transmission Of HTLV-III In The Hospital Setting**

  Wisconsin Division of Health, AIDS/HIV Program
  Special Audiences; $3.00; 1988.
  ▲ For Ordering Information, see p. 231

- **Preventing The Transmission Of HTLV-III In The Prison Setting**

  Wisconsin Division of Health, AIDS/HIV Program
  Public Safety And Support Workers; $2.75; 1988.
  ▲ For Ordering Information, see p. 231

- **Preventing The Transmission Of HTLV-III In The Jail Setting**

  Wisconsin Division of Health, AIDS/HIV Program
  Public Safety And Support Workers; $2.50; 1988.
  ▲ For Ordering Information, see p. 231

- **Preventing The Transmission Of HTLV-III In The School Setting**

  Wisconsin Division of Health, AIDS/HIV Program
  Parents, Educators, And Administrators; $2.00; 1988.
  ▲ For Ordering Information, see p. 231

- **Preventing The Transmission Of HTLV-III In The Nursing Home Setting**

  Wisconsin Division of Health, AIDS/HIV Program
  Health Care Professionals; $3.25; 1988.
  ▲ For Ordering Information, see p. 231

- **Preventing The Transmission Of HTLV-III In The Pre-Hospital Emergency Medical Care Setting**

  Wisconsin Division of Health, AIDS/HIV Program
  Public Safety And Support Workers; $3.00; 1988.
  ▲ For Ordering Information, see p. 231

- **Preventing The Transmission Of HTLV-III In The Work Place**

  Wisconsin Division of Health, AIDS/HIV Program
  Workplace; $2.25; 1988.
  ▲ For Ordering Information, see p. 231

- **Prevention Of Disease Transmission In Schools - AIDS**

  Connecticut Department of Health Services AIDS Program
  Parents, Educators, And Administrators; cost not specified; 1986.
  ▲ For Ordering Information, see p. 218

- **Prospects For Vaccines Against HIV Infection**

  Institute of Medicine, National Academy of Sciences
  Policy Makers And Lawyers; free, limited copies; 1988.
  ▲ For Ordering Information, see p. 221

- **Psychological, Neuropsychiatric, And Substance Abuse Aspects Of AIDS, Vol. 44, Advances In Biochemical Psychopharmacology**

  National Clearinghouse for Alcohol and Drug Information
  Health Care Professionals; free; 1988.
  ▲ For Ordering Information, see p. 223

- **Psychosocial Impact Of AIDS On Women**

  The Feminist Institute Clearinghouse
  Women; $6.40; special rates / discounts; 1988.
  ▲ For Ordering Information, see p. 229

- **Reaching Ethnic Communities In The Fight Against AIDS**

  San Francisco AIDS Foundation
  General Community; $5.00; 1986.
  ▲ For Ordering Information, see p. 227

- **Reducing Risk: A School Leader's Guide To AIDS Education**

  National School Boards Association
  Parents, Educators, And Administrators; free; 1989.
  ▲ For Ordering Information, see p. 224

- **Report Of The Child Welfare League Of America Task Force On Children And HIV Infection Initial Guidelines**

  Child Welfare League of America
  Psychologists And Social Workers; cost not specified.
  ▲ For Ordering Information, see p. 217

- **Report On Discrimination Against PWA's And People Perceived To Have AIDS**

  New York City Commission on Human Rights/AIDS Discrimination
  General Community; free; 1987.
  ▲ For Ordering Information, see p. 225

● **Reports On AIDS Published In The MMWR, Volume 1, June 1981 - May 1986; Volume 2, June 1986 - May 1987**

U.S. Government,
  Department of Health and Human Services
  Centers for Disease Control
Health Care Professionals; cost not specified; 1987.
▲ For Ordering Information, see p. 230

● **Review Of The Public Health Service's Response To AIDS**

Office of Technology Assessment, U.S. Congress
Policy Makers And Lawyers; $5.50; 1985.
▲ For Ordering Information, see p. 225

● **SIDA - Una Cartilla**

Truckee Meadows Community College
  AIDS Education Project
Latino Community; free, limited copies; 1987.
▲ For Ordering Information, see p. 230

● **State Statutes And Regulations On AIDS: Confidentiality, Discrimination And Public Health Control Measures**

AIDS Policy Center IHPP,
  George Washington University
Policy Makers And Lawyers; $30.00; Mar 1988.
▲ For Ordering Information, see p. 213

● **Status Report On AIDS**

United Way of America
General Community; cost not specified; Jan 1988.
▲ For Ordering Information, see p. 230

● **Summary Of AIDS Laws: 1986 Session**

AIDS Policy Center IHPP,
  George Washington University
Policy Makers And Lawyers; $30.00; Jan 1987.
▲ For Ordering Information, see p. 213

● **Summary Of AIDS Laws: 1987 Session**

AIDS Policy Center IHPP,
  George Washington University
Policy Makers And Lawyers; $30.00; Jan 1988.
▲ For Ordering Information, see p. 213

● **Summary Of AIDS Laws: 1988 Session**

AIDS Policy Center IHPP,
  George Washington University
Policy Makers And Lawyers; $30.00; Jan 1989.
▲ For Ordering Information, see p. 213

● **Summary Report: Public Health Task Force On Acquired Immune Deficiency Syndrome (AIDS)**

Wisconsin Division of Health, AIDS/HIV Program
Policy Makers And Lawyers; $3.00; 1988.
▲ For Ordering Information, see p. 231

● **A Synopsis Of State AIDS Related Legislation**

George Washington University
  Intergovernmental Health Policy Project
Policy Makers And Lawyers; cost not specified; 1987.
▲ For Ordering Information, see p. 220

● **A Synopsis Of State AIDS Related Legislation, 1983 - 1987**

AIDS Policy Center IHPP,
  George Washington University
Policy Makers And Lawyers; $80.00; Oct 1988.
▲ For Ordering Information, see p. 213

● **Teens And AIDS: Opportunities For Prevention**

Children's Defense Fund
Parents, Educators, And Administrators; $4.50;
special rates / discounts; 1988.
▲ For Ordering Information, see p. 217

● **Women And AIDS: Promoting Healthy Behaviors**

U.S. Government,
  Department of Health and Human Services
  National Institute of Mental Health
Women; cost not specified.
▲ For Ordering Information, see p. 230

VIDEOS / FILMS

● AIDS And Health Care Workers

U.S. Government,
  Department of Health and Human Services Office
  of the Assistant Secretary for Health
Health Care Professionals; free, limited copies; 1988.
▲ For Ordering Information, see p. 230

● AIDS Care Beyond The Hospital - Attendant Care

San Francisco AIDS Foundation
Health Care Professionals; $95.00; 1984.
▲ For Ordering Information, see p. 227

● AIDS Care Beyond The Hospital - Case Management

San Francisco AIDS Foundation
Health Care Professionals; $95.00; 1984.
▲ For Ordering Information, see p. 227

● AIDS Face-To-Face: A Phil Donahue Show

Films for the Humanities & Sciences, Inc.
General Community; $75.00.
▲ For Ordering Information, see p. 219

● AIDS: Facts Over Fears

ABC Television
General Community; $200.00; 1987.
▲ For Ordering Information, see p. 213

● AIDS Infection Control Procedures

American Academy of Dermatology
Health Care Professionals; $65.00; Dec 1987.
▲ For Ordering Information, see p.

● AIDS: The Surgeon General's Update

Videolearning Systems, Inc.
General Community; $95.00; rental fee: $75.00;
special rates / discounts; 1988.
▲ For Ordering Information, see p. 231

● AIDSAFE

Polaris Research and Development
General Community; $100.00; $35.00/2 Weeks; 1987.
▲ For Ordering Information, see p. 226

● Ain't No Justice

Gay Men's Health Crisis, Inc.
General Community; $79.95; special rates / discounts; 1988.
▲ For Ordering Information, see p. 219

● Doctors, Liars, And Women

Gay Men's Health Crisis, Inc.
General Community; $79.95; special rates / discounts; 1988.
▲ For Ordering Information, see p. 219

● Front Page NJ: A Special Issue On AIDS

New Jersey Network
General Community; $75.00; $50.00/2 Weeks;
special rates / discounts; 1988.
▲ For Ordering Information, see p. 225

● Handwashing

Medfilms, Inc.
Health Care Professionals; $190.00;
special rates / discounts; 1987.
▲ For Ordering Information, see p. 222

● The Helms Amendment

Gay Men's Health Crisis, Inc.
Policy Makers And Lawyers; $39.95; special rates / discounts; 1987.
▲ For Ordering Information, see p. 219

● HIV/AIDS In The Dental Office: Management And Treatment

NYU Regional Education and Training Center
Health Care Professionals; $29.95; 1988.
▲ For Ordering Information, see p. 225

● An Institutional Response To AIDS

Carle Medical Communications
Health Care Professionals; $385.00; $65.00/3 Days; special rates / discounts; 1984.
▲ For Ordering Information, see p. 216

● The National AIDS Awareness Test

Metropolitan Life Insurance Company
General Community; free; Sep 1987.
▲ For Ordering Information, see p. 223

● **Neuropsychiatric Manifestations, Long-Term Management And Community Support**

NYU Regional Education and Training Center
Health Care Professionals; $29.95; 1988.
▲ For Ordering Information, see p. 225

● **New Jersey AIDS Helpline**

New Jersey Network
General Community; $150.00; $100.00/2 Weeks;
special rates / discounts; 1988.
▲ For Ordering Information, see p. 225

● **Nightline: A National Town Meeting On AIDS**

ABC Video Enterprises, Inc.
c/o Coronet/MTI Film & Video
General Community; $250.00; 1987.
▲ For Ordering Information, see p. 213

● **NOVA: Can AIDS Be Stopped?**

Public Broadcast System
c/o Coronet MTI Film & Video
General Community; $350.00; 1986.
▲ For Ordering Information, see p. 227

● **On The Record**

New Jersey Network
General Community; $95.00; $50.00/2 Weeks;
special rates / discounts; 1988.
▲ For Ordering Information, see p. 225

● **Remarks Of Admiral Watkins To AFT On AIDS**

American Federation of Teachers
Parents, Educators, And Administrators; special rates / discounts; 1988.
▲ For Ordering Information, see p. 214

● **The Right To Die - The Choice Is Yours**

Society for the Right to Die
General Community; $31.45; 1987.
▲ For Ordering Information, see p. 228

● **Rights And Reactions**

Tapestry Productions
General Community; $395.00; rental fee: $95.00; Oct 1987.
▲ For Ordering Information, see p. 229

● **The Ryan White Story**

Landsburg Company
General Community; $49.95; special rates / discounts; 1988.
▲ For Ordering Information, see p. 222

● **Virology, Transmission, And Clinical Expression**

NYU Regional Education and Training Center
Health Care Professionals; $29.95; 1988.
▲ For Ordering Information, see p. 225

● **Women With AIDS - A Phil Donahue Show**

Films for the Humanities & Sciences, Inc.
General Community; cost not specified; 1987.
▲ For Ordering Information, see p. 219

● **Women, Children And AIDS**

San Francisco AIDS Foundation
General Community; cost not specified.
▲ For Ordering Information, see p. 227

NATIONAL RESOURCE ORGANIZATIONS

AIDS Action Council
729 Eighth Street, SE
Suite 200
Washington, D.C. 20003
(202) 547-3101

American Red Cross National Headquarters
AIDS Education Office
1730 E Street, NW
Washington, D.C. 20006
(202) 693-3223

Centers For Disease Control
AIDS Information Office
1600 Clifton Road, NE
Atlanta, GA 30333
(404) 329-2891

Coalition of Hispanic Health and Human Services
Organizations (COSSMHO)
1030 15th Street, NW
Washington, D.C. 20005
(202) 371-2100

George Washington University
Intergovernmental Health Policy Project
2011 I Street, NW, Suite 200
Washington, D.C. 20006
(202) 872-1445

Lambda Legal Defense and Education Fund
666 Broadway, 12th Floor
New York, NY 10012
(212) 995-8585

National AIDS Hotline
(800) 342-AIDS (2437)
(7 days a week, 24 hours a day)

National AIDS Information Clearing House
P.O. Box 6003
Rockville, MD 20850
(800) 458-5231

National AIDS Network (NAN)
2033 M Street, NW
8th Floor
Washington, D.C. 20036
(202) 293-2437

National Association of People With AIDS (NAPWA)
2025 I Street, NW
Suite 415
Washington, D.C. 20006
(202) 429-2856

National Gay and Lesbian Task Force
1517 U Street, NW
Washington, D.C. 20009
(202) 332-6483

National Hemophilia Foundation
SoHo Building
110 Greene Street, Room 406
New York, NY 10012
(212) 219-8180

National Leadership Coalition on AIDS
1150 17th Street, Suite 202
Washington, D.C. 20036
(202) 429-0930

National Minority AIDS Council
714 G Street, SE
Washington, D.C. 20003
or
P.O. Box 28547
Washington, D.C. 20038
(202) 544-1076

U.S. Conference of Mayors
AIDS Program
1620 Eye Street, NW
4th Floor
Washington, D.C. 20006
(202) 293-7330

STATE AIDS AGENCIES AND HOTLINES

Alabama Department of Health
AIDS Program
State Office Building, Room 662
434 Monroe Street
Montgomery, AL 36130
(205) 261-5017
(800) 228-0469

Alaska Department of Health
AIDS Health Program
3601 C Street
Anchorage, AK 99524
(907) 561-4406

Arizona Department of Health
Office of Health Education
431 North 24th Street
Phoenix, AZ 85008
(602) 230-5836
(800) 334-1540

Arkansas Department of Health
AIDS Activities
4815 West Markham
Little Rock, AR 72205
(501) 661-2135
(800) 445-7720

California Department of Health
Office of AIDS
P.O. Box 160146
Sacramento, CA 95816
(916) 445-0553
(800) 367-2437 (Northern CA)

Colorado Department of Health
AIDS Education Risk
Reduction Program
4210 East 11th Street
Denver, CO 80220
(303) 331-8320

Connecticut Department of Health
AIDS Program
150 Washington Street
Hartford, CT 06106
(203) 566-2048
(203) 566-1157

Delaware Department of Health and
Social Services
AIDS Program Office
3000 Newport Gap Pike
Building G
Wilmington, DE 19808
(302) 995-8422

D.C. Commission of Public Health
Division of AIDS Education
1875 Connecticut Avenue, NW
Room 838-C
Washington, DC 20009
(202) 673-3425
(202) 332-AIDS (2437)

Florida Department of Health and
Rehabilitation
Health Education and
Risk Reduction
1317 Winewood Blvd.
Building 6, Room 453
Tallahassee, FL 32399
(904) 487-2478
(800) FLA AIDS (352-2437)

Georgia Department of
Human Resources
STD Control Program
878 Peachtree Street, NE
Atlanta, GA 30309
(404) 894-5304
(800) 551-2728

Hawaii Department of Health
Public Health Education
3627 Kilauea Avenue
Honolulu, HI 96816
(808) 735-5303
(808) 922-1313

Idaho Department of Health
and Welfare
AIDS Program
Statehouse Mall
Boise, ID 83720
(208) 334-5930

Illinois Department of Health
Infectious Diseases,
AIDS Activity Section
525 West Jefferson
Springfield, IL 62761
(217) 524-5983
(800) 243-2437

Indiana Department of Health
Office of AIDS Activity
1330 West Michigan
Indianapolis, IN 46206
(317) 633-8406

Iowa Department of Public Health
AIDS Education
Lucas Building
3rd Floor
Des Moines, IA 50319
(515) 281-4938
(800) 532-3301

Kansas Department of Health
and Environment
Office of Health Education
Forbes Field Building 321
Room 13
Topeka, KS 66620
(913) 296-5587
(800) 232-0040

Kentucky Department for
Health Services
AIDS Health Education
275 E. Main Street
Frankfort, KY 40621
(502) 564-4804
(800) 654-AIDS (2437)

Louisiana Office of Prevention
Medicine and Public Health
Services
325 Loyola Avenue
Room 615
New Orleans, LA 70012
(504) 568-5005
(800) 999-4379

Maine Bureau of Health
Office on AIDS
Station House, Station 11
Augusta, ME 04333
(207) 289-3591
(800) 851-AIDS (2437)

Maryland Department of Health and
Mental Hygiene Epidemiology
201 West Preston Street
Baltimore, MD 21201
(301) 225-6707
(800) 638-6252

Massachusetts Department of
Public Health
AIDS Health Education
150 Tremont Street
Boston, MA 02111
(617) 727-0368
(800) 235-2331

Michigan Department of Health
Special Office of AIDS Prevention
3500 N. Logan
Lansing, MI 48909
(517) 335-8371
(800) 872-AIDS (2437)

Minnesota Department of Health
AIDS Program
717 S.E. Delaware Street
Minneapolis, MN 55440
(612) 623-5698
(800) 248-AIDS (2437)

Mississippi Department of Health
AIDS Education Program
2423 N. State Street
Jackson, MS 39215
(601) 960-7725
(800) 826-2961

Missouri Department of Health
AIDS Program
P.O. Box 570
Jefferson City, MO 65102
(314) 751-6438

Montana Department of Health and
Environmental Services
AIDS Program
Cogswell Building
Helena, MT 59260
(406) 444-2457

Nebraska Department of Health
AIDS Prevention Program
P.O. Box 95007
Lincoln, NE 68509
(402) 471-2937
(800) 782-2437

Nevada State Health Division
Department of Human Resources
505 East King Street, Room 200
Carson City, NV 89710
(702) 885-4800

New Hampshire Department of
Health and Welfare
6 Hazen Drive
Concord, NH 03301
(603) 271-4490

New Jersey Department of Health
AIDS Division
C.N. 360, 363 West State Street
Trenton, NJ 08625
(609) 984-6000
(800) 624-2377

New Mexico Department of Health
and Environment Epidemiology
P.O. Box 968
Santa Fe, NM 87504
(505) 827-0086

New York State Department
of Health
AIDS Institute
1315 Empire State Plaza
25th Floor, Room 2580
Albany, NY 12237
(518) 474-8160
(800) 462-1884

North Carolina Health Department
AIDS Control Program
P.O. Box 2091
Raleigh, NC 27602
(919) 733-7301

North Dakota Department of Health
AIDS Project
State Capitol Building
Bismark, ND 58505
(701) 224-8378
(800) 592-1861

Ohio Department of Health
AIDS Activity Unit
246 North High Street
Columbus, OH 43266
(614) 466-5480
(800) 332-AIDS (2437)

Oklahoma Department of Health
STD Division
P.O. Box 53551
Oklahoma City, OK 73152
(405) 271-5601

Oregon Department of Health
AIDS Program
1400 Southwest 5th Street
Room 710
Portland, OR 97201
(503) 229-5792

Pennsylvania Department of Health
Disease Control
P.O. Box 90
Harrisburg, PA 17108
(717) 787-3350
(800) 692-7254

Sexually Transmitted Disease
Control Program
Call Box STD
Caparra Heights Station
San Juan, PR 00922
(809) 754-8118

Rhode Island Department of Health
AIDS Control Program
75 Davis, Room 105
Providence, RI 02908
(401) 277-2362
(401) 277-6502

South Carolina Deparment of Health
AIDS Project
2600 Bull Street
Columbia, SC 29201
(803) 734-5482
(800) 322-AIDS (2437)

South Dakota Department of Health
AIDS Program
523 East Capital
Pierre, SD 57501
(605) 773-3357
(800) 472-2180

Tennessee Department of Health and
Environment-Disease Control
100 9th Avenue North
Nashville, TN 37219
(615) 741-7387

Texas Department of Health
Epidemiology-Health Promotion
100 West 49th Street
Austin, TX 78756
(512) 458-7405

Utah Department of Health
Epidemiology
288 North, 1460 West
P.O. Box 16660
Salt Lake City, UT 84116
(801) 538-6191
(801) 466-9976
(800) 843-9388

Vermont Department of Health
AIDS Education
60 Main Street
P.O. Box 70
Burlington, VT 05402
(802) 863-7245
(800) 882-AIDS (2437)

Virgin Island Department of Health
AIDS Committee
P.O. Box 7309
St. Thomas, VI 00801
(809) 776-8311

Virginia Department of Health
AIDS Activity Program
109 Governor Street
Room 722
Richmond, VA 23219
(804) 225-4844
(800) 533-4148

Washington Department of Health
Epidemiology-AIDS Program
1610 Northeast 150th Street
Seattle, WA 98155
(206) 361-2888

West Virginia Department of Health
151 11th Avenue
South Charleston, WV 25303
(304) 348-2950
(800) 624-8244

Wisconsin Department of Health
and Social Services
AIDS Program
1 West Wilson Street
P.O. Box 309
Madison, WI 53701
(608) 267-5287
(800) 334-AIDS (2437)

Wyoming Division of Health and
Medical Services
AIDS Program
Hathaway Building
4th Floor
Cheyenne, WY 82002
(307) 777-7953

WORLD HEALTH ORGANIZATION

BOOKS / MANUALS

- **AIDS Prevention And Control**

  World Health Organization,
  Global Programme on AIDS
  Health Care Professionals; $24.00; special rates / discounts;
  1988.
  ▲ For Ordering Information, see p. 221

BROCHURES

- **AIDS Discrimination And Public Health**

  World Health Organization,
  Global Programme on AIDS
  Policy Makers And Lawyers; free; 1988.
  ▲ For Ordering Information, see p. 221

PERIODICALS

- **AIDS Health Promotion Exchange**

  World Health Organization,
  Global Programme on AIDS
  Health Care Professionals; free.
  ▲ For Ordering Information, see p. 221

- **GPA Digest**

  World Health Organization,
  Global Programme on AIDS
  Special Audiences; free.
  ▲ For Ordering Information, see p. 221

POLICY STATEMENTS / GUIDELINES

- **AIDS Information For Travellers**

  World Health Organization,
  Global Programme on AIDS
  General Community; free; 1987.
  ▲ For Ordering Information, see p. 221

- **Blood Transfusion Guidelines For International Travellers**

  World Health Organization,
  Global Programme on AIDS
  General Community; free; 1988.
  ▲ For Ordering Information, see p. 221

- **Consensus Statement From Consultation On Sexually Transmitted Diseases As Risk Factor For HIV Transmission**

  World Health Organization,
  Global Programme on AIDS
  Health Care Professionals; free; 1989.
  ▲ For Ordering Information, see p. 221

- **Consultation On Nursing And HIV Infection**

  World Health Organization,
  Global Programme on AIDS
  Policy Makers And Lawyers; free; 1988.
  ▲ For Ordering Information, see p. 221

- **Counseling In HIV Infection And Disease**

  World Health Organization,
  Global Programme on AIDS
  Policy Makers And Lawyers; free; 1988.
  ▲ For Ordering Information, see p. 221

- **Guidelines For Nursing Management Of People Infected With HIV**

  World Health Organization,
  Global Programme on AIDS
  Health Care Professionals; $7.20; special rates / discounts;
  1988.
  ▲ For Ordering Information, see p. 221

- **Guidelines For The Development Of A National AIDS Prevention And Control Programme**

  World Health Organization,
  Global Programme on AIDS
  Policy Makers And Lawyers; $6.40; special rates / discounts;
  1988.
  ▲ For Ordering Information, see p. 221

- **Guidelines For Treatment Of Acute Blood Loss**

  World Health Organization, Global Programme on AIDS
  Health Care Professionals; free; 1988.
  ▲ For Ordering Information, see p. 221

- **Guidelines On Sterilization And High-Level Disinfection Methods Effective Against HIV**

  World Health Organization, Global Programme on AIDS
  Health Care Professionals; $3.20; special rates / discounts; 1988.
  ▲ For Ordering Information, see p. 221

- **Report Of The Meeting On Criteria For HIV Screening Programmes**

  World Health Organization, Global Programme on AIDS
  Health Care Professionals; free; 1987.
  ▲ For Ordering Information, see p. 221

- **Screening And Testing In AIDS Prevention And Control Programmes**

  World Health Organization, Global Programme on AIDS
  Policy Makers And Lawyers; free; 1988.
  ▲ For Ordering Information, see p. 221

- **Statement From The Consultation On Prevention And Control Of AIDS In Prison**

  World Health Organization, Global Programme on AIDS
  Policy Makers And Lawyers; free; 1987.
  ▲ For Ordering Information, see p. 221

- **Statement On Breast-Feeding/Breast Milk And HIV**

  World Health Organization, Global Programme on AIDS
  Policy Makers And Lawyers; free; 1987.
  ▲ For Ordering Information, see p. 221

- **Statement On Consultation On AIDS And The Workplace**

  World Health Organization, Global Programme on AIDS
  Policy Makers And Lawyers; free; 1988.
  ▲ For Ordering Information, see p. 221

- **Statement On HIV And Routine Childhood Immunization**

  World Health Organization, Global Programme on AIDS
  Policy Makers And Lawyers; free; 1987.
  ▲ For Ordering Information, see p. 221

- **Statement On Screening Of International Travellers For Infection With HIV**

  World Health Organization, Global Programme on AIDS
  Policy Makers And Lawyers; free; 1988.
  ▲ For Ordering Information, see p. 221

- **WHO Against AIDS Discrimination: Resolution Of The 41st World Health Assembly**

  World Health Organization, Global Programme on AIDS
  Policy Makers And Lawyers; free; 1988.
  ▲ For Ordering Information, see p. 221

- **World Summit Of Ministers Of Health: London Declaration On AIDS Prevention**

  World Health Organization, Global Programme on AIDS
  Policy Makers And Lawyers; free; Jan 1988.
  ▲ For Ordering Information, see p. 221

REPORTS / MONOGRAPHS

● **Global Programme On AIDS: Progress Report No. 4**

World Health Organization, Global Programme on AIDS
Policy Makers And Lawyers; free; 1988.
▲ For Ordering Information, see p. 221

● **Report Of A WHO Informal Consultation On Animal Models For HIV Infection And AIDS**

World Health Organization, Global Programme on AIDS
Special Audiences; free; Mar 1988.
▲ For Ordering Information, see p. 221

● **Report Of An Informal Discussion On The "WHO AIDS Reagent Project"**

World Health Organization, Global Programme on AIDS
Special Audiences; free; 1988.
▲ For Ordering Information, see p. 221

● **Report of Consultation On International Travel And HIV Infection**

World Health Organization, Global Programme on AIDS
Policy Makers And Lawyers; free; 1987.
▲ For Ordering Information, see p. 221

● **Report of Consultation On the Neuropsychiatric Aspects Of HIV Infection**

World Health Organization, Global Programme on AIDS
Policy Makers And Lawyers; free; 1988.
▲ For Ordering Information, see p. 221

● **Tabular Information On Legal Instruments Dealing With AIDS And HIV Infection**

World Health Organization, Global Programme on AIDS
Policy Makers And Lawyers; free; 1988.
▲ For Ordering Information, see p. 221

VIDEOS / FILMS

● **AIDS - A Worldwide Effort Will Stop It**

World Health Organization, Global Programme on AIDS
General Community; $18.00; special rates / discounts; 1988.
▲ For Ordering Information, see p. 221

● **A World United Against AIDS**

World Health Organization, Global Programme on AIDS
General Community; $44.00; 1988.
▲ For Ordering Information, see p. 221

Producer and Distributor Information

All producers whose materials appear in this Directory are listed in this chapter in alphabetical order. Each entry identifies the pages on which the producer's products appear and includes the producer's address and telephone number. Below is a sample item.

National Native American AIDS
Prevention Center
6239 College Ave., #201
Oakland, CA 94618
(415) 658-2051
▲ See pages 178, 182, 185

ORGANIZATIONS

A. C. Croft, Inc.
Personnel Journal
245 Fischer Avenue, B-2
Cosa Mesa, CA 92626
(714) 751-1883
▲ See page 181

Abbott Laboratories
Public Affairs, Dept. 383
Abbott Park, IL 60064
(312) 937-8521
▲ See pages 20, 47

ABC Television
c/o Coronet/MTI Film & Video
108 Wilmot Rd.
Deerfield, IL 60015
(312) 940-1260
▲ See page 202

ABC Video Enterprises, Inc.
c/o Coronet/MTI Film & Video
108 Wilmot Road
Deerfield, IL 60015
(312) 940-1260
▲ See pages 63, 203

ABT Books, Inc.
146 Mt. Auburn St.
Cambridge, MA 02138
(617) 661-1300
▲ See pages 172, 173

ACLU National Prison Project
1616 P St., NW, #340
Washington, D.C. 20036
(202) 331-0500
▲ See page 148

**Addison-Wesley Publishing
Company, Inc.**
Jacob Way
Reading, MA 01867
(617) 944-3700
▲ See page 172

Advanced Imaging, Inc.
22 Southview Dr.
Wallingford, CT 06492
(203) 284-1224
▲ See page 75

**African Americans Taking Action
Against AIDS Council**
c/o American Red Cross
Hawkeye Chapter
2530 University Ave.
Waterloo, IA 50701
(319) 234-6831
▲ See pages 5, 182

AID Atlanta, Inc.
1132 West Peachtree St., NW
Atlanta, GA 30309-3624
(404) 872-0600
▲ See pages 44, 90, 111, 155

**AIDS Action Committee of
Massachusetts, Inc.**
661 Boylston St.
Boston, MA 02116
(617) 437-6200
▲ See pages 68, 81, 104, 133

**AIDS Administration for the State of
Maryland**
Maryland C.A.R.E.S.
201 West Preston Street
Baltimore, MD 21201
(301) 225-5025
▲ See pages 36, 41, 50, 52, 68, 74, 99, 139, 140, 157

**AIDS Council of Northeastern
New York**
307 Hamilton Street
Albany, NY 12210
(518) 434-4686
▲ See page 140

AIDS Foundation Houston, Inc.
3927 Essex Lane
Houston, TX 77027
(713) 623-6796
▲ See pages 4, 44, 46, 88, 97, 104, 131

AIDS Housing of Washington
93 Pike St., #312
Seattle, WA 98101
(206) 623-8292
▲ See pages 196, 198

AIDS Legal Referral Panel
25 Hickory St.
San Francisco, CA 94102
(415) 864-8186
▲ See pages 171, 173

AIDS Ministries Program
1335 Asylum Ave.
Hartford, CT 06105-2295
(203) 233-4481
▲ See pages 119, 182, 184

**AIDS Policy Center IHPP,
George Washington University**
2021 K St., NW
Washington, D.C. 20006
(202) 676-8144
▲ See pages 189, 197, 201

AIDS Prevention Project
Dallas County Health Department
1936 Amelia Ct.
Dallas, TX 75235
(214) 920-7916
▲ See pages 4, 15, 26, 90, 105, 109, 113, 136

**AIDS Prevention Project for Dental
Health Professionals**
University of California
Dental School
707 Parnassus, Box 0754
San Francisco, CA 94143-0754
(415) 476-9879
▲ See page 188

AIDS Project Los Angeles
6721 Romaine St.
Los Angeles, CA 90038
(213) 380-2000
▲ See pages 47, 57, 60, 61, 62, 81, 87, 89, 103, 106

AIDS Project of the East Bay
400 40th Street, Suite 200
Oakland, CA 94609
(415) 420-8181
▲ See pages 95, 187

**AIDS Research and Education Project,
Psychology Department
California State University at
Long Beach**
1250 Bellflower Blvd.
Long Beach, CA 90840
(213) 985-7508
▲ See pages 35, 65, 107, 133, 177

AIDS Services of Austin
P.O. Box 4874
Austin, TX 78765
(512) 458-3505
▲ See page 152

AIDS Task Force of Central New York
P.O. Box 1911
Syracuse, NY 13201
(315) 475-2430
▲ See pages 38, 96, 121, 137

AIDS Task Force of Winston-Salem
P.O. Box 2982
Winston-Salem, NC 27102
(919) 723-5031
▲ See page 48

AIDS Treatment News
P.O.Box 411256
San Francisco, CA 94141
(415) 255-0588
(415) 255-0588
▲ See page 186

AIDS Virus Education and Research Institute (AVERI)
P.O. Box 31562
San Francisco, CA 94131
(415) 239-5200
▲ See page 183

AIDS-Related Community Services
214 Central Park Avenue, Lower Lev.
White Plains, NY 10606
(914) 993-0606
▲ See page 53

AIDSCOM/Academy for Educational Development
1255 23rd Street, NW
Suite 400
Washington, D.C. 20037
▲ See page 173

AIDSFILMS
50 West 34th St., Suite 6B6
New York, NY 10001
(212) 629-6288
▲ See page 145

Albert Einstein College of Medicine AIDS Family Care Center
1300 Morris Park Ave.
Room F-401
New York, NY 10461
(212) 430-3652
▲ See pages 107, 112, 115, 120

Alliance 7 Buyer's Club
3115 Gregory St.
San Diego, CA 92104
(619) 281-5360
▲ See page 177

Allstate Insurance Company Allstate Forum on Public Issues
Allstate Plaza F-3
Northbrook, IL 60062
(312) 291-5974
▲ See page 183

American Academy of Dermatology
1567 Maple Ave., P.O. Box 3116
Evanston, IL 60174
(312) 869-3954
▲ See pages 69, 184, 202

American Academy of Optometry
5530 Wisconsin Ave. NW
Suite 1149
Washington, D.C. 20815
(301) 652-0905
▲ See page 190

American Alliance for Health, Physical Education, Recreation, Dance
1900 Association Dr.
Reston, VA 22091
(703) 476-3480
▲ See page 17

American Association for the Advancement of Science
1333 H St., NW
Washington, D.C. 20005
(202) 326-6400
▲ See pages 170, 175

American Association of Blood Banks National Office
1117 North 19th St., Suite 600
Arlington, VA 22209
(703) 528-8200
▲ See pages 10, 11, 50

American Association of Physicians for Human Rights (AAPHR)
2940 16th St.
Suite 309
San Francisco, CA 94103
(415) 558-9353
▲ See page 199

American Association of School Administrators
1801 North Moore St.
Arlington, VA 22209
(703) 528-0700
▲ See page 114

American Bar Association
1800 M St., NW
Washington, D.C. 20036
(202) 331-2248
▲ See page 171

American Civil Liberties Union Foundation
132 West 43rd St.
New York, NY 10036
(212) 944-9800
▲ See pages 174, 181, 194, 195

American College Health Association
15879 Crabbs Branch Way
Rockville, MD 20855
(301) 963-1100
▲ See pages 34, 88, 135, 136, 154, 170, 191

American College of Physicians
655 15th Street, NW
Suite 425
Washington, D.C. 20005
(202) 393-1650
▲ See page 193

American Correctional Health Services Association
5530 Wisconsin Avenue, NW
Suite 1149
Chevy Chase, MD 20815
(301) 652-1172
▲ See page 187

American Council of Life Insurance
1001 Pennsylvania Ave., NW
Washington, D.C. 20004-2599
(202) 624-2372
▲ See page 26

American Council on Science and Health
1995 Broadway
New York, NY 10023
(212) 362-7044
▲ See page 54

American Dental Association Division of Communications
211 East Chicago Ave.
Chicago, IL 60611
(312) 440-2500
▲ See pages 52, 183, 191

American Federation of Teachers
555 New Jersey Ave., NW
Washington, D.C. 20001
(202) 879-4490
▲ See pages 73, 112, 118, 203

American Health Care Association
1200 15th St. NW
Washington, D.C. 20005
(202) 778-3304
▲ See page 169

American Health Consultants
67 Peachtree Park Drive
Atlanta, GA 30309
(404) 351-4523
▲ See page 185

American Hospital Association
840 North Lake Shore Drive
Chicago, IL 60611
(312) 280-6000
▲ See pages 78, 165, 190, 195

American Indian Health Care Association
245 East Sixth St., #499
St. Paul, MN 55101
(612) 293-0233
▲ See page 149

American Institute for Teen AIDS Prevention, Inc.
P.O. Box 10852
Fort Worth, TX 76114
(817) 237-0230
▲ See pages 13, 31

American Management Association AMACOM Briefings and Surveys
135 W. 50th
New York, NY 10010
(212) 586-8100
▲ See page 196

American Medical Record Association
875 North Michigan Ave., #1850
Chicago, IL 60611
(312) 787-2672
▲ See page 184

American Podiatric Medical Association
9312 Old Georgetown Road
Bethesda, MD 20814
(301) 571-9200
▲ See page 175

American Public Health Association
1015 15th St., NW
Washington, D.C. 20005
(202) 789-5688
▲ See pages 172, 187, 197,

American Red Cross
National Headquarters
1730 E St., NW
Washington, D.C. 20006
(202) 639-3223
▲ See pages 10, 14, 21, 39, 45, 47, 49, 65, 82, 88, 95, 103, 112, 113, 120, 135, 154, 155, 161, 163, 176

Columbus Area Chapter
995 East Broad Street
Columbus OH, 43205
(614) 253-7981
▲ See pages 24, 160

Hawkeye Chapter
2530 University
Waterloo, IL 50701
(319) 234 6831
▲ See page 170

St. Paul Area Chapter
100 South Robert Street
St. Paul, MN 55107
(612) 291-6789
▲ See pages 18, 185

American Social Health Association
P.O.Box 13827
Research Triangle Park, NC 27709
(919) 361-2742
▲ See page 14, 20, 46

American Society of Electroneurodiagnostic Technologists
Sixth St. at Quint
Carroll, IA 51401
(712) 792-2978
▲ See page 192

American Technavision, Inc.
3624 North Hills Dr., C103
Austin, TX 78731
(512) 346-5860
▲ See page 80

AMI Television
c/o Coronet/MTI Film & Video
108 Wilmot Rd.
Deerfield, IL 60015
(312) 940-1260
▲ See page 75

Anne Arundel County Public Schools
2644 Riva Rd.
Annapolis, MD 21401
(301) 224-5415
▲ See pages 13, 44

Arizona Department of Health Services Office of Health Promotion and Education
3008 North Third St., Room 103
Phoenix, AZ 85102
(602) 230-5838
▲ See pages 45, 114

Association for Drug Abuse Prevention and Treatment (ADAPT)
85 Bergen Street
Brooklyn, NY 11201
(718) 834-9585
▲ See pages 94, 96, 98, 106

Association of State and Territorial Health Officials
6728 Old McLean Village Drive
McLean, VA 22101
(703) 556-9222
▲ See page 189

Audio-Video Digest Foundation
1577 E. Chevy Chase Drive
Glendale, CA 91206
(213) 245-8505
▲ See page 183

Bantam Books, Inc.
666 Fifth Ave.
New York, NY 10103
(212) 765-6500
▲ See page 173

Bay Area Physicians for Human Rights
P.O. Box 14546
San Francisco, CA 94114
(415) 558-9353
▲ See pages 89, 90

Bebashi, Inc.
1319 Locust St.
Philadelphia, PA 19107
(215) 546-4140
▲ See pages 3, 6, 103

Being Alive
4222 Santa Monica Blvd., #105
Los Angeles, CA 90029
(213) 667-3262
▲ See pages 82, 85, 187

Beth Israel Medical Center
317 East 17th St., Fierman Hall
Room 715
New York, NY 10003
(212) 420-4184
▲ See page 95

BioData Publishers
P.O. Box 66020
Washington, D.C. 20035-6020
(202) 393-2437
▲ See pages 177, 179, 185

BIOSIS
2100 Arch St.
Philadelphia, PA 19103-1399
(215) 587-4800
▲ See pages 177, 186

Birmingham AIDS Outreach, Inc.
P.O. Box 550070
Birmingham, AL 35255
(205) 930-0440
▲ See page 59

Black Community AIDS Program
2215 West McFadden, Suite K
Santa Ana, CA 92704
(714) 543-3441
▲ See page 5

Black Women's Health Council, Inc.
225 Harry S. Truman Dr., #22
Upper Marlboro, MD 20772
(301) 350-4251
▲ See page 4

Blacks Against AIDS
P.O.Box 7732
Atlantic City, NJ 08404
(609) 347-1645
▲ See pages 4, 6

Blue Cross and Blue Shield Association
676 North Saint Clair St.
Chicago, IL 60611
(312) 440-6000
▲ See page 50

Body Positive of New York
208 West 13th St.
New York, NY 10011
(212) 633-1782
▲ See page 187

Boston Public Schools
The School Committee of the
City of Boston
26 Court St.
Boston, MA 02108
(617) 726-6200
▲ See page 19

Brookline Health Department;
Brookline School Department
11 Pierce St.
Brookline, MA 02146
(617) 730-2335
▲ See page 190

Brooklyn AIDS Task Force
22 Chapel St.
Brooklyn, NY 11201
(718) 596-4781
▲ See pages 6, 57, 99

Brotherhood Press
279 South Beverly Dr., #185
Beverly Hills, CA 90212
(213) 395-5667
▲ See page 171

Buraff Publications, Inc.
1231 25th St., NW
Washington, D.C. 20037
(202) 452-7889
▲ See page 186

California Association of AIDS Agencies
1900 K Street, #201
Sacramento, CA 95814
(916) 448-2437
▲ See page 187

California Firefighter Foundation
300 T Street
Sacramento, CA 95814
(916) 441-7650
▲ See page 172

California Nurses Association
1855 Folsom St., #670
San Francisco, CA 94103
(415) 864-4141
▲ See pages 68, 69

California Prostitutes Education Project
(CAL-PEP)
333 Valencia St., #213
San Francisco, CA 94103
(415) 558-0450
▲ See page 71

California Rural Indian Health
Board, Inc.
2020 Hurley Way, #155
Sacramento, CA 95825
(916) 929-9761
▲ See pages 146, 149

Camden County Health Department
AIDS Program
1800 Pavilion West, Rm. 603
2101 Ferry Ave.
Camden, NJ 08104
(609) 757-8606
▲ See page 179

Capitol Publications
1101 King Street, Suite 444
Alexandria, VA 22314
(703) 683-4100
▲ See page 170

Caremark Homecare
455 Knightsbridge Parkway
4th Floor, 4-28
Lincolnshire, IL 60069
(312) 215-3860
▲ See pages 174, 175, 185

Carle Medical Communications
110 West Main St.
Urbana, IL 61801
(217) 384-4838
▲ See pages 65, 78, 79, 80, 122, 128, 202

Carolina Biological Supply Company
2700 York Rd.
Burlington, NC 27215
(919) 584-0381
▲ See pages 15, 31, 36, 37, 74, 77, 80, 115, 185

Cascade AIDS Project
408 SW 2nd, #412
Portland, OR 97204
(503) 223-5907
▲ See pages 38, 42, 50, 88

Catholic Health Association of the
United States
4455 Woodson Rd.
St. Louis, MO 63134
(314) 427-2500
▲ See page 77

CD Resources / Libraries-To-Go
1123 Broadway, #902
New York, NY 10010
(212) 929-8044
▲ See page 178

CDC AIDS Program Technical
Information Activity
1600 Clifton Rd., NE (MS-G29)
Atlanta, GA 30333
(404) 639-3311
▲ See page 190

CDC AIDS Weekly
P.O. Box 5528
Atlanta, GA 30307-0528
(404) 377-8895
▲ See pages 178, 180, 187

CDC National AIDS Information and
Education Program
1600 Clifton Rd.
Atlanta, GA 30333
(404) 639-3311
▲ See pages 8, 27, 48, 51, 59, 61, 101, 104, 108,
117, 122, 140, 141, 142, 143, 144, 145, 157, 158,
159

Celestial Arts Publishing
P.O.Box 7327
Berkeley, CA 94707
(415) 524-1801
▲ See page 172

Center for AIDS and Substance Abuse
Training
5205 Leesburg Pike, #400
Falls Church, VA 22041
(703) 820-2424
▲ See pages 126, 127, 128.

Center for Community Action to
Prevent AIDS
Hunter College
425 East 25th St., Box 633
New York, NY 10010
(212) 481-7672
▲ See page 70

Center for Excellence in Addiction
Treatment Research
401 Haddon Ave., #261
Camden, NJ 08103-1505
(609) 757-7808
▲ See page 172

**Center for Indian Youth Program
Development**
U. New Mexico, School of Medicine
Deptartment of Pediatrics
Albuquerque, NM 87131
(505) 277-5551
▲ See page 150

Center for Population Options
1012 14th St., NW, #1200
Washington, D.C. 20005
(202) 347-5700
▲ See pages 12, 13, 111, 177, 189, 191, 197

Center One Anyone In Distress
370 East Prospect Rd.
Ft. Lauderdale, FL 33334
(305) 561-0316
▲ See pages 54, 132

Centre Productions
c/o Barr Films
P.O. Box 7878
Irwindale, CA 91706-7878
(800) 234-7879
▲ See page 66

Century House Publications, Inc.
20432 S. Santa Fe, Suites J and K
Carson, CA 90810
(213) 631-5117
▲ See page 174

Channing L. Bete Co., Inc.
200 State Rd.
S. Deerfield, MA 01373
(800) 628-7733
▲ See pages 25, 26, 33, 41, 55, 56, 64, 73, 97, 129, 156, 164

Chelsea Psychotherapy Associates
80 Eighth Ave., Suite 1305
New York, NY 10011
(212) 206-0045
▲ See page 120

**Chicago Department of Health
AIDS Program**
50 West Washington St.
Chicago, IL 60602
(312) 744-4372
▲ See page 45

**Chicago Public Schools
Bureau of Science**
1819 West Pershing Rd. 6C(se)
Chicago, IL 60609
(312) 890-7977
▲ See pages 20, 182

Child Welfare League of America
440 First St., NW, #310
Washington, D.C. 20016
(202) 638-2952
▲ See pages 173, 197, 184, 200

Children's Defense Fund
122 C St., NW, #400
Washington, D.C. 20001
(202) 628-8787
▲ See page 201

**Children's Hospital National Medical
Center**
111 Michigan Ave., NW
Washington, D.C. 20010
(202) 745-5400
▲ See page 136

**Children's Hospital of New Jersey
Children's Hospital AIDS Program
(CHAP)**
15 South Ninth St.
Newark, NJ 07107
(201) 268-8273
▲ See pages 121, 184

Children's Hospital of Philadelphia
2101 Chestnut St., 3rd Fl.
Philadelphia, PA 19103
(215) 557-4500
▲ See page 83

Childrens Press
5440 North Cumberland Ave.
Chicago, IL 60656
(312) 693-0800
▲ See page 23

Churchill Films
662 North Robertson Blvd.
Los Angeles, CA 90069
(213) 657-5110
▲ See pages 28, 29, 31, 32, 64, 76, 83

**Cinema Group Home Video
For Apex Productions**
1875 Century Park East, 3rd Floor
Los Angeles, CA 90067
(213) 785-3100
▲ See page 66

CIRID at UCLA
10833 Le Conte Ave.
Los Angeles, CA 90024-1793
(213) 825-1510
▲ See pages 72, 170

**Citizens Commission on AIDS for New
York City and Northern
New Jersey**
121 Sixth Ave., 6th Fl.
New York, NY 10013
(212) 779-0311
▲ See pages 193, 195

Classroom Connections, Inc.
P.O. Box 2208
Merced, CA 95344
(209) 383-1008
▲ See pages 16, 185

College Satellite Network
#2 Communications Complex, #215
Irving, TX 75039
(214) 869-1102
▲ See page 35

**Colorado Department of Health
AIDS Education & Risk Reduction
Program**
4210 East 11th Ave.
Denver, CO 80220
(303) 331-8320
▲ See pages 82, 89, 96

**Columbia University
Graduate School of Journalism
Seminars on Media and Society**
475 Riverside Dr., Suite 248
New York, NY 10115
(212) 280-3666
▲ See page 63

Columbus AIDS Task Force
1500 West Third Ave., #329
Columbus, OH 43212
(614) 488-2437
▲ See pages 38, 42, 49, 58, 59, 85, 141

Communication Technologies
140 Second St., #600
San Francisco, CA 94105
(415) 541-9551
▲ See page 197

**Community Outreach Risk Reduction
Education Program (CORE)**
7740 1/2 Santa Monica Blvd.
W. Hollywood, CA 90046
(213) 656-8201
▲ See pages 38, 39, 40, 105, 137

Concern for Dying
250 West 57th St., Room 831
New York, NY 10107
(212) 246-6962
▲ See pages 172, 175

Connecticut Department of Education
25 Industrial Park Rd.
Middletown, CT 06457
(203) 638-4227
▲ See pages 19, 20

Connecticut Department of Health Services
AIDS Program
150 Washington St.
Hartford, CT 06106
(203) 566-2048
▲ See pages 45, 52, 63, 91, 94, 179, 200

Connecticut State Department of Health
150 Washington St.
Hartford, CT 06106
(203) 566-1157
▲ See pages 27, 52, 100, 141, 143

Consumer Reports Books
51 East 42nd St., #800
New York, NY 10017
(212) 983-8250
▲ See page 12

Cook County Hospital
AIDS Service
1835 West Harrison St.
Chicago, IL 60612
(312) 633-7810
▲ See pages 48, 88, 93, 134, 132

Coronado Neighborhood Council
1501 Florida Ave.
Richmond, CA 94804
(415) 233-3244
▲ See page 24

County of Riverside
Department of Health
4065 County Circle Drive
Riverside, CA 92503
(714) 358-5307
▲ See page 48

Cowley Publications
980 Memorial Drive
Cambridge, MA 02138
(617) 876-3507
▲ See page 172

Coyote
333 Valencia St., #213
San Francisco, CA 94103
(415) 558-0450
▲ See page 193

Creative Media Group
Health Alert Division
123 4th St., NW
Charlottesville, VA 22901
(804) 296-6138
▲ See page 28

Cristo AIDS Ministry
1029 East Turney Ave.
Phoenix, AZ 85014
(602) 265-2831
▲ See pages 44, 45, 48, 49, 50, 87

Current-Rutledge
614 Twelfth Ave. East
Seattle, WA 98102
(206) 324-7530
▲ See page 37

Dallas County Health Department
1936 Amelia Court
Dallas, TX 75235
(214) 920-7916
▲ See page 47

Damien Ministries
P.O.Box 10202
Washington, D.C. 20018
(202) 387-2926
▲ See page 51

Dartmouth College
Department of Health Education
7 Rope Ferry Rd.
Hanover, NH 03755
(603) 646-5449
▲ See pages 35, 37, 175

Dartnell Corporation
4660 Ravenswood Ave.
Chicago, IL 60640
(312) 561-4000
▲ See page 162

D.C. Commission of Public Health
1660 L St., NW, #700
Washington, D.C. 20036
(202) 673-3676
▲ See pages 4, 5, 7, 38, 41, 47, 88, 97, 99, 103, 107

D.C. Public Schools
AIDS Education Office
Lovejoy School 12th & D Sts., NE
Washington, D.C. 20002
(202) 724-4008
▲ See pages 13, 18

Delaware Department of Health and Social Services
Division of Public Health,
AIDS Program Office
3000 Newport Gap Pike, Building G
Wilmington, DE 19808
(302) 995-8422
▲ See page 192

Denver Disease Control Service
605 Bannock St.
Denver, CO 80204-4507
(303) 893-6300
▲ See pages 46, 87, 88, 132

Development Associates
2924 Columbia Pike
Arlington, VA 22204
(703) 979-0100
▲ See page 69

Development Through Self-Reliance, Inc.
9650 Santiago Rd., #10
Columbia, MD 21045
(301) 964-0037
▲ See page 44

Dimension Communications Network (DCN) / RAMSCO Publishing Co.
P.O. Box N
Laurel, MD 20707
(301) 953-3699
▲ See pages 12, 46, 47, 94, 152

Division of Education and Ministry
National Council of Churches Task Force on AIDS
475 Riverside Drive, Ste. 705
New York, NY 10115
▲ See page 176

Dixwell Preventive Health Program
226 Dixwell Ave.
New Haven, CT 06511
(203) 562-2178
▲ See pages 147, 192

Durrin Films / New Day Films
1748 Kalorama Rd., NW
Washington, D.C. 20009
(202) 387-6700
▲ See pages 9, 29

Educational Productions
4925 Southwest Humphrey Park Crest
Portland, OR 97221
(503) 292-9234
▲ See page 77

**Elsevier Science Publishing
Company, Inc.**
52 Vanderbilt Avenue
New York, NY 10017
(212) 370-5520
▲ See pages 169, 170

Employee Benefits Review
715 Eighth St., SE, #300
Washington, D.C. 20003
(202) 546-3394
▲ See page 160

Enslow Publishers
Bloy St. & Ramsey Ave. Box 77
Hillside, NJ 07205
(201) 964-4116
▲ See page 12

Equitable Life Assurance Society of U.S.
787 7th Ave.
New York, NY 10023
(212) 554-2345
▲ See page 164

Eroticus Publications
P.O. Box 410503
San Francisco, CA 94141-0503
(415) 543-3470
▲ See pages 40, 137

ETR Associates/Network Publications
P.O.Box 1830
Santa Cruz, CA 95061-1830
(408) 438-4080
▲ See page 14, 19, 34, 51, 52, 113, 114, 131, 132, 133, 135, 137, 154, 169

**Eugene Public Schools
School District 4J**
200 North Monroe
Eugene, OR 97402
(503) 687-3321
▲ See page 16

Exploring AIDS
2880 Folsom, Suite 104
Boulder, CO 80302
(303) 447-8777
▲ See page 169

Family Health International
P.O. Box 13950
Research Triangle Park, NC 27709
(919) 549-0517
▲ See page 174

**Family Planning Council of Western
Massachusetts, Inc.**
16 Center St.
Northampton, MA 01060
(413) 586-2016
▲ See page 30

Fanlight Productions
47 Halifax Street, Box A
Boston, MA 02130
(617) 524-0980
▲ See page 123

Fenway Community Health Center
93 Massachusetts Ave.
Boston, MA 02115
(617) 267-0900
▲ See pages 88, 155

Filmakers Library, Inc.
133 East 58th St.
New York, NY 10022
(212) 355-6545
▲ See page 122

**Films for the Humanities &
Sciences, Inc.**
P.O. Box 2053
Princeton, NJ 08543
(800) 257-5126
▲ See pages 63, 164, 202, 203

**Florida Association of Pediatric Tumor
Programs, Inc.**
1105 W. University Ave., #200
P.O. Box 13372, University Station
Gainesville, FL 32604
(904) 375-6848
▲ See pages 10, 12

**Florida Department of Education
Florida Prevention Center**
Knott Building
Tallahassee, FL 32399
(904) 487-1077
▲ See pages 180, 191

**Florida Department of Health and
Rehabilitative Services**
1317 Winewood Blvd.
Building 6, Room 453-A
Tallahassee, FL 32399-0700
(904) 487-2478
▲ See pages 103, 169, 192

**Florida Mental Health Institute,
Department of Community
Mental Health**
13301 Bruce B. Downs Blvd.
Tampa, FL 33612
(813) 974-4632
▲ See page 186

Focal Point Productions
33 Buchanan
Sausalito, CA 94965
(415) 332-8088
▲ See pages 101, 130

Focus International
14 Oregon Dr.
Huntington, NY 11746
(516) 549-5320
▲ See pages 43, 145

Fortune Magazine
Time and Life Building
Rockefeller Center
New York, NY 10020
(212) 522-1212
▲ See page 197

Foundation for Public Communication
P.O.Box 5176
New York, NY 10150
(212) 371-8502
▲ See page 187

Future Vision
P.O. Box 801
Tulsa, OK 74101
(918) 494-0202
▲ See pages 63, 117

**Gay and Lesbian Community Center
of Orange County
AIDS Response Program**
12832-E Garden Grove Blvd.
Garden Grove, CA 92643
(714) 534-0961
▲ See page 14

**Gay and Lesbian Community
Services Center**
1213 North Highland Ave.
Los Angeles, CA 90038
(213) 464-7400
▲ See pages 38, 40, 46, 103, 104, 136, 178, 182

Gay Community AIDS Project
P.O.Box 713
Champaign, IL 61820
(217) 351-2437
▲ See pages 10, 13, 38, 48, 49, 81, 88, 95, 133, 153

Gay Men's Health Crisis, Inc.
129 West 20th St.
New York, NY 10011
(212) 807-7517
▲ See pages 5, 39, 42, 43, 55, 66, 84, 86, 104, 131, 134, 135, 136, 155, 160, 172, 180, 182, 187, 189, 190, 199, 202

Genesis House
911 West Addison
Chicago, IL 60613
(312) 281-3917
▲ See pages 146, 147

George Washington University
School of Medicine and Health Sciences
2300 I St., NW
Washington, D.C. 20037
(202) 994-2945
▲ See page 183

Intergovernmental Health Policy
Project
2011 I St., NW
Washington, D.C. 20006
(202) 872-1445
▲ See pages 179, 197, 201

**Georgetown University, Kennedy
Institute of Ethics
National Reference Center for
Bioethics Literature**
1437 37th St. N.W., Pulton Hall 210
Washington, D.C. 20057
(202) 687-6738
▲ See page 176

Georgia Department of Corrections
Room 854, East Tower
2 Martin Luther King, Jr. Drive, NE
Atlanta, GA 30334
(404) 656-4601
▲ See page 129

**Georgia Department of Human
Resources**
878 Peachtree Street, NE,
Room 109
Atlanta, GA 30309
(404) 894-5304
▲ See pages 49, 90, 134, 154, 161, 171, 194

Globe Book Company, Inc.
50 West 23rd St.
New York, NY 10010
▲ See page 17

Good Samaritan Project
3940 Walnut
Kansas City, MO 64111
(816) 561-8784
▲ See pages 5, 13, 93, 136

Goodday Video, Inc.
115 North Esplanade
Cuero, TX 77954
(800) 221-1426
▲ See page 17

**Greater Cincinnati AIDS Task Force
University of Cincinnati
Medical Center**
231 Bethesda Ave., M.L. 563
Cincinnati, OH 45267-0563
(513) 558-4701
▲ See page 48

Greenwich Department of Health
101 Field Point Road
Greenwich, CT 06836
(203) 622-6496
▲ See page 85

Haight Asbury Free Medical Clinic
1696 Haight
San Francisco, CA 94117
(415) 751-4221
▲ See pages 94, 95

**Haitian & Caribbean Foundation for
Education and Development**
10 East 87th St.
New York, NY 10128
(212) 427-8100
▲ See pages 120, 147, 149

Haitian Women's Program/AFSC
15 Rutherford Pl.
New York, NY 10003
(212) 598-0965
▲ See pages 148, 151

Harris County Health Department
P.O. Box 25249
Houston, TX 77265
(713) 526-1841
▲ See pages 177, 180

**Harris County Medical Society
Houston Academy of Medicine**
1133 M.D. Anderson Blvd., Suite 400
Houston, TX 77030
(713) 790-1838
▲ See pages 30, 117, 169

**Hartford Health Department
AIDS Prevention Program**
80 Coventry St.
Hartford, CT 06112
(203) 722-6742
▲ See page 146

Hawaii Council of Churches
1300 Kailua Road
Kailua, HI 96734
(808) 263-9788
▲ See page 190

**Hawaii State Department of Health
STD/AIDS Prevention Program**
3627 Kilauea Ave., #304
Honolulu, HI 96816
(808) 735-5303
▲ See pages 45, 46, 60, 88, 95, 113, 120, 138, 153

Hazelden Educational Materials
P.O.Box 176
Center City, MN 55012-0176
(612) 257-4010
▲ See pages 97, 101, 171

Health Alert Press
P.O. Box 2060
Cambridge, MA 02238
(617) 497-4190
▲ See page 174

Health and Education Resources
4733 Bethesda Ave.
Bethesda, MD 20814
(301) 656-3178
▲ See page 183

**Health Councils of Pasco-Pinellas and
West-Central Florida, Inc.**
9887 North Gandy Blvd., #200
St. Petersburg, FL 33702
(813) 576-7772
▲ See page 54

Health Education Consultants
1284 Manor Park
Lakewood, OH 44107
(216) 521-1766
▲ See page 18

**Health Education Learning
Programs, Inc.**
P.O. Box 568
Jericho, NY 11753
(516) 364-4974
▲ See page 58

**Health Education Resource
Organization (HERO)**
101 West Read St., Suite 812
Baltimore, MD 21201
(301) 685-1180
▲ See pages 6, 8, 12, 46, 68, 70, 73, 91, 92, 96, 98, 134, 135, 141, 144, 155

Health Information Network
P.O.Box 30762
Seattle, WA 98103
(206) 784-5655
▲ See pages 175, 176, 177, 180,

Health Issues Taskforce of Cleveland
2250 Euclid Ave.
Cleveland, OH 44115
(216) 621-0766
▲ See pages 4, 39, 52, 57, 124

Health Matters, Inc.
4 Harding Ave.
Delmar, NY 12054
(518) 439-9078
▲ See pages 62, 183

Healthcare Network, Inc.
2500 Airport Road South, #106
Naples, FL 33962
(813) 775-9999
▲ See page 74

Hennepin County Administration
2308A Government Center
Minneapolis, MN 55487
(612) 348-4466
▲ See pages 27, 164

**Hispanic AIDS Committee for
Education and Resources, Inc.
(HACER)**
1139 W. Hildebrand, #B
San Antonio, TX 78201
(512) 732-3108
▲ See page 105

Hispanic Health Alliance
1608 North Milwaukee, #912
Chicago, IL 60647
(312) 252-6888
▲ See page 108

Hispanic Health Council
98 Cedar St., #3A
Hartford, CT 06106
(203) 527-0856
▲ See page 106

Hispanos Unidos Contra SIDA/AIDS
c/o New Haven Health Department
One State Street
New Haven, CT 06511
(203) 777-5833
▲ See pages 93, 103

Howard Brown Memorial Clinic
945 West George St.
Chicago, IL 60657
(312) 871-5777
▲ See pages 38, 50, 77, 87, 96, 140, 141, 142, 160, 189

Human Interaction Research Institute
1849 Sawtelle Blvd., #102
Los Angeles, CA 90025
(213) 479-3028
▲ See pages 176, 178

Human Relations Media
175 Tompkins Ave.
Pleasantville, NY 10570
(800) 431-2050
▲ See pages 31, 37

**Idaho Department of Health
and Welfare
AIDS Program**
Statehouse Mall
Boise, ID 83702
(208) 334-5937
▲ See pages 47, 49, 59, 89

**Illinois Alcoholism and Drug
Dependence Association**
859 West Wellington
Chicago, IL 60657
(217) 528-7335
▲ See pages 15, 51, 50, 84, 90, 91, 94, 95, 96, 97, 98, 121, 153

**Illinois Department of Public Health
AIDS Facts for Life**
AIDS Activity Section
525 W. Jefferson, 1st Floor
Chicago, IL 62761
(312) 917-4846
▲ See pages 13, 53, 69, 70, 170, 192

Illinois State Medical Society
20 North Michigan Ave., Ste. 700
Chicago, IL 60602
(312) 782-1654
▲ See pages 15, 169, 174

Indiana Department of Education
State House
Student Services Unit, Room 229
Indianapolis, IN 46204-2798
(317) 232-9111
▲ See page 193

Indiana State Board of Health
1330 West Michigan
Indianapolis, IN 46206-1964
(317) 663-0600
▲ See pages 26, 27, 61, 65, 97, 117, 140, 144, 165

**Indiana University
Audio-Visual Center**
Bloomington, IN 47405-5901
(812) 335-8087
▲ See page 63

Industrial Biotechnology Association
1625 K St., NW, Suite 1100
Washington, D.C. 20006
(202) 857-0244
▲ See page 184

InfoMedix
12806 Garden Grove Blvd., Suite F
Garden Grove, CA 92643
(714) 530-3454
▲ See page 177

Inglewood Physicians Association
P.O. Box 2126
Inglewood, CA 90305
(213) 603-8166
▲ See page 5

Institute For Development Training
P.O.Box 2522
Chapel Hill, NC 27514
(919) 967-0563
▲ See page 71

**Institute of Medicine,
National Academy of Sciences**
2101 Constitution Ave., NW
Washington, D.C. 20418
(202) 334-2453
▲ See pages 171, 195, 200

**Instituto Familiar De La Raza -
Latino AIDS Project**
2515 24th St., #2
San Francisco, CA 94110
(415) 647-5450
▲ See pages 106, 109, 197

Instructional Media Institute
Affiliate of Weston Woods Inst.
Village Market Square, Lower Plaza
Wilton, CT 06897
(800) 243-5020
▲ See page 118

**International Working Group on
AIDS and IV Drug Use
Narcotic and Drug Research, Inc.**
11 Beach St.
New York, NY 10013
(212) 966-8700
▲ See pages 177, 188

Iowa AIDS Legislature Task Force
321 E. First St.
Iowa City, IA 52240
(319) 351-0140
▲ See page 193

Iowa Department of Education
Grimes State Office Building
Des Moines, IA 50319
(515) 281-4804
▲ See page 182

John Canalli
182-B Castro St.
San Francisco, CA 94114
(415) 861-0843
▲ See page 65

Kaiser Permanente

Audio Visual Services
825 Colorado Blvd., Room 319
Los Angeles, CA 90041
(213) 259-4546
▲ See page 75

Medical Care Program
1 Kaiser Plaza, 21st Floor
Oakland, CA 94612
(415) 271-6334
▲ See pages 190, 191

**Kansas Department of Health
and Environment
Bureau of Epidemiology AIDS**
Mills Building, Suite 605
109 S.W. Ninth
Topeka, KS 66612-1271
▲ See pages 176, 180

Keats Publishing, Inc.
27 Pine Street, Box 876
New Canaan, CT 06840
(203) 966-8723
▲ See page 170

221

Kent County Health Department
700 Fuller Ave., NE
Grand Rapids, MI 49503
(616) 774-3030
▲ See pages 194

Krames Communications
312-90th St.
Daly City, CA 94015
(415) 994-8800
▲ See pages 51, 45, 136, 137, 138

**Lambda Legal Defense and
Education Fund, Inc.**
666 Broadway, 12th Fl.
New York, NY 10012
(212) 995-8585
▲ See pages 85, 170, 186

Landsburg Company
11811 West Olympic Blvd.
Los Angeles, CA 90064
(213) 478-7878
▲ See page 203

Latin Americans United
1520 Merritt Dr.
El Cajon, CA 92020
(619) 440-4335
▲ See page 195

Lerner Publications Co.
241 First Ave. N.
Minneapolis, MN 55401
(612) 332-3344
▲ See page 20

Light Video Television, Inc.
21 Highland Circle
Needham, MA 02194
(617) 449-7770
▲ See page 62

**Long Island Association For
AIDS Care, Inc.**
Box 2859
Huntington Sta., NY 11746
(516) 385-2451
▲ See pages 40, 57, 58, 99, 188

**Los Angeles Centers for
Alcohol & Drug Abuse**
2701 North Main St.
Los Angeles, CA 90031
(213) 221-3939
▲ See pages 59, 68, 104, 107

**Los Angeles County Dept.
of Health Services
AIDS Program Office**
2901 South Hope St. Annex
Los Angeles, CA 90007
(213) 744-3837
▲ See pages 6, 9, 13, 89, 94, 104, 109, 110, 121

Los Angeles County Medical Association
1925 Wilshire Blvd.
Los Angeles, CA 90057
(213) 483-1581
▲ See page 91

Los Angeles Unified School District
450 North Grand Ave., G390
Los Angeles, CA 90012
(213) 625-6432
▲ See page 19

**Louisville and Jefferson County
Board of Health**
400 East Gray St.
Louisville, KY 40201-1704
(502) 625-5601
▲ See pages 64, 179

Macro Systems, Inc.
3 Corporate Sq., #370
Atlanta, GA 30329
(404) 321-3211
▲ See pages 174, 195

Madison AIDS Support Network
P.O. Box 731
Madison, WI 53701
(608) 255-1711
▲ See pages 4, 34, 39, 192

**Maine Department of Human Services
Office on AIDS**
State House Station 11
157 Capitol St.
Augusta, ME 04333
(207) 289-3747
▲ See pages 56, 81, 87, 131, 133

Manisses Communications Group, Inc.
P.O. Box 3357, Wayland Square
Providence, RI 02906-0357
(401) 831-6020
▲ See pages 93, 187

Marin AIDS Support Network
4 G St., Suite 1
San Rafael, CA 94901
(415) 457-2437
▲ See page 132

**Mariposa Education And Research
Foundation**
4545 Park Blvd., #207
San Diego, CA 92116
(619) 542-0088
▲ See page 122

Mary Ann Liebert Inc., Publishers
1651 Third Ave., #301
New York, NY 10128
(212) 289-2300
▲ See page 186

**Maryland Department of Health
and Mental Hygiene
AIDS Administration**
201 West Preston St.
Baltimore, MD 21201
(301) 225-6707
▲ See pages 5, 48, 49, 52, 55, 82

**Massachusetts Department of
Public Health**
150 Tremont St., 11th Fl.
Boston, MA 02111
(617) 727-0368
▲ See pages 3, 6, 13, 19, 45, 46, 57, 90, 94, 98, 99,
113, 133, 134, 138, 155, 179, 180, 191, 193

Massachusetts Hospital Association
5 New England Executive Pk.
Burlington, MA 01803
(617) 272-8000
▲ See pages 169, 189

Maternity Center Association
48 East 92nd St.
New York, NY 10128
(212) 369-7300
▲ See page 131

**Mayor's Task Force On AIDS,
New Haven**
1 State St.
New Haven, CT 06511
(203) 787-6957
▲ See pages 153, 158

**McGraw-Hill Healthcare
Information Center**
1120 Vermont Ave. NW, #1200
Washington, D.C. 20005
(202) 463-1600
▲ See page 188

Medcom, Inc.
12601 Industry St.
Garden Grove, CA 92641
(714) 891-1443
▲ See page 76

Medfilms, Inc.
6841 North Cassim Pl.
Tucson, AZ 85704
(602) 575-8900
▲ See pages 74, 78, 80, 122, 202

Medical Action Group, Inc.
c/o Freeman Marketing
P.O. Box 685
Chanute, KS 66720
(316) 839-5593
▲ See page 62

Medical Data Exchange
445 South San Antonio Road
Los Altos, CA 94019
(415) 941-3600
▲ See page 179

Medical Surveillance, Inc.
MED-ED Productions
P.O. Box 1629
West Chester, PA 19380
(215) 436-8881
▲ See pages 54, 62

Medical Video Productions
859 Vistavia Circle
Decatur, GA 30033
(404) 634-9955
▲ See pages 75, 145

Memphis / Shelby County
Health Department
814 Jefferson Ave.
Memphis, TN 38104
(901) 576-7714
▲ See page 38

Merced County Health Department
240 East 15th St.
Merced, CA 95340
(209) 385-7709
▲ See pages 46, 132

Metropolitan Life Insurance Company
One Madison Avenue
New York, NY 10010
(212) 578-7273
▲ See pages 56, 202

Michigan Department of Education
P.O. Box 30008
Lansing, MI 48909
(517) 373-2589
▲ See pages 18, 19, 192

Michigan Department of Public Health
Special Offices on AIDS Prevention
3500 North Logan St.
P.O. Box 30035
Lansing, MI 48909
(517) 335-8371
▲ See page 53

Milestone Productions
1565 16th Ave.
San Francisco, CA 94122
(415) 641-8436
▲ See page 32

Minnesota AIDS Project
2025 Nicollet Ave. S.
Minneapolis, MN 55404
(612) 870-7773
▲ See pages 23, 24, 85, 115, 125, 135, 137, 161, 179, 188

Minnesota American Indian AIDS Task
Force
c/o The Minneapolis Indian
Health Board
1315 East 24th Street
Minneapolis, MN 55404
(612) 721-7425
▲ See page 150

Minnesota Department of Health
(MDH)
AIDS Program Unit
717 S.E. Delaware St.
P.O. Box 9441
Minneapolis, MN 55440
(612) 623-5698
▲ See pages 175, 193, 194

Minority AIDS Project
5149 West Jefferson Blvd.
Los Angeles, CA 90016
(213) 936-4949
▲ See pages 6, 7, 8

Mississippi State Department of Health
2423 North State St., P.O. Box 1700
Jackson, MS 39215-1700
(601) 960-7725
▲ See pages 14, 49, 52, 83, 89, 90

Monmouth Ocean AIDS Information
Group, Inc.
P.O. Box 834
Neptune, NJ 07753
(201) 758-0077
▲ See page 179

Montana Department of Health &
Environmental Sciences
Montana AIDS Program
Cogswell Bldg.
Helena, MT 59620
(404) 444-2457
▲ See pages 51, 81, 88, 134

Montefiore Medical Center
Department of Social Medicine,
AIDS Education Project
111 East 210th St.
Bronx, NY 10467
(212) 920-6741
▲ See page 93

Multicultural Prevention Resource
Center (MPRC)
1540 Market St., Suite 320
San Francisco, CA 94102
(415) 861-2142
▲ See pages 9, 25, 95, 96, 99, 101, 108, 146

National Academy Press
2101 Constitution Ave., NW
Washington, D.C. 20418
(202) 334-3180
▲ See page 171

National AIDS Network (NAN)
2033 M St., NW, 8th Fl.
Washington, D.C. 20036
(202) 293-2437
▲ See pages 120, 125, 173, 181, 187, 188, 196

National AIDS Prevention Institute
P.O. Box 2500, 205 South East St.
Culpeper, VA 22701
(703) 825-4040
▲ See pages 55, 111, 186

National Association of Manufacturers
1331 Pennsylvania Ave., NW #1500
North Lobby
Washington, D.C. 20004
(202) 637-3124
▲ See page 164

National Association of Protection
and Advocacy Systems
220 I St., NE, #150
Washington, D.C. 20001
(202) 546-8202
▲ See pages 188, 197

National Association of PWA's
(NAPWA)
2025 "I" St., NW, Suite 415
Washington, D.C. 20006
(202) 429-2856
▲ See page 188

National Association of Social Workers
7981 Eastern Avenue, Fourth Floor
Silver Spring, MD 20910
(301) 565-0333
▲ See pages 61, 173, 189, 190, 192,

National Association of State
Boards of Education
1012 Cameron St.
Alexandria, VA 22314
(703) 684-4000
▲ See page 191

National Clearinghouse For
Alcohol And Drug Information
P.O. Box 2345
Rockville, MD 20852
(301) 468-2600
▲ See page 200

National Coalition of Advocates for Students
100 Boylston St., #737
Boston, MA 02116
(617) 357-8507
▲ See pages 116, 190, 191

National Coalition of Black Lesbians and Gays
P.O. Box 2420
Washington, D.C. 20013
(202) 265-7117
▲ See page 4

National Coalition of Hispanic Health and Human Services Organizations (COSSMHO)
1030 15th Street, N.W., Suite 1053
Washington, D.C. 20005
(202) 371-2100
▲ See page 180

National Committee for Clinical Laboratory Standards (NCCLS)
771 E. Lancaster Avenue
Villanova, PA 19085
(215) 525-2435
▲ See page 193

National Education Association (NEA) Health Information Network
100 Colony Square
Suite 200
Atlanta, GA 30361
(404) 875-8819
▲ See page 198

National Gay Rights Advocates
540 Castro Street
San Francisco, CA 94114
(415) 863-9156
▲ See pages 170, 183, 184, 188, 189, 195, 196

National Health Publishing
99 Painters Mill Rd.
Owings Mills, MD 21117
(301) 363-6400
▲ See pages 76, 169, 170

National Hemophilia Foundation
110 Greene St., Soho Bldg., #406
New York, NY 10012
(212) 219-8180
▲ See pages 25, 156, 186, 192

National Institute on Drug Abuse ORC
5600 Fishers Lane, Rm.10A-054
Parklawn Bldg.
Rockville, MD 20857
(301) 443-1124
▲ See pages 95, 100, 101

National Lawyers Guild AIDS Network
558 Capp Street
San Francisco, CA 94110
(415) 824-8884
▲ See pages 171, 187

National Leadership Coalition on AIDS
1150 17th St., NW, #202
Washington, D.C. 20036
(202) 429-0930
▲ See page 164

National Legal Research Group, Inc.
2421 Fry Road
P.O. Box 7187
Charlottesville, VA 22901
(804) 977-5690
▲ See page 185

National Lesbian and Gay Health Foundation
1638 R St., NW, #2
Washington, D.C. 20009
(202) 797-3708
▲ See page 173

National Library of Medicine
8600 Rockville Pike, Rm.1W22
Bethesda, MD 20894
(301) 496-6097
▲ See pages 176, 177, 178

National Native American AIDS Prevention Center
6239 College Ave., #201
Oakland, CA 94618
(415) 658-2051
▲ See pages 178, 182, 185

National Organization of Black County Officials, Inc.
440 First St., NW, #500
Washington, D.C. 20001
(202) 347-6953
▲ See pages 177, 181, 182

National PTA
700 North Rush St.
Chicago, IL 60611
(312) 787-0977
▲ See page 112

National Safety Council
444 North Michigan Ave.
Chicago, IL 60611
(312) 526-4800
▲ See pages 22, 106, 111, 161

National School Boards Association
1680 Duke St.
Alexandria, VA 22314
(703) 838-6722
▲ See pages 182, 190, 195, 200

National Sheriffs' Association
1450 Duke St.
Alexandria, VA 22314
(800) 424-7827
▲ See pages 54, 129, 150, 170

National Women's Health Network
1325 G St., NW
Washington, D.C. 20005
(202) 347-1140
▲ See pages 152, 156

Native American Women's Health Education Resource Center
P.O. Box 572
809 High St.
Lake Andes, SD 57356
(605) 487-7072
▲ See pages 146, 148, 149, 198

Nebraska Department of Education
301 Centennial Mall South
Lincoln, NE 68509
(402) 471-2295
▲ See page 15

Neon Street Center for Youth
3227 North Sheffield
Chicago, IL 60657
(312) 528-7767
▲ See page 13

Nevada AIDS Foundation
P.O. Box 478
Reno, NV 89504
(702) 329-2437
▲ See pages 54, 188

New Dimension Media, Inc.
85895 Lorane Hwy.
Eugene, OR 97405
(503) 484-7125
▲ See pages 29, 30

New England Corporate Consortium for AIDS Education
150 Coulter Drive
Concord, MA 01742
(508) 264-1418
▲ See page 164

New Focus Films, Inc.
Division of Northern Lights Alternatives
2170 Broadway, #3286
New York, NY 10024
(212) 727-7614
▲ See page 85

New Haven Health Department
1 State St.
New Haven, CT 06511
(203) 787-8189
▲ See pages 98, 196

New Jersey Department of Health
AIDS Education Unit
CN 360, 363 West State St.
Trenton, NJ 08625-0360
(609) 984-6000
▲ See page 129

New Jersey Network
1573 Parkside Ave., CN777
Trenton, NJ 08625-0777
(609) 530-5015
▲ See pages 8, 65, 66, 109, 202, 203

New Mexico AIDS Services, Inc.
124 Quincy Northeast
Albuquerque, NM 87108
(505) 266-0911
▲ See pages 13, 47, 94, 131

New Mexico State
Department of Education
Education Building
Santa Fe, NM 87501-2786
(505) 827-6570
▲ See page 194

New York City Commission on Human
Rights/AIDS Discrimination
52 Duane St.
New York, NY 10007
(212) 566-1826
▲ See pages 45, 195, 200

New York City Department of Health
AIDS Education Training Unit
311 Broadway, 4th Floor
New York, NY 10007
(212) 285-4626
▲ See pages 7, 14, 26, 44, 46, 48, 49, 60, 81, 87, 96,
98, 102, 116, 132, 133, 138, 139, 141, 142, 146,
154, 179

New York City Parents and Friends of
Lesbians and Gay Men, Inc.
P.O. Box 553, Lenox Hill Station
New York, NY 10021
(212) 463-0629
▲ See page 184

New York State Department of Health
Empire State Plaza
Corning Tower, Room 1084
Albany, NY 12237
(518) 474-5370
▲ See pages 24, 32, 46, 55, 57, 87, 103, 107, 108,
110, 116, 129, 131, 134, 139, 145, 153, 155, 158,
159, 160, 184

New York State Department of
Social Services,
Office of Human Resource
Development
40 North Pearl St.
Albany, NY 12243
(518) 473-8966
▲ See pages 125, 171, 186

Newmarket Press
18 East 48th St.
New York, NY 10017
(212) 832-3575
▲ See page 111

NO/AIDS Task Force
P.O. Box 2616
New Orleans, LA 70126
(504) 891-3732
▲ See pages 3, 14, 47, 67, 82, 94, 113, 120, 132, 152,
161, 174

North Carolina AIDS Control Program
P.O.Box 2091
Raleigh, NC 27602-2091
(919) 733-7301
▲ See pages 4, 51, 82, 89, 114, 124, 134, 153, 191,
192, 193

North Central Florida AIDS Network
1103 Southwest Second Ave.
Gainesville, FL 32601
(904) 372-4370
▲ See pages 47, 93, 131, 155, 160

Northern Lights Alternatives, Inc.
1811 North Wilton St.
Los Angeles, CA 90028
(213) 461-0261
▲ See pages 169, 178, 181

Northwest AIDS Foundation
1818 East Madison
Seattle, WA 98122
(206) 329-6923
▲ See pages 41, 42, 52, 140

Northwest University Medical School
AIDS Mental Health Education and
Evaluation Project
303 E. Superior, Passavant 538
Chicago, IL 60611
(312) 908-9191
▲ See page 180

Novela Health Foundation
2524 16th Ave. South
Seattle, WA 98144
(206) 325-9897
▲ See pages 32, 77, 78, 105

NYU Regional Education and
Training Center
532 Shimkin Hall, 50 West 4th St.
New York, NY 10003
(212) 998-5332
▲ See pages 202, 203

O.D.N. Productions, Inc.
74 Varick St., Suite 304
New York, NY 10013
(212) 431-8923
▲ See pages 32, 33

Oak Lawn Counseling Center
AIDS Program
3000 Turtle Creek Plaza, Suite 204
Dallas, TX 75219
(214) 521-5144
▲ See pages 49, 57

Office of Technology Assessment,
U.S. Congress
U.S. Congress, Health Programs
Washington, D.C. 20510-8025
(202) 228-6590
▲ See pages 195, 197, 198, 201

Office Sterilization and Asepsis
Procedures Research Found.
U. of Texas Health Science Ctr.
Dental School at San Antonio
7703 Floyd Curl Dr.
San Antonio, TX 78284
(512) 567-3333
▲ See pages 79, 199

Ohio AIDS Foundation
P.O. Box 12126
Columbus, OH 43212-0126
(614) 275-6339
▲ See pages 181, 186

Ohio Department of Health - AIDS Unit
246 North High St.
Columbus, OH 43266-0588
(614) 466-5480
▲ See pages 3, 17, 50, 112, 136, 154, 183

Orange County Health Care Agency
AIDS Community Education Project
1725 West 17th St., Rm. 116-C
Santa Ana, CA 92706
(714) 834-8700
▲ See page 105

Oregon Council for Hispanic
Advancement
621 S.W. Morrison, #729
Portland, OR 97205
(503) 228-4131
▲ See page 180

Oregon Department of Human Resources, Oregon Health Division, AIDS Education Program
P.O. Box 231
Portland, OR 97207
(503) 229-5792
▲ See pages , 192

Oregon Health Division, HIV Program
1400 SW Fifth, #209
Portland, OR 97201
(503) 229-5792
▲ See pages 16, 27, 58, 137

The Oryx Press
2214 North Central at Encanto
Phoenix, AZ 85004
(602) 254-6156
▲ See pages 175, 179

Outsider Productions
929 14th St.
San Francisco, CA 94114
(415) 626-6203
▲ See page 122

Pacifica Program Service and Radio Archive
5316 Venice Blvd.
Los Angeles, CA 90019
(213) 931-1625
▲ See page 169

Panel Publishers, Inc.
14 Plaza Rd.
Greenvale, NY 11548
(516) 484-0006
▲ See page 186

Pennsylvania Medical Society Educational and Scientific Trust
20 Erford Rd.
Lemoyne, PA 17043
(800) 228-2823
▲ See page 73

People of Color Against AIDS Network
105 14th Ave., #2D
Seattle, WA 98122
(206) 322-7061
▲ See pages 3, 4, 24, 96, 134, 146, 153

Perennial Education, Inc.
930 Pitner Ave.
Evanston, IL 60202
(312) 328-6700
▲ See pages 28, 29

Performance Matters, Inc.
c/o Printed Matter, Inc.
P.O. Box 15246
Atlanta, GA 30333
(404) 523-6522
▲ See page 62

Pergrine Productions
330 Santa Rita
Palo Alto, CA 94301
(415) 328-4843
▲ See page 29

Pharmaceutical Manufacturers Association
1100 15th St. NW
Washington, D.C.
(202) 835-3400
▲ See page 189

Philadelphia AIDS Task Force
P.O. Box 53429
Philadelphia, PA 19101
(215) 545-8686
▲ See pages 39, 50, 68

Philadelphia Commission on AIDS at University of Pennsylvania
Davis Inst. of Health Economics
3641 Locust Walk
Philadelphia, PA 19104
(215) 898-4750
▲ See page 193

Philadelphia Sciences Group
774 North 24th St.
Philadelphia, PA 19130
(215) 232-8687
▲ See page 196

Pima County Health Department
150 West Congress St.
Tucson, AZ 85701
(602) 792-8315
▲ See page 144

Pittsburgh AIDS Task Force, Inc.
Stevenson Pl.
141 South Highland Ave.
Pittsburgh, PA 15206
(412) 363-6500
▲ See pages 42, 182, 189

Planned Parenthood
Alameda / San Francisco
815 Eddy St., #300
San Francisco, CA 94109
(415) 441-7858
▲ See pages 14, 154

Federation of America
810 Seventh Ave.
New York, NY 11215
(212) 603-4626
▲ See page 54, 116, 178

Central Oklahoma
Education Department
619 Northwest 23rd St.
Oklahoma City, OK 73103
(405) 525-0344
▲ See page 136

Maryland
610 North Howard St.
Baltimore, MD 21201
(301) 576-1400
▲ See page 62

Metropolitan Washington D.C.
1108 16th St., NW
Washington, D.C. 20036
(202) 347-8500
▲ See page 71

N.E. Pennsylvania
112 North 13th St.
Allentown, PA 18102
(215) 439-8008
▲ See page 114

New York City
380 Second Ave.
New York, NY 10014
(212) 777-2002
▲ See pages 50, 90, 156, 184

San Diego and Riverside Counties
210 5th Ave.
San Diego, CA 92101
(619) 231-6820
▲ See page 118

South Palm Beach and Broward Counties
455 NW 35th St.
Boca Raton, FL 33431
(407) 394-3540
▲ See page 147

Pocket Books
1230 Avenue of the Americas
New York, NY 10020
(212) 698-7000
▲ See page 172

Polaris Research and Development
185 Berry St., #6600
San Francisco, CA 94107
(415) 777-3229
▲ See pages 174, 197, 202,

Portnoy Enterprises
17408 Oak Drive
Detroit, MI 48221
(313) 861-4783
(313) 494-1240
▲ See page 26

Positive Promotion
222 Ashland Place
Brooklyn, NY 11217
(718) 858-4199
▲ See page 133

Premier Hospitals Alliance, Inc.
1 Westbrook Corporate Ctr.
Westchester, IL 60153
(312) 531-8220
▲ See page 186

Prima Publishing
P.O. Box 1260
Rocklin, CA 95677
(916) 624-5718
▲ See page 172

Pro - Ed Publishing
5341 Industrial Oaks Boulevard
Austin, TX 78735
(512) 892-3142
▲ See pages 20, 22,

Professional Training Systems, Inc.
1201 Peachtree St., N.E.
Bldg 400, Suite 1525
Atlanta, GA 30361
(404) 872-9700
▲ See page 80

Project Inform
347 Dolores St., #301
San Francisco, CA 94110
(415) 558-8669
▲ See pages 174, 189

PSI Associates, Inc.
1000 Vermont Ave., NW, #300
Washington, D.C. 20005
(202) 842-2790
▲ See page 20

Public Affairs Committee, Inc.
381 Park Ave. South
New York, NY 10016-8884
(212) 683-4331
▲ See page 45

Public Broadcast System
c/o Coronet MTI Film & Video
108 Wilmot Road
Deerfield, IL 60015
(312) 940-1260
▲ See page 203

Public Health Foundation
1220 L Street, NW, #350
Washington, D.C. 20005
(202) 898-5600
▲ See page 191

PWA (People With AIDS) Coalition, Inc.
31 West 26th St., 5th Fl.
New York, NY 10010
(212) 532-0290
▲ See pages 173, 188

Pyramid Film and Video
2801 Colorado Ave.
Santa Monica, CA 90404
(213) 828-7577
▲ See page 64

R & E Research, Inc.
P.O.Box 2008
Saratoga, CA 95070
(408) 866-6303
▲ See pages 20, 67, 115, 174, 175, 176

Random House, Inc., Vintage Books
201 East 50th
New York, NY 10022
(212) 751-2600
▲ See page 173

Regnery Gateway, Inc.
1130 17th St., NW
Washington, D.C. 20036
(202) 457-0978
▲ See page 15

Resource Technical Services, Inc.
P.O.Box 2882
Toledo, OH 43606
(419) 535-5743
▲ See page 72

Rhode Island Department of Health AIDS Program
75 Davis St., Room 105
Providence, RI 02908-5097
(401) 277-2362
▲ See pages 87, 111, 136, 154, 181, 182, 186, 189

Rhode Island Hospital
593 Eddy St.
Providence, RI 02903
(401) 277-5617
▲ See page 175

Richmond City Health Department
500 North 10th St., Room 114
Richmond, VA 23219
(804) 780-4365
▲ See page 174

Riverside County Department of Health AIDS Activities Program
3575 11th Street Mall
Riverside, CA 92501
(714) 369-4308
▲ See pages 82, 90, 174

Roanoke AIDS Project
920 South Jefferson St.,#518
Roanoke, VA 24003
(703) 985-0131
▲ See page 182

Rutgers University Press
109 Church Street
New Brunswick, NJ 08901
(201) 932-7765
▲ See page 170

Sacramento AIDS Foundation
1900 K St., #201
Sacramento, CA 95814
(916) 448-2437
▲ See pages 5, 41, 45, 155

San Diego Department of Health Services
P.O.Box 85222
San Diego, CA 92138-5222
(619) 236-2705
▲ See pages 69, 94, 103, 135, 160

San Francisco AIDS Foundation
333 Valencia St.
P.O. Box 6182
San Francisco, CA 94101-6182
(415) 861-3397
▲ See pages 25, 39, 43, 46, 49, 53, 59, 81, 84, 91, 93, 94, 96, 97, 98, 99, 104, 113, 115, 121, 133, 135, 137, 139, 147, 152, 162, 170, 174, 187, 197, 198, 199, 200, 202, 203

San Francisco General Hospital Medical Center
Medical Special Care Unit for Treatment of AIDS
995 Potrero Ave., 5A
San Francisco, CA 94110
(415) 821-8153
▲ See page 186

San Francisco Human Rights Commission
AIDS Discrimination Unit
1095 Market St., Suite 501
San Francisco, CA 94103
(415) 558-4901
▲ See page 81

San Mateo County AIDS Project
225 West 37th Ave.
San Mateo, CA 94403
(415) 573-2588
▲ See pages 47, 84, 94, 131, 135, 138, 152

**Santa Barbara County Health
Care Services**
300 San Antonio Road
Santa Barbara, CA 93110
(805) 681-5120
▲ See pages 186, 179

Scholastic, Inc.
730 Broadway
New York, NY 10003
(212) 505-3019
▲ See page 16

**Seattle-King County
Department of Public Health**
1116 Summit Ave.
Seattle, WA 98101
(206) 296-4649
▲ See pages 17, 50, 67, 87, 104, 107, 111, 112, 135, 154

**Sequoia YMCA
Youth Development Department**
609 Price Ave., Suite 202
Redwood City, CA 94132
(415) 366-8408
▲ See page 147

**Service Employees International,
AFL-CIO, CLC**
1313 L St., NW
Washington, D.C. 20005
(202) 898-3200
▲ See pages 68, 160

**Sex Information And Education
Council Of The United States**
32 Washington Pl.
New York, NY 10003
(212) 673-3850
▲ See pages 112, 172, 173, 175, 189

**Sexually Transmitted Diseases Control
Program**
Call Box STD, Caparra Heights Sta.
San Juan, PR 00922
(809) 754-8118
▲ See pages 68, 89, 104, 108, 120

Shiprock Community Health Center
P.O.Box 1734
Shiprock, NM 87420
(505) 368-5181
▲ See pages , 146, 147,

Simon & Schuster, Inc.
Simon & Shuster Building
1230 Avenue of the Americas
New York, NY 10020
▲ See page 173

**SIRS - Social Issues Resources
Series, Inc.**
P.O.Box 2348
Boca Raton, FL 33427
(800) 327-0513
▲ See page 169

**Social Security Administration
Department of Health and
Human Services**
518B East Main Street
Riverhead, NY 11901
(800) 234-5772
▲ See page 184

Society for the Right to Die
250 West 57th St.
New York, NY 10107
(212) 246-6973
▲ See pages 174, 175, 203

**South Carolina Dept. of Health and
Environmental Control
Bureau of Preventive Health Services**
2600 Bull St., Mills Bldg.
Columbia, SC 29201
(803) 737-4110
▲ See pages 49, 67, 153, 155, 181

Southeastern Massachusetts University
Old Wesport Rd.
N. Dartmouth, MA 02747
(508) 999-8584
▲ See page 70

**Southern California Women
for Understanding**
9054 Santa Monica Blvd., Suite 103
West Hollywood, CA 90064
(213) 274-1086
▲ See page 135

**Special Immunology Service,
Children's Hospital**
111 Michigan Ave., NW
Washington, D.C. 20010
(202) 745-3495
▲ See pages 14, 15, 113

St. Louis Efforts for AIDS
4050 Lindell Blvd.
St. Louis, MO 63108
(314) 531-2847
▲ See pages 39, 48, 133, 155

St. Martin's Press
175 Fifth Ave.
New York, NY 10010
(212) 674-5151
▲ See pages 171, 173

St. Paul Division of Public Health
555 Cedar St.
St. Paul, MN 55101
(612) 292-7238
▲ See page 48

**Stanford University
Cowell Student Health Center**
606 Campus Dr.
Stanford, CA 94305-8580
(415) 723-2300
▲ See page 132

**State of Florida Department of Health
and
Rehabilitative Services - Broward
County Public Health Unit**
2421 Southwest Sixth Ave.
Ft. Lauderdale, FL 33315
(305) 467-4807
▲ See page 24

**State of New Mexico
AIDS Prevention Program
Health & Environment Department**
1190 St. Francis Dr.
Santa Fe, NM 87503
(505) 827-0090
▲ See pages 16, 109, 194

**State of Wyoming, Division of Health
and Medical STD/AIDS**
Hathaway Building, Room 483
Cheyenne, WY 82002-0710
(307) 777-7953
▲ See pages 179, 185

**State University of New York at Stony
Brook - Dept of Allied
Health Professions,
SUNY AIDS Education Project**
Health Sciences Center - L2-052
Stony Brook, NY 11794-8204
(516) 444-3246
▲ See page 34

**Statewide Minority Advocacy Group
for Alcohol and Drug
Prevention, Inc.**
P.O. Box 54677
Atlanta, GA 30308
(404) 894-4795
▲ See page 182

Stop AIDS Resource Center
(Stop AIDS Project)
347 Dolores, #118
San Francisco, CA 94110
(415) 621-7177
▲ See pages 182, 198, 199

Substance Abuse Education, Inc.
670 South 4th St.
P.O. Box 13738
Edwardsville, KS 66113
(913) 441-1868
▲ See pages 20, 40

Sunburst Communications, Inc.
39 Washington Ave.
Pleasantville, NY 10570-2898
(914) 769-5030
▲ See page 29

Sweetwater Union High School District
1130 Fifth Ave.
Chula Vista, CA 92011
(619) 691-5536
▲ See page 16

Syndistar, Inc.
648 Hickory Ave.
New Orleans, LA 70123
(800) 841-9532
▲ See page 129

Syntex Corporation
3401 Hillview Ave.
Palo Alto, CA 94304
(415) 852-1000
▲ See page 195

T.H.E. Clinic
Asian Health Project
3860 West King Blvd.
Los Angeles, CA 90008
(213) 295-6571
▲ See page 54

Tampa AIDS Network
P.O.Box 8333
Tampa, FL 33674-8333
(813) 221-6420
▲ See pages 40, 93, 174, 181

Tapestry Productions
942 Broadway
New York, NY 10010
(212) 677-6007
▲ See page 203

Tennessee Department of Health
and Environment
100 Ninth Ave., North CDC-3
Nashville, TN 37219
(615) 741-7387
▲ See pages 48, 179

Teschuba
6038 Brann St.
Oakland, CA 94605
(415) 568-2838
▲ See pages 7, 8

Testing The Limits Collective
31 West 26th St., 4th Fl.
New York, NY 11222
(212) 545-7120
▲ See page 66

Texas Commission on Alcohol and
Drug Abuse
1705 Guadalupe
Austin, TX 78701-1214
(512) 463-5510
▲ See pages 67, 194

Texas Department of Health
Bureau of AIDS and STD Control
1100 West 49th St.
Austin, TX 78756
(512) 458-7207
▲ See pages 3, 51, 60, 94, 152, 160, 179, 182

Texas Medical Association
Committee on Sexually Transmitted
Diseases
1801 North Lamar Blvd.
Austin, TX 78701
(512) 477-6704
▲ See page 49

The Access Group
4 Cielo Lane, #4D
Novato, CA 94949
(415) 883-6111
▲ See page 183

The Center for Attitudinal Healing
19 Main St.
Tiburon, CA 94920
(415) 435-5022
▲ See page 121

The Exodus Trust
1523 Franklin St.
San Francisco, CA 94109
(415) 928-1133
▲ See pages 37, 77, 86, 91, 117, 128, 131, 159

The Feminist Institute Clearinghouse
P.O.Box 30563
Bethesda, MD 20814
(301) 951-9040
▲ See pages 156, 200

The Foundation Center
79 Fifth Ave.
New York, NY 10003
(212) 620-4230
▲ See pages 179, 195, 199

The J. Gary Mitchell Film Company
c/o Coronet/MTI Film & Video
108 Wilmot Rd.
Deerfield, IL 60015
(312) 940-1260
▲ See page 33

The Johns Hopkins Health System
Office of Public Affairs
550 North Broadway
Baltimore, MD 21205
(301) 955-4949
▲ See pages 74, 75, 76

The Knowledge Well
P.O. Box 1598
Levittown, PA 19058-1598
(215) 945-0222
▲ See page 54

The Kupona Network
4611 South Ellis Ave.
Chicago, IL 60653
(312) 536-3000
▲ See page 4

The National Coalition of Gay
Sexually Transmitted Disease
Services
P.O.Box 239
Milwaukee, WI 53201-0239
(414) 277-7671
▲ See page 38

The National Foundation for
Infectious Diseases
4733 Bethesda Avenue, Suite 750
Bethesda, MD 20814
(301) 656-0003
▲ See page 190

The New York Business
Group on Health
622 Third Avenue, 34th Floor
New York, NY 10017
(212) 808-0550
▲ See page 190

The State Education Department
Bureau of Curriculum Development
Washington Ave.
Albany, NY 12234
(518) 474-5897
▲ See page 18

The Stop AIDS Project
40 Plympton St.
Boston, MA 02118
(617) 542-9189
▲ See page 174

United Way of America
701 North Fairfax St.
Alexandria, VA 22314
(703) 836-7100
▲ See pages 164, 201

Universal Fellowship of Metropolitan
Community Churches
5300 Santa Monica Blvd, Suite 304
Los Angeles, CA 90029
(213) 464-5100
▲ See pages 119, 187

University Hospitals of Cleveland
2074 Abington Rd.
Cleveland, OH 44106
(216) 844-3196
▲ See page 47

University of California at Irvine
P.O. Box 19556
Irvine, CA 92713
(714) 856-7309
▲ See page 178

University of California at San
Francisco
AIDS Health Project
Box 0884
San Francisco, CA 94143-0884
(415) 476-6430
▲ See pages 67, 69, 78, 79, 92, 120, 169, 187, 194
Institute for Health Policy Studies,
AIDS Resource Program
1326 Third Avenue
San Francisco, CA 94143-0936
(415) 476-8263
▲ See page 176

University of California, Berkeley:
The Library
Room 386 Library
University of California
Berkeley, CA 94720
(415) 642-5339
▲ See page 176

University of Louisville
Department of Psychiatry
School of Medicine
Louisville, KY 40292
(502) 588-5394
▲ See page 177

University of Massachusetts
Medical Center
55 Lake Ave. North
Worcester, MA 01655
(508) 856-2176
▲ See page 31

University of Pittsburgh
P.O. Box 7319
Pittsburgh, PA 15213
(412) 624-5046
▲ See page 184

University of Texas Health Services
Center,
AIDS Working Group
P.O. Box 20186
Houston, TX 77006
(713) 792-4400
▲ See page 186

University Publishing Group
107 East Church St.
Frederick, MD 21701
(301) 694-8531
▲ See pages 171, 172, 177, 185

Up Front Drug Information
5701 Biscayne Blvd., Suite 602
Miami, FL 33137
(305) 757-2566
▲ See pages 97, 189

Vida Latina
3305 West Lafayette
Detroit, MI 48216
(313) 964-0890
▲ See page 105

Video Services, University of Maryland
32 South Greene St.
Baltimore, MD 21201
(301) 328-7720
▲ See pages 74, 75, 77, 78, 79

Videolearning Systems, Inc.
354 West Lancaster Ave.
Haverford, PA 19041
(215) 896-6600
▲ See page 202

Virginia Department of Health
AIDS Program
109 Governor St., #722
Richmond, VA 23219
(804) 225-4844
▲ See pages 3, 46, 68, 88

Visiting Nurses and Hospice of
San Francisco
1390 Market St., #510
San Francisco, CA 94102
(415) 861-8705
▲ See pages 67, 171

W.B. Saunders
1250 6th Ave.
San Diego, CA 92101
▲ See page 170

Walt Disney Educational
Media Company
c/o Coronet/MTI Film & Video
108 Wilmot Rd.
Deerfield, IL 60015
(312) 940-1260
▲ See pages 28, 118

Walter Reed Army Institute of Research
Washington, D.C. 20307-5100
(202) 576-2106
▲ See page 130

Washington State Office on HIV\AIDS
Airdustrial Pk.,Bldg.14, Stp.LP-20
Olympia, WA 98504
(206) 586-0426
▲ See pages 44, 51, 54, 115

Wellness Networks, Inc. - Flint
P.O. Box 1046
Royal Oak, MI 48072
(313) 876-3582
▲ See pages 38, 39, 51, 83, 82, 89

West Virginia Department of Health
AIDS Prevention Program
151 11th Ave.
S. Charleston, WV 25303
(304) 348-2950
▲ See page 134

Westover Consultants, Inc.
500 E St., SW, #910
Washington, D.C. 20024
(202) 863-0962
▲ See page 147

Whitehall Press-Budget Publications
Rt. 1, Box 603
Sondersville, GA 31082
(912) 552-7455
▲ See pages 172, 173

Whitman-Walker Clinic
1407 S St., NW
Washington, D.C. 20009
(202) 797-3500
▲ See pages 38, 39, 40, 82, 93

Willamette AIDS Council
329 West 13th, Suite D
Eugene, OR 97401
(503) 345-7089
▲ See page 41

WIN Project Foundation
4119 Los Feliz Blvd., #10
Los Angeles, CA 90027
(213) 663-0088
▲ See page 178

**Wisconsin Division of Health,
AIDS/HIV Program**
P.O.Box 309
1 West Wilson St.
Madison, WI 53701-0309
(608) 267-3733
▲ See pages 24, 48, 68, 73, 96, 136, 139, 198, 199, 200, 201

**Women and AIDS Resource Network
(WARN)**
55 Johnson St.,Bldg.G, Rm.303
Brooklyn, NY 11202
(718) 596-6007
▲ See page 185

Women's Action Alliance
370 Lexington Ave.
New York, NY 10017
(212) 532-8330
▲ See page 181

**Workplace Health Communications
Corporation**
110 Wolf Rd.
Albany, NY 12205
(518) 438-9141
▲ See page 163

**World Health Organization, Global
Programme on AIDS**
1211 Geneva 27,
Switzerland,
▲ See pages 204 - 206

World Hemophilia AIDS Center
2400 South Flower St.
Los Angeles, CA 90007-2697
(213) 742-1357
▲ See pages 183, 187

Worthington Associates Worldwide
345 West 21st St., #3D
New York, NY 10011-3059
(212) 243-5883
▲ See pages 180, 194, 198

Yale University Press
92A Yale Station
New Haven, CT 06511
(203) 432-0940
▲ See page 169

Year Book Medical Publishers
200 North Lasalle St.
Chicago, IL 60601
(312) 726-9733
▲ See pages 171, 169

Young Adult Institute
460 West 34th St., 11th Fl.
New York, NY 10001
(212) 563-7474
▲ See page 105

INDICES

Three indices are provided

1. Alphabetical index

2. Product Type Index

3. Non-English Language Index

All product titles (along with designation of product type) listed alphabetically.

All titles listed alphabetically under appropriate product type.

Titles only of non-English language products listed alphabetically under appropriate language category (e.g., Spanish).

233

INDEX ONE: TITLE INDEX

A

239

P

Q

T

INDEX TWO: PRODUCT TYPE INDEX

■ AUDIO TAPES

■ BOOKS / MANUALS

■ BROCHURES

CATALOGS / BIBLIOGRAPHIES

COMPUTER INFORMATION SERVICES

DIRECTORIES

■ INSTRUCTIONAL PROGRAMS

■ MICROFILMS / SLIDES

■ MULTICOMPONENT PROGRAMS

■ PAMPHLETS

PERIODICALS

■ POLICY STATEMENTS / GUIDELINES

◼ POSTERS

■ PUBLIC SERVICE ADS (TV, RADIO, PRINT)

REPORTS / MONOGRAPHS

■ VIDEOS / FILMS

266

INDEX THREE: PRODUCTS IN LANGUAGES OTHER THAN ENGLISH

TAGALOG

THAI

VIETNAMESE

VISAYAN

NOTES

NOTES

Available from AmFAR:

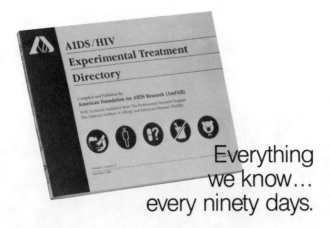

Everything we know... every ninety days.

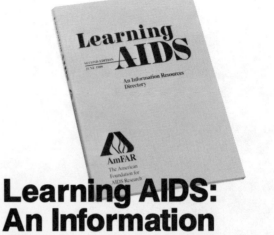

AIDS/HIV Experimental Treatment Directory

Every ninety days, AmFAR's editorial staff queries hundreds of drug companies and clinical investigators to track down new information on experimental treatments for AIDS.

Our continuous review of the medical literature and coverage of key research conferences puts you on the cutting edge of AIDS drug development.

Comprehensive information on clinical trials for treatment of all stages of HIV infection is presented in a "user friendly" format for primary care physicians and people with HIV disease.

Each edition includes AmFAR's "Stage-by-Stage Clinical Trial Index," and a special table of approved and experimental treatments for opportunistic infections.

Each listing includes a physical description of the drug, mechanism of action, results of clinical studies and pre-clinical investigations. Investigators and institutions participating appear with each trial.

Learning AIDS: An Information Resources Directory

"AmFAR has provided a tool that will soon become as integral a part of every human service agency and AIDS organization as its telephone or copier machine..."

Larry Kessler, Executive Director
AIDS ACTION Committee/Massachusetts
Member of National AIDS Commission

Organized by specialized target audiences, over 1000 educational brochures, instructional programs, videos, posters, public service ads have been abstracted and reviewed, giving you an overview of the educational efforts of hundreds of agencies and organizations nationwide.

Products reviewed have been assessed by an independent expert review panel for medical accuracy, appropriateness for its intended audience, and for the quality of its production.

Our reference section provides listings on policy statements, guidelines, studies, and other valuable resources, along with listings of state agencies and hotlines for AIDS/HIV information.

We also include a complete listing of the producers whose materials appear in the directory, giving you ready access to those organizations involved in AIDS/HIV education.

Learning AIDS is the only tool that can help you rapidly identify materials best suited to your organization, school or community.

AmFAR-sponsored publications

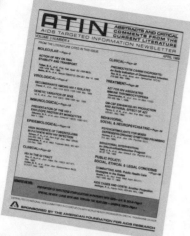

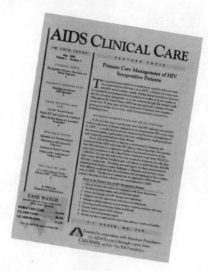

AIDS Targeted Information Newsletter (ATIN)

"ATIN bridges the gaps between the information needs of the research specialist and the informed lay person."

Dr. James B. Wyngaarden
Director, National Institute of Health

Published by Williams & Wilkins, ATIN is designed to target important AIDS/HIV literature and organize it for you in a form you can rapidly assimilate and use. Each issue provides abstracts and citations for literature in 7 areas of study: molecular, virological, immunological, epidemiological, clinical, treatment, and public policy. ATIN reviews the contents of hundreds of journals for each issue, every 30 days.

Each month you will be alerted to key findings, questionable data, and important case observations. Commentaries on individual articles are given by our expert editorial advisory board—you will have the benefit of at least one minireview each month that will put you in touch with the important new developments and perspectives on the HIV epidemic.

With over 400 articles cited each month, ATIN will bring you up-to-date on the latest published findings on AIDS/HIV.

AIDS Clinical Care

This new monthly publication is designed to give health care providers ready access to the most up-to-date information on techniques for the diagnosis, clinical management, and support of patients with HIV infection.

If you are already providing care and services for people with AIDS/HIV, AIDS Clinical Care is an invaluable resource that will keep you current with the latest techniques. If you or your institution have yet to encounter patients infected with the AIDS virus, AIDS Clinical Care can help you plan and prepare to cope with the HIV health crisis.

Created by the Massachusetts Medical Society (publishers of the New England Journal of Medicine) and sponsored by AmFAR, this newsletter draws upon the hard-won AIDS clinical management experience of an outstanding panel of medical managers. AIDS Clinical Care puts current, scientifically accurate information into your hands every 30 days.

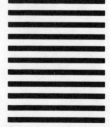

NO POSTAGE
NECESSARY
IF MAILED
IN THE
UNITED STATES

BUSINESS REPLY MAIL
FIRST CLASS MAIL   PERMIT NO. 936   NEW YORK, NY

POSTAGE WILL BE PAID BY ADDRESSEE

American Foundation for AIDS Research
1515 Broadway
Suite 3601
New York, NY 10109-0732